ANNUAL REVIEW OF GERONTOLOGY AND GERIATRICS

VOLUME 38, 2018

Editors

Annual Review of Gerontology and Geriatrics

Environments in an Aging Society: Autobiographical Perspectives in Environmental Gerontology

VOLUME 38, 2018

Volume Editors

HABIB CHAUDHURY, PhD

FRANK OSWALD, PhD

Series Editor

TONI C. ANTONUCCI, PhD

SPRINGER PUBLISHING COMPANY
NEW YORK

Springer Publishing Company, LLC
11 West 42nd Street
New York, NY 10036
www.springerpub.com

Acquisitions Editor: Sheri W. Sussman
Compositor: Exeter Premedia Services Private Ltd.

ISBN: 978-0-8261-7986-9
e-book ISBN: 978-0-8261-7987-6
ISSN: 0198-8794
Online ISSN: 1944-4036

17 18 19 20 / 5 4 3 2 1

Contents

About the Volume Editors vii
Habib Chaudhury
Frank Oswald

Contributors ix

Previous Volumes in the Series xi

Preface xiii

Acknowledgments xvii

1. In the Rearview Mirror: Personal Reflections in Environmental Gerontology 1
Habib Chaudhury and Frank Oswald

PART 1—Conceptual Evolution in Environmental Gerontology

2. The Environment as Developmental Context: In All Ages But Certainly in Old Age 17
Hans-Werner Wahl

3. Being There: Personal Reflection on a Quest for Understanding the Meaning of Place in Environmental Gerontology 39
Graham D. Rowles

4. Intellectual Origins of Residential Normalcy Theory 57
Stephen M. Golant

5. Personal Biography and the Development of Gerontological Environmental Theory 73
Robert L. Rubinstein

PART 2—Home and Neighborhood

6. Reflections on a Professional Journey to Making Home Life Better for Older Adults and Families 89
Laura N. Gitlin

7. From Occupational Therapy to Environmental Gerontology 109
Susanne Iwarsson

8. Home Thoughts 131
Sheila Peace

9. Housing for Older Adults: A Personal Journey in Environmental Gerontology 147
Jon Pynoos

10. The Role of Community and the Environment in the Lives of Older People: Understanding Local and Global Social Change 165
Chris Phillipson

11. A "Good Fit": Professionally Aging in Small Kansas Towns 183
Rick J. Scheidt

PART 3—Care Environments: Housing With Support Services and Long-Term Care Settings

12. Finding Place: An Intellectual Journey 201
Benyamin Schwarz

13. The Art of Questioning 217
Margaret P. Calkins

14. A Compelling Societal Problem Makes for a Good Professional Life 239
Victor Regnier

15. Discovering Environment–Behavior Studies: A Personal Adventure 257
John Zeisel

16. A Career Outside the Mainstream 277
Edward Steinfeld

Index 303

About the Volume Editors

Habib Chaudhury, PhD, is Chair and Professor in the Department of Gerontology at Simon Fraser University, Vancouver, Canada. Dr. Chaudhury has conducted research and consulting work in the area of Environmental Gerontology for the last two decades. His research interests are: physical environment for people with dementia in long-term care facilities, memories of home and personhood in dementia, community planning and urban design for active aging, and design in acute-care settings. Published books: *Remembering Home: Rediscovering the Self in Dementia* (Johns Hopkins University Press, 2008) and coedited volume *Home and Identity in Later Life: International Perspectives* (with G. D. Rowles; Springer Publishing Company, 2005). Dr. Chaudhury conducts research consulting with various national and international organizations in the areas of planning and design of seniors' housing and long-term care facilities. He is Associate Editor of the *Journal of Housing for the Elderly* and serves on the Editorial Board of the *Journal of Aging Studies.* He is also affiliated with the Centre for Research on Personhood in Dementia at the University of British Columbia, Vancouver and Alzheimer Catalonia, Barcelona, Spain.

Frank Oswald, PhD, is Professor for Interdisciplinary Ageing Research, Vice Dean of the faculty of Educational Sciences and Chair of the Frankfurt Forum for Interdisciplinary Ageing Research at the Goethe University Frankfurt, Germany. He is a psychologist by training and author or coauthor of several articles in the areas of gerontology and psychology. His research interests are contexts of adult development, issues of person–environment transaction and transitions in old age, housing, ageing in place, relocation, and the role of technologies in later life. He is coauthor of the book *Umwelten des Alterns: Wohnen, Mobilität, Technik und Medien [Environments of aging: Housing, mobility, technology and media]* (with C. Claßen, M. Doh, U. Kleinemas, and H.-W. Wahl; Kohlhammer, 2014) and coeditor of the volume *Aging Independently: Living Arrangements and Mobility* (with K.W. Schaie, H.-W. Wahl, and H. Mollenkopf; Springer Publishing Company, 2003). He has conducted research in Environmental Gerontology since two decades on local, national and international (European) levels. He is associate editor of the *Zeitschrift für Gerontologie und Geriatrie [Journal of Gerontology and Geriatrics]*.

Contributors

Margaret P. Calkins, PhD, MArch, Executive Director, The Mayer-Rothschild Foundation, Chicago, IL

Habib Chaudhury, PhD, Professor, Department of Gerontology, Simon Fraser University, Vancouver, Canada

Laura N. Gitlin, PhD, Isabel Hampton Robb Distinguished Scholar, Professor, School of Nursing, School of Medicine, Director, Center for Innovative Care in Aging, John Hopkins University, Baltimore, MD

Stephen M. Golant, PhD, Professor, Department of Geography, University of Florida, Gatesville, FL

Susanne Iwarsson, PhD, Professor, Department of Health Sciences, Lund University, Lund, Sweden

Frank Oswald, PhD, Professor, Interdisciplinary Aging Research, Faculty of Educational Sciences, Goethe University, Frankfurt, Germany

Sheila Peace, BA, PhD, FAcSS, Emeritus Professor of Social Gerontology, School of Health, Wellbeing & Social Care, Faculty of Wellbeing, Education and Languages, The Open University, Milton Keyes, UK

Chris Phillipson, PhD, Professor of Sociology and Social Gerontology, School of Social Sciences, The University of Manchester, Manchester, UK

Jon Pynoos, MCP, PhD, UPS Foundation Professor of Gerontology, Policy and Planning, Leonard Davis School of Gerontology, University of Southern California, Los Angeles, CA

Victor Regnier, FAIA, ACSA Distinguished Professor, Professor of Architecture and Gerontology, School of Architecture, University of Southern California, Los Angeles, CA

Graham D. Rowles, PhD, Professor, Graduate Center for Gerontology, University of Kentucky, Lexington, KY

Robert L. Rubinstein, PhD, Professor, Department of Sociology, Anthropology, and Health Administration and Policy, University System of Maryland (UMBC), Baltimore, MD

Benyamin Schwarz, PhD, Professor, Department of Architectural Studies, University of Missouri, Columbia, MO

Rick J. Scheidt, PhD, Professor, School of Family Studies and Human Services, Kansas State University, Manhattan KS

Edward Steinfeld, ArchD, SUNY Distinguished Professor, Department of Architecture, University at Buffalo, SUNY, Buffalo, NY

Hans-Werner Wahl, PhD, Director, Network Aging Research of Heidelberg University, Heidelberg University, Heidelberg, Germany

John Zeisel, PhD, HonDSc, Hearthstone Alzheimer Care & The I'm Still Here Foundation, Woburn, MA

Previous Volumes in the Series

Vol. 37, 2017: Contemporary Issues and Future Directions in Lesbian, Gay, Bisexual, and Transgender Aging

Editors: Kristina M. Hash, PhD, LICSW, and Anissa Rogers, PhD, MSW, MA, LCSW

Vol. 36, 2016: Optimizing Physical Activity and Function Across All Settings

Editors: Barbara Resnick, PhD, CRNP, FGSA, FAANP, and Marie Boltz, PhD, RN, GNP-BC, FGSA, FAAN

Vol. 35, 2015: Subjective Aging: New Developments and Future Directions

Editors: Manfred Diehl, PhD; Hans-Werner Wahl, PhD

Vol. 34, 2014: Genetics

Editor: Richard Sprott, PhD

Vol. 33, 2013: Healthy Longevity: A Global Approach

Editors: Jean-Marie Robine, DEA, DED, Carol Jagger, PhD, and Eileen M. Crimmins, PhD

Vol. 32, 2012: Emerging Perspectives on Resilience in Adulthood and Later Life

Editors: Bert Hayslip Jr., PhD, Gregory C. Smith, PhD

Vol. 31, 2011: Pathways Through Transitions of Care for Older Adults

Editors: Peggye Dilworth-Anderson, PhD, Mary H. Palmer, PhD

Vol. 30, 2010: Biobehavioral Perspectives on Health in Later Life

Editor: Keith E. Whitfield, PhD

Vol. 29: Life-Course Perspectives on Late Life Health Inequalities

Editors: Toni C. Antonucci, PhD, James S. Jackson, PhD

Vol. 28: Gerontological and Geriatric Education

Editors: Harvey L. Sterns, PhD and Marie A. Bernard, MD

Vol. 27: Biopsychosocial Approaches to Longevity

Editors: Leonard W. Poon, PhD, DPhil, and Thomas T. Perls, MD, MPH

Vol. 26: The Crown of Life Dynamics of the Early Postretirement Period

Editors: Jacquelyn Boone James, PhD, and Paul Wink, PhD

Vol. 25: Aging Health Care Workforce Issues

Editors: Toni Miles, MD, PhD, and Antonio Furino, PhD, JD

Vol. 24: Focus on Intergenerational Relations Across Time and Place

Editors: Merril Silverstein, PhD, and K. Warner Schaie, PhD

Vol. 23: Focus on Aging in Context: Socio-Psysical Environments

Editors: Hans Werner Wahl, PhD, Rick J. Scheidt, PhD, and Paul G. Windley, PhD

Vol. 22: Focus on Economic Outcomes in Later Life

Editors: Stephen Crystal, PhD, and Dennis Shea, PhD

Vol. 21: Focus on Modern Topics in the Biology of Aging

Editors: Vincent C. Cristofalo, PhD, and Richard Adelman, PhD

Preface

This edition of the *Annual Review of Gerontology and Geriatrics* has been inspired by an edited volume (Birren & Schroots, 2000) entitled, *The History of Geropsychology in Autobiography*, which is an excellent collection of autobiographically reflective essays by critical figures in the field of geropsychology, including Paul B. Baltes, James E. Birren, M. Powell Lawton, and many others. In elucidating the value of autobiographical histories, the coeditors of that volume, Birren and Schroots noted in their introductory chapter:

> *Autobiographies can reveal how chance and accidents help determine the flow of events and choices, as do the shifting balances of resources and the interests of institutional administrators, family members, and peers. Autobiographies reveal different career paths to contributions and achievements and perhaps to lingering disappointments. The details of individual careers are often left out of histories of fields and overlooked are the decisions individuals make in the process of shaping their careers and that contribute to the creation of a new field.*

As knowledge in the growing multidisciplinary field of Environmental Gerontology proliferates, and as increasingly mature theory and applied knowledge are developed, this volume is a timely endeavor to take a step back and examine the evolution of this field through the unique experiences and intellectual development of a selected group of its pioneers and leaders, who have made (and continue to do so) crucial contributions to the field in the last several decades. We are witnessing in a promising resurgence of conceptual, methodological, and empirical development in the field of Environmental Gerontology after it went through a "languishing state" (Parmelee & Lawton, 1990; Wahl & Weisman, 2003), and we believe that it is time to take account of the field as a collective body of knowledge and practice. This volume addresses that objective with a unique perspective, which is through a set of *self-reflective* essays that assist us in gaining a contextually grounded and nuanced understanding of this important area within gerontology. The growth and evolution of any given field of study are based on individual scholars' and researchers' contributions over several decades, and understanding their intellectual roots, personal motivations, interpersonal exchange, and influencing factors can not only broaden our understanding of their scholarly contributions, but also deepen our appreciation of the nature of their academic journey over multiple decades.

As a precursor to this volume, we organized a symposium on this topic at the 67th Annual Meeting of the Gerontological Society of America in Washington, D.C., in 2014 (Chaudhury & Oswald, 2014). Four individual presentations were made by influential scholars (Hans-Werner Wahl, Graham D. Rowles, Sheila Peace, and Stephen M. Golant) in Environmental Gerontology along with discussion by a notable scholar (Laura N. Gitlin). The session was well received with critical positive feedback from the contributors and from the audience. The success of the conference symposium, in part, prompted the value of a volume that will present a collection of essays from a wider range of disciplinary perspectives and a larger group of scholars in this field, although nevertheless limited to the length and scope of a book.

We take this opportunity to gratefully acknowledge the early pioneers in this field who fundamentally spearheaded its birth and critical growth, including M. Powell Lawton, Frances Carp, Eva Kahana, and Leon Pastalan in the 1960s, 1970s, and early 1980s. These first-generation environmental gerontologists broke the ground with the vision to see the importance of understanding the role of the environment and places in older people's lives in both conceptual and empirical terms, which included conceptualizations of person-environment interaction, congruence and fit, ecological view of environment and aging, empirical findings in specified housing and mainstream living environments for older adults. They laid the groundwork for a new interdisciplinary subfield within gerontology to emerge in its own right. Over the next several decades, the field has grown to expand within and from the original disciplines that include, among others, psychology, geography, sociology, anthropology, occupational therapy, educational science, urban planning, architecture, rehabilitation science, and nursing.

As the field of Environmental Gerontology moves forward, researchers, (early- and late-career) graduate students, and related practitioners need to address the issue of making this field more relevant for the broader field of gerontology and public policy, programs and services relevant for improving the quality of life in older adults. As there is a need for critical self-reflection to take stock of personal and collective scholarly achievements and underlying limitations, we should also take the charge of conscious self-projection to reach out to the community at large with the goal to more effectively relate to, connect with and contribute to gerontology itself, for example, as it is typical from a transdisciplinary research approach. Ultimately the challenge is to keep the balance of maintaining the focus of the field to "understand, explain, and optimize the interaction between older adults and their environment" (Schwarz, 2012, p. 5) and making the connections with other areas of gerontology to more effectively and meaningfully demonstrate the importance of the socio-physical environment in the understanding of the neurological, individual, social, collective and institutional factors of the aging phenomenon and the related societal discourses at large.

Habib Chaudhury and Frank Oswald

REFERENCES

Birren, J. E., & Schroots, J. J. F. (Eds.). (2000). *A history of geropsychology in autobiography*. Washington, DC: American Psychological Association.

Chaudhury, H., & Oswald, F. (2014, November). *Advances and challenges in Environmental Gerontology: Autobiographical perspectives*. Symposium at the 67th Annual Scientific Meeting of the Gerontological Society of America, Washington, DC.

Parmelee, P. A., & Lawton, M. P. (1990). The design of special environments for the aged. In J. Birren & K. W. Schaie (Eds.), *Handbook of the psychology of aging* (3rd ed., pp. 464–488). New York, NY: Academic Press.

Schwarz, B. (2012). Environmental gerontology: What now? *Journal of Housing for the Elderly, 26*(1), 4–19.

Wahl, H.-W., & Weisman, J. (2003). Environmental gerontology at the beginning of the new millennium: Reflections on its historical, empirical, and theoretical development. *The Gerontologist, 43*(5), 616–627.

Acknowledgments

We are sincerely grateful to Sheri W. Sussman and Mindy Chen for assistance in effectively guiding us through the process of publication of this volume. Special thanks to Sheri for initiating the possibility of utilizing this series as the venue for this collection of reflective essays. A big thank-you to our Editorial Assistant Riley Malvern for her capable assistance in this project. Finally and most importantly, we are deeply fortunate to have received the enthusiasm, support and professionalism from all our contributors. We sincerely appreciate their commitment to make a contribution in a timely manner amidst their highly demanding schedules. It has been our honor and pleasure to have worked with them on this project.

Editors

ANNUAL REVIEW OF GERONTOLOGY AND GERIATRICS

VOLUME 38, 2018

CHAPTER 1

In the Rearview Mirror

Personal Reflections in Environmental Gerontology

Habib Chaudhury and Frank Oswald

ABSTRACT

The chapter outlines the relevance and value of professional autobiographical reflections by pioneers and senior scholars for a richer and grounded understanding of theories and substantive scholarship in the field of Environmental Gerontology. We argue that critical self-reflection would reveal a better insight into these individual professional contributions to the field and personal career paths, as well as the professional paths not taken and potential shortcomings in one's intellectual contributions, and missed opportunities. As we appreciate the key scientific contributions of the notable scholars in these chapters, we also recognize the "humanistic" nature of the process that worked behind the outcomes. Salient issues and topics from the chapters are presented to highlight the significance of each contribution, as well as brief summative commentaries on the state-of-the-art in the categories of conceptual developments, and substantive understanding in the areas of home and neighborhood, and care environments. Finally, three broader emergent issues are identified for consideration, which include issues of the unpredictable nature of career paths, diversity in research methodologies, and the importance of mentoring. This volume has brought to the surface the personal stories behind the scholarship in this field. We hope that it will inspire early career researchers to learn from the self-reflections; particularly

http://dx.doi.org/10.1891/0198-8794.38.1

the focus, persistence, determination, mentorship, peer-support, and commitment that are clearly evident in the veteran scholars' professional journeys.

THE FIELD OF ENVIRONMENTAL GERONTOLOGY: VALUE OF SELF-REFLECTIONS

This introductory chapter provides the volume's rationale, scope, coverage, and expected outcomes. Our aim is to highlight the relevance and value of autobiographical reflections by pioneers, senior researchers, and influential scholars to gain a richer and contextual understanding of major theoretical developments, substantive findings and policy implications in the field of Environmental Gerontology. Moreover, we identify key emergent issues from the contributions to serve as a guide for the readers to fully appreciate the messages and wisdom in the chapters of this volume.

The saying of Socrates, "An unexamined life is not worth living," is perhaps stark and binary in its appeal, but it does present itself as a decree coming down from above, one that we are hard-pressed to face. Nevertheless, the value of examining one's life, and for that matter, one's professional life, is a topic that is worth at least a brief examination. A focused and voluntary self-reflection on the origins of a professional career would provide the opportunity to revisit earlier life circumstances, goals, plans, influences, networks, opportunities, initiatives, and chances in some combination or other. At one level, self-reflections on individual professional careers provide glimpses on the trajectory of career development and self-presentation of the scientific contributions. At another level, the collective reflections build a mosaic of understanding on the various overlaps, linkages, and chronological build-ups of scientific knowledge in a specific research area, as well as shed light on common threads of influences and circumstances, along with the uncommon or unique trajectories. An academic and scientific field of study is most often, and rightfully, understood and studied in analytical rigor and conceptual insights, and that is how we build and advance a body of knowledge. Within this paradigm, the practice of formal and/or informal as well as public self-reflection among scholars and academics tends to remain ignored and unaccounted for. We believe this oversight of personal history and self-selection of one's scientific/scholarly contribution is a missed opportunity to provide a more in-depth and nuanced understanding of a given field, as well as acknowledging the importance of the content and network—institutions and people that had shaped an individuals' intellectual growth, evolution, and scholarly contributions.

From a personal standpoint (going back to the Socratic quote), there are potential gains for the scholar engaging in a self-reflection endeavor. This is an opportunity to engage in a "guided reminiscence" to understand and explain the professional decisions made, the "significant others" in the career journey, the institutions and places to connect the dots and develop a comprehensive tapestry of professional life where the profession and person intersect. Note, however, that we did not provide any "guidelines" for such a better understanding with our invitation to contribute to this volume. At the same time, a critical self-reflection can reveal the paths not taken, the potential shortcomings and "fault-lines" in one's intellectual contributions, and missed opportunities. Even without engaging in a pseudo-clinical professional "life review" inspired by Robert N. Butler's (1963) work, a semiformal critical view on one's own contributions can prove to be a healthy exercise toward self-improvement, development, and refinement. As well established in life-span psychology (e.g., Baltes, 1987), the opportunity for growth and change are ever present in one's life trajectory including its professional track. Also, the idea of a reflective narrative as a summative professional legacy can be a tantalizing idea. As science builds upon itself in the normative path of building upon previous research, so can our understanding of individual scholar's own version of the key contributions to the field and the process behind it as outlined with professional milestones and circumstances. One of the most intriguing contemporary examples in this regard might be Didier Eribon's book *Returning to Reims* (Eribon, 2013). This represents a legacy of not only the *what* (scientific knowledge) but the *how* and *why* of its coming into existence. This background information of the individual researchers' intellectual and professional journey make the legacy personal and relatable for early career researchers, graduate students, and others engaged in the field. In the limited scope of our own pathways through research it was always our observation (if not our bias) that the field of Environmental Gerontology has been particularly influenced by the personalities or personal views and biographies of its scholars, and it would be a worthwhile endeavor to carve out the potential from this.

The following factors were taken into consideration in selection of the contributors' research focus and background: (a) research/scholarship in Environmental Gerontology in diverse scales/contexts in the physical/built environment, for example, home environment, neighborhood, cityscape, long-term care facilities; (b) multiple geographic regions and/or countries at least addressing some international balance between North America and Europe; (c) diversity of disciplinary backgrounds represented by related social sciences, health sciences, and environmental design; and (d) basic/theoretical and applied/policy-oriented research. Of course, the list of these contributors is impacted by the reality of this volume's length and scope. There are several other scholars in the field of Environmental Gerontology who could have enriched this reflective collection. Perhaps there will be an opportunity for us or others to revisit this approach of self-reflective essays and another similar volume project envisioned at an opportune time in the future.

We believe that this collection of autobiographical reflections will provide better understanding and insights on multiple levels: (a) origins and development of this domain of gerontology as a whole addressing the question: What is the individual scholar's scientific contribution to the field of Environmental Gerontology?; (b) individual autobiographical accounts of intellectual development as a method to interpret the collective knowledge addressing the question: How is the biography of each author linked to the development of the field?; (c) an understanding of the institutional and societal discourse factors that might have influenced and shaped the generated knowledge and scholarship; and (d) a contribution to the intellectual heritage of the field of Environmental Gerontology at large.

Have we succeeded with this plan in mind? Basically, yes. First, from a process standpoint, we were gratified to receive positive response from majority of the contributors to the premise of this volume. Admittedly, the scope and format of the contribution is a departure from the normative writing of a theoretical essay or empirical findings-based paper. The personal nature of autobiographical writing task could elicit reluctance on at least two grounds. All contributors we approached are currently highly active in their research, and in a way, one could view their own professional life as still being constructed. In general, the prevailing perception is that a self-reflection is timely at or near the "end" (self-determined and/or externally defined) of one's academic career. Also, for some scholars, the premise of a self-reflective essay represents unnecessary self-exposure and possible self-indulgence. In the end, as editors, we are deeply grateful that all contributors were fully convinced and appreciative of this exercise and engaged in the process with full commitment.

Second, most of the contributions provide answers to the questions we had raised earlier. Although not every chapter speaks to all questions and not all chapters address the field of Environmental Gerontology in the same way, it is the collection of various topics, perspectives, individual pathways as well as the connectivity of all chapters that may give an answer to the question how this field of research has developed over the last few decades. The professional "self-portraits" of the contributors are, in our opinion, not only excellent portrayals of the professional life courses of the scholars, but collectively, they present summative insights into the highlights of our current state of knowledge in key subdomains of Environmental Gerontology. The reader has the opportunity to learn about a considerable number of key topics, theoretical orientations and concepts, findings and implications in the home, community/neighborhood and care environments, along with a broader conceptualization for the field as a whole. Finally, with this colorful picture in mind, the reader might better address the role of Environmental Gerontology for aging research at large. We believe this broad, yet integrative scope of the individual chapters and in turn, the collective pictures are uniquely helpful for us to take stock of what has been achieved and where do we go from here.

STRUCTURE OF THE VOLUME

The contributions in this volume are categorized into three sections, addressing mainly: (a) conceptual evolution in Environmental Gerontology; (b) the fundamental environment of the home, the neighborhood, and the community context as fundamental sections of the environment; and (c) care environments, particularly emphasizing housing with support services and long-term care settings. It is important to note that the authors are by no means limited to the section in which their contributions appear; nevertheless, we thought that it would be useful for the reader to follow this classical segment of Environmental Gerontology. Here, we briefly highlight the premise and content for each section.

Section I—Conceptual Evolution in Environmental Gerontology

This section focuses on the influential and predominantly theoretical contributions by four scholars in this field. The conceptual origins of Environmental Gerontology from M. Powell Lawton's seminal work over three decades made a major influence on the theoretical development of our understanding of the interaction of socio-spatial environment and older person from a psychological, geographical, sociological/anthropological, and architectural background. Subsequently, a few scholars' work have not only expanded and enriched the Environmental Gerontology theories and frameworks, but have also influenced empirical research in multiple domains, such as seniors' housing, aging in place, geographical experience, housing decision making, long-term care, and so forth. The chapters in this section will trace four such researchers' intellectual roots, highlight their contributions in the theoretical body of work, and direct our attention to future potential. Influenced and stimulated by the classical Lawton and Nahemow press-competence model (1973) and subsequent extensions of environmental docility and press toward environmental proactivity and richness by M. Powell Lawton, many of the contributors to this book—and the four scholars in this section in particular—followed different pathways to extend this seminal model in sophisticated ways. Note, however, that all examples of theory development in this section are based on systematic collections of a variety of empirical evidence. One way toward a better understanding of person–environment exchange is Graham Rowles' auto-ethnographic route of searching for personal meaning of place as a biographical experience following the question (among others) how people "make and remake places" across the life span. Also rooted in a deep anthropological curiosity and a biographical approach toward evidence to better understand human culture, Robert Rubinstein follows the question how "individuals with identities" can, following Lawton's ideas, better combine press and competence "in a larger meaningful cultural context," exemplified by experiences of (spatial) miniaturization, for instance in situations when people live alone in later life. While the authors in these two chapters deal to a great extent with personal experience of place and space not only (but also) from an adaptation perspective to maintain autonomy and to deal with perceived changes in the balance of the older adult and his/her environment (e.g., at home), Stephen Golant more explicitly emphasizes on the process of environmental decision making in later life based on a broad variety of personal (psychological) resources to cope with the situation in order to maintain or reestablish residential normalcy. Emphasizing on a clearly stated selected set of options and outcomes within this complex process, he offers a model to be either tested from a scientific perspective, or to be used from a more practical or applied perspective on everyday living in later life. Finally, following the idea to better address changing processes of person–environment exchange over time (i.e., agency and belonging) but also to value and to categorize the multiple empirical findings and various pieces of empirical evidence from different methodological backgrounds, Hans-Werner Wahl introduced (among other findings) how his (and Frank Oswald's) idea of a comprehensive model of person–environment transaction occurred, enriched by empirical findings from the European context. Now the four chapters are introduced briefly in the order of appearance.

In his chapter, Hans-Werner Wahl identifies several scholars as key influencers in shaping his thinking and focus, including Margret M. Baltes, M. Powell Lawton, and Vern L. Bengtson. It is fascinating to learn how his early research career moved toward aging and its social context at the beginning, and eventually, toward physical-spatial environment by scholars and circumstances. The chapter provides an integrative and reflective summary of Hans-Werner's scholarly contributions in establishing the importance of social and physical environments against the background of life-span development theories. Moreover, he integrated conceptualizations of person–environment transaction and several related subdomains, which provides a rich theoretical foundation in Environmental Gerontology.

Graham Rowles rigorously adopts an auto-ethnographic methodological approach in his reflective-analytic essay where his professional career is interspersed with his environmental history. The first three decades of frequent moves played a palpable role in his desire to stay in one place and to understand place itself. The three phases of his career trajectory represent a full circle through engagement, expansion, and realization, where the inquiring and personal selves worked together to understand and realize the meaning of place in the aging experience. Graham's rich conceptualization of person–environment transaction has provided the field deeply meaningful conceptual building blocks of action, orientation, feeling, fantasy, insideness (and its variations), and being in place, among others.

The importance of surreptitious events in influencing most of the contributor's research focus is exemplified by Stephen Golant's identification of a series of events and intersections with people who shaped his interests and career path. These events included his early introduction to the topic of prediction of human responses to natural hazards (as a PhD student), joining the University of Chicago's Department of Geography as a faculty member, and receiving an invitation to work with Bernice Neugarten on a project on aging in urban settings. Arguably, Golant's most important scholarly contribution thus far is the theoretical model of residential normalcy, which delves into the complexities and richness of person–environment congruence by bringing together several rich concepts including residential comfort and residential mastery. The process of adaption conceptualized in this model, along with its broader appeal, has been very well received in the field.

In his chapter, Robert Rubinstein traces his cultural anthropological roots to cultural ecology (analysis of the interrelationship among ecology, cultural meaning, ritual, and social life), structuralism (culturally situated pan-human construction of binary oppositions of cultural categories), symbolic anthropology (the study of key cultural symbols), and Clifford Geertz's classic work. His reflections on his research on the island of Malo focusing on the interaction/transaction of person, place, and object with the backdrop of psychoanalytic versus cultural construction is revealing of the powerful influence of place and people. Among the rich array of concepts and conceptualizations that represent Rubinstein's work in Environmental Gerontology, the crucial ones that he self-identifies are: the biographical approach, the culture of living alone, miniaturization, and personal meaning system.

Section II—Home and Neighborhood

The home and neighborhood environment are critically important settings or geographic scales for older adults' health, attachment, functioning, and wellbeing on a private and community level of quality of life. Over the last few decades, substantial empirical research has been conducted in these areas, which includes issues of accessibility and barriers, home modifications, aging in place, physical functioning, meaning of home, perceived aspects of home, housing-health connection, assisted living, home care, retirement communities, and so forth.

This does not preclude research rooted in theoretical concepts or development of new methods to assess seniors' housing options. In addition, research and policy work on broader socio-psychological dimensions of the community, such as social inclusion, community participation, economic inequality, and sense of belonging, have contributed to a more comprehensive understanding of the importance of the neighborhood as a place on both group and individual levels. In general, home and neighborhood have been looked upon in the extant literature as distinct research foci maintaining an analytic differentiation. Given that home is a complex phenomenon with its objective and subjective relevance for daily activities, family and social life, self-expression, and identity, it has been a critically important topic in the field for the last several decades, particularly with respect to the outcome of daily independence and autonomy. Community-dwelling elders are by definition able to maintain independent living at home. Giving up their own home may thus clearly indicate giving up daily independence. On the other hand, interest in the importance of neighborhood for older adults is relatively recent in Environmental Gerontology, and arguably, with an emphasis on associated health-related outcomes for older adults. There is a growing recognition and evidence-base in the literature on several aspects of the neighborhood environment, including walkability, accessibility, services and amenities, open spaces, transportation, recreation, age-friendliness, and so forth. Neighborhood and community are now part of the broader definition and understanding of the aging-in-place topic. Nevertheless, the interrelation between the two settings point out the need for examination of both home setting and neighborhood in the same study, which will provide an opportunity for study designs to more effectively understand the nature of the interrelation and interdependence as it influences the quality of life for older adults; for example, with respect to the future need to better create and maintain caring communities. With this in mind, we present essays by six scholars who have made a significant impact on our understanding of the nature, characteristics, and processes of older adults' experience of and in the home and the neighborhood environments. This section presents the scholarly work in these research domains through reflective contributions of a notable group of individuals.

Laura Gitlin identifies the broad influence of two overarching frameworks from Lawton ("environmental press and competence model" and "quality of life") on her work. Her distinctly applied orientation in intervention research has been remarkably consistent with five themes related to: (a) a bio-psycho-social-environmental approach of health care, (b) environmental context of behavior, (c) adaptive psychosocial-environmental processes and family involvement, (d) team approaches engaging interprofessional and community partners, and (e) theoretically based action-oriented research. Gitlin's research has made major advancements in the areas of socio-psychological-environmental approaches in dementia care, family caregiving, and physical functioning, particularly in the context of the home environment. The reader will appreciate the early influences of living in a family with chronic and life-threatening illnesses, exceptional mentors (most importantly, M. Powell Lawton) over the professional career, supportive institutional applied and research environments have all contributed in shaping the research journey in important ways.

For Susanne Iwarsson, the early influences include witnessing environmental challenges for her disabled grandmother related to multiple sclerosis and the adaptations made to address them. Her professional life as a practicing Occupational Therapist also impacted a life-long interest in home, health, and disability interrelations. Susanne Iwarsson's strong interdisciplinary and user-oriented research can be traced back to early mentors at Lund University's Department of Community Health. Her most notable contribution to the field includes the instrument Housing Enabler which has broken new grounds in providing a systematic method to link accessibility based on objective assessment of both environmental barriers and individual competence, strongly linked to M. Powell Lawton's press-competence model as well. In her chapter, among other contributions, she highlights the ENABLE-AGE project serving as a landmark study on examining housing and health links with a cross-national scope in Europe. The chapter also provides an insightful discussion of emergent questions and challenges for future research in the housing and home environment domain.

Sheila Peace reflects on her early first-hand experiences of aging and place as a community volunteer and visiting Mrs. E in her home as well as her work at Percy Garden's Old People's Home in London Borough. Her academic and research career spans multiple projects and settings, ranging from quality of life of older people in care homes, self-identity and environment, seniors' housing options, intergenerational interaction, environmental autobiographies, among others. Peace draws from her own earlier work to identify future challenges for theoretical development which include: better integration of environmental docility and proactivity, temporality, physical and social environments, ongoing cohort dynamics, and so forth. Certainly, these remain among the highlights of research threads for current and future Environmental Gerontologists.

In his chapter, Jon Pynoos recalls his early encounters and exposure to the meaning and richness of home environment and the challenges of living independently in later life from his older adult neighbor Mrs. Benton. Pynoos' illustrious career as an academic in seniors' housing started with diverse and rich experiences in housing planning and policy with multiple community-based agencies, which perhaps shaped his strong commitment to translational and interdisciplinary research. His research contributions in seniors' housing, aging in place, home modifications and fall prevention have not only advanced our substantive understanding in these areas, but have also actively contributed to public policy changes and program interventions at local and state levels.

Chris Phillipson's chapter title succinctly captures his research contributions in understanding the role of community and environment in older people's lives. His work has significantly advanced our knowledge of the importance of both local social contexts and globalization in shaping the community life of older adults. For Phillipson, the early influences included his time as a volunteer at a psychiatric hospital in the UK, which provided an exposure to the challenges of "institutional" care for older adults and in parallel, the importance of understanding social issues in shaping social construction of individual pathology. His chapter provides an excellent overview and summary of the multiple substantive threads in his research, including development of "critical gerontology," local impact of macro social-economic forces, social exclusion and community life, transnational migration and globalization, belonging and identity in the context of global changes, development of age-friendly cities, and so forth.

With a foundational training in clinical and social psychology, Rick Scheidt revisits his spark of interest in environmental psychology by Roger Barker's on "Behavior Setting." The interest in understanding behavior-in-milieu was perhaps focused on rural communities by the sheer fact of being in the Midwest. These personal interests were enhanced while he was at the Andrus Centre in California with Environmental Gerontology and life-span human development. Scheidt's productive and positive research collaborations with Paul Windley and Lyn Norris-Baker come through strongly in his essay. As a major researcher in rural aging and community, Scheidt's work has advanced conceptual understanding and substantive knowledge of rural aging on many levels, including environmental, psychological, and demographic predictors of mental health, service utilization, and activity profiles among residents with diverse psychological statuses, and adaptive strategies of residents of small rural towns experiencing significant decline.

Section III—Care Environments: Housing With Support Services and Long-Term Care Settings

The final section presents essays from five scholars who have made critical contributions in research, practice, and policy on environmental issues in housing with support services (e.g., supportive housing, assisted living), long-term care facilities (e.g., nursing homes/residential care, special care units) and/or (universal) design guidelines and accessibility assessments at large, again from different disciplinary backgrounds including architecture and design. The role of the physical environment in congregate service-based housing or institutional care settings on the quality of life in physically and/or cognitively declined elders has received substantial research attention. The extant literature in this area demonstrates the effect of the physical environment as inhibitor or facilitator of various indicators of quality of life in a congregate setting, including mobility, accessibility, social interaction, autonomy, comfort, and identity. One key component in the context of service-based housing options and long-term care facilities is the role of the service provider organization. The organizational philosophy, mission, care approach, staffing models, care practices, and so forth, have tremendous impact on the physical planning and design decisions, quality of care and social interactions, older adults' autonomy and quality of life. Arguably, the organization or provider's pivotal role signifies the threshold that represents a primary shift of emphasis in control and autonomy from the person to an organization. On a broader scale, emphasizing organizations or at least including them in Environmental Gerontology opens up the discussion to the institutional and policy levels, as well as the societal discourse level (e.g., culture of long-term care, older adults' civic participation) often neglected in a narrow or individualistic point of view. As the care needs of older adults increase across these setting types, in general, the operating system and organizational culture become more prominent with an associated decline in older persons' ability to exercise choice, preference and decision making. An ongoing challenge in research is to isolate the influence of organizational policies and practices from that of the physical environment on older adult's functioning, health, and wellbeing. The complexity of intertwined nature of individual, social, and organizational factors have resulted in more comprehensive conceptual approaches, multimethod and mixed-method strategies and more explicit attempts at knowledge translation efforts. The chapters in this section revisit the key developments in this domain over the last few decades, as reflected through the autobiographical reflections of five key figures in this area.

Benyamin Schwarz recollects his remarkable family history in which his parents migrated from Czechoslovakia to Israel in 1948, and settled in the multigenerational kibbutz community. The gaps between the ideals and reality of these early years influenced his values to work to address such gaps in purpose-built communities for seniors in the United States. His professional practice as an architect designing housing units and a day-care center for elders in the Jordan Valley was the formative phase for him to understand the importance of the environment for seniors' quality of life. Schwarz's academic career in the United States and scholarly contributions in Environmental Gerontology is marked by three themes: his inclination for applied research and evidence-based practice, balance between autonomy and security in long-term care, and significance and meaning of place in later life. The contradictions and challenges in innovative models for housing and care for older adults in the chapter are apt reminders of how much work needs to be done in this field.

Margaret Calkins' interest in dementia care settings was prompted by a single question raised by an administrator of a care home in the early 1980s, making us realize and appreciate the motivating power of a question to launch a life-long career. Calkins has been at the forefront of design for people with dementia in long-term care facilities. Starting with the first book on this topic in the late 1980s, she has been a pioneer, advocate, researcher, and educator in the area of responsive physical environments for people with dementia. Her passion and strong commitment to address the gap between research and practice in design professions is exemplified through several noteworthy projects and initiatives, which include founding the IDEAS Institute, developing "Culture Change Proposals," research consulting service with many care provider organizations, development of creative design solutions, and so forth. Without a doubt, her most recent engagement with the Mayer-Rothschild Foundation to support applied environmental research will result in much needed systemic changes in the long-term care sector in North America.

Architect and researcher Victor Regnier reflects on his highly productive professional career focusing on applied research in the area of senior's housing and long-term care. Perhaps the "extreme work ethic" from his childhood instilled a passion in Regnier for work that would have a common tangible good. Undoubtedly, Regnier is a pioneer in developing design guidelines for multiple seniors' housing options in North America inspired by the innovative models in Scandinavia. His three books in this area are considered among the most used and notable for design professionals. Among his contributions, the advocacy for community-based residential alternatives to long-term care through his books, projects, and teaching have clearly positively shaped the planning and design of housing in North America. We look forward to his forthcoming publication on community and neighborhood.

John Zeisel addresses in his chapter how much his professional path has been driven by his interest and passion to improve the world. In his search for new adventures he significantly impacted the field of Environment-Behavior research methods by his milestone publication *Inquiry by Design*, giving him as well the chance to organize his professional life somewhat beyond classical academic career patterns. Based on a broad scope of methodological perspectives, he introduced and optimized assessment strategies in the design process including theoretical knowledge and empirical evidence from various disciplines (including neuroscience).

In his essay, we can trace Edward Steinfeld's sensitivity to social issues of design back to his early childhood that instilled the value of the older generation. As his academic training, a social action approach to the architectural profession resonated, which eventually led to his doctoral education that was broad based and socially inclined. Steinfeld's pioneering contribution in developing both a strong body of knowledge in universal design and developing building standards impacted the building industry with barrier-free and accessible built environments has fundamentally shifted this domain of design practice and built environmental outcomes. From the "New ANSI Standard Project," (the first major study on accessibility issues), ADA Accessibility Guidelines, Principles of Universal Design, and several other guidelines and standards are examples of his highly impactful contributions. His established Center for Inclusive Design and Environmental Access at SUNY Buffalo is a major enterprise for research, education, and practice in this domain of accessibility standards in the built environment.

The reader may appreciate that the individual contributors could belong in a different section of the volume, for example, authors in the second section on housing and neighborhood could have been categorized in Section 1 or 3. Laura Gitlin, for instance, argues from a strong theoretical background and addresses dementia care environments. The categorization of the chapters in various sections serves to provide a preliminary structure in this volume, but not meant to restrict the individual author to one of the three topics.

EXPECTED IMPACT OF THIS VOLUME

Given the broad interdisciplinary approach of this volume, we believe that this edition of the *Annual Review of Gerontology and Geriatrics* will appeal to a broad audience of academics, practitioners, administrators, and graduate students in gerontology, social and behavioral sciences (e.g., psychology, sociology, geography), health-related sciences (e.g., nursing, occupational therapy, and medical behavioral science), and environmental design disciplines (e.g., architecture, urban planning). The individual scholars' reflections and the collective "big picture" on the historical evolution of the field of Environmental Gerontology will attract readers on multiple levels. The emergence and intellectual development of this subfield of gerontology, as presented in the contributions, is very useful to understand in its initial roots, landmarks in conceptual and substantive growth, and overall trajectory, while the personal accounts of the key scholars' career paths provide insights on how diverse factors influence individual intellectual growth, professional decisions, and career progressions. We believe that the book has the potential to inform public policy and key applied areas in Environmental

Gerontology; that is, planning and design of seniors' housing issues, aging in place, public transportation, and age-friendly communities.

EMERGENT ISSUES FOR EDUCATION AND RESEARCH IN ENVIRONMENTAL GERONTOLOGY

The authors of this volume reflect a broad variety of individual professional contributions and biographically rooted lifestyles. Although we would argue that there is no need to categorize or evaluate this variety of individual contributions, we would nevertheless like to underpin some common observations that might help the reader (and/or early career researcher) to value her/his independent thinking and intellectual approach.

Reliability of the unforeseeable: Individual professional biographies can vary based on professional background, program/institutional expectations and personal inclinations, including classic academic career pathways, design research consulting and professional practice. The authors in this volume reflect a multiplicity of career trajectories as well as biographies with individual turning points, breaks, and even happenstances or changes in disciplines and diverse foci of interests. In general, it seems that most of them are aware that, in hindsight, professional academic life appears as an amalgamation of achievement-related behaviors, social support, circumstances, chance encounters/life events, and a portion of opportunities and serendipities. The tapestry of the professional reflections suggests the importance of the dynamics between personal goals/ambitions and external influences, especially mentors and academic cultures. Eventually, it should particularly encourage early career researchers in the field that although this is not surprising, it is worthwhile to note the value of consistent focus that is required to build upon one's own work and beliefs over time to develop a coherent body of scholarship, but also to remain open for external influences as well. We witness this consistency and focus demonstrated in all scholars' essays. All these scholars were focused on certain primary substantive area with occasional secondary area(s) with a commitment to build and evolve on one's own work toward a mature and substantial body of scholarship.

Diversity of methods: With respect to the scope of methodological approaches, utilized methods, and understanding of empirical evidence, the variety of orientations across different chapters is considerably large as well. The reader can find practice-building projects and useful guidelines for design processes, as well as qualitative in-depth case studies, measurement developments, conceptual reflections, literature reviews, or rigorous quantitative surveys and intervention studies. These reflect a robust approach of methodological approaches in Environmental Gerontology, but as several authors have noted, there is a need for greater attention in multiple areas, including the application of a more effective use of mixed methods, theory-guided empirical research, use of innovative and emergent methods, participatory research with marginalized and vulnerable population groups, and public policy research. As the field of gerontology is itself interdisciplinary with researchers from multiple social and health sciences joining in, the subfield of "Environmental" Gerontology is even more interdisciplinary (or even transdisciplinary) given the nature and understanding of the "Environment" drawing design professions and academics in the mix as well.

Value of mentoring in academic career: The scholars of Environmental Gerontology in this volume reflect a broad variety of disciplines and/or interdisciplinary/transdisciplinary approaches in their professional lives. However, the critical role of their mentors in the progression of their career paths (e.g., focus of research, institution of employment, relocation) is clearly evident. In some cases, the mentors' influences had a fundamental impact on the research direction of these scholars, and in many cases, there is mention of larger-than-life mentors, such as M. Powell Lawton, who by his personal input and interactions made a significant and lasting impact on several of these scholars. In addition, in their own careers, most if not all scholars in this volume reflect on the value and importance of their own role as mentors to their graduate students and young researchers. Perhaps for some, this is a conscious or subconscious effort to "pay it forward" because of a positive experience with their own mentors. Regardless of the internal motivations, the significance and positive influence of mentoring come across strongly in all these essays, which point out the need for continuation of this time-honored tradition in academia. We would argue that the role of mentoring is even more important for a field like Environmental Gerontology which needs to attract "new recruits" from students and young scholars to grow its rank and file.

CONCLUDING THOUGHTS

As editors, we were privileged to have had the opportunity to work on this volume with an unconventional premise and to have contributions from the pioneers and front-line scholars in this field. The volume is a collection of profiles that emerged at the intersection of individual scholar's professional journeys and their scholarly contributions. It is clearly evident in these essays that an individual researcher's scholarly contribution in a given field is as much a product of societal, cultural, and academic contexts, as it is a product of personal inclinations and focus. On a related note, it is important to point out that there are several scholars and researchers in Environmental Gerontology who are not part of this volume—a fact that does not reflect in any way on the merit of their scholarly work, but rather the limits of a single volume's length. Those notable scholars include (in alphabetic order) Neil Charness, Uriel Cohen, Malcolm Cutchin, Sara Czaja, Carole Després, Arthur Fisk, Lyn Geboy, Allen Glicksman, Norah Keating, Frieder Lang, Atiya Mahmood, Keith Diaz Moore, Susan Rodiek, Wendy Rogers, Jon Sanford, Tom Scharf, Andrew Scharlach, Ruth Brent Tofle, Gerald Weisman, and many others. We anticipate that there will be a sequel of this volume in the future to capture these and other scholars' reflective essays in Environmental Gerontology.

We hope this volume will help bring forward the topic of Environmental Gerontology to the forefront of the field of Gerontology. As a collective group of gerontologists, we will be better served to acknowledge, incorporate and address the interrelated nature of aging experience and the important role of the environment in shaping that experience. This volume brings to surface the latent personal stories behind the scholarship in this area, and by doing so, we hope that it will inspire early career researchers to learn from the focus, persistence, determination, mentorship, peer-support, and commitment evident in the scholars' lives. Learning from others' thoughtful reflections who are ahead of ourselves in the career trajectory remains a valuable pathway for self-growth and intellectual development.

REFERENCES

Baltes, P. B. (1987). Theoretical propositions of life-span developmental psychology: On the dynamics between growth and decline. *Developmental Psychology, 23*(5), 611–626.

Butler, R. N. (1963). The life review: An interpretation of reminiscence in the aged. *Psychiatry, 26*, 65–76.

Eribon, D. (2013). *Returning to Reims* (M. Lucey, Trans.). Cambridge, MA: MIT-Press.

Lawton, M. P. & Nahemow, L. (1973). Ecology and the aging process. In C. Eisdorfer & M. P. Lawton (Eds.), *The psychology of adult development and aging* (pp. 619–674). Washington, DC: American Psychological Association.

CHAPTER 2

The Environment as Developmental Context

In All Ages But Certainly in Old Age

Hans-Werner Wahl

ABSTRACT

The biographical account underlying this chapter starts in the midst of the 1980s in Berlin, after my first job as a research associate in an epidemiology and aging project at Heidelberg University had ended. The real breakthrough toward becoming a scientist with a serious interest in behavioral aging came when I received the opportunity to work with Margret M. Baltes at the Free University of Berlin, and later also with Paul B. Baltes in the context of the Berlin Aging Study. At the time, my emerging focus on the ecology of aging was much infused by Margret's research on social ecologies of aging as well as the work of M. Powell Lawton at the Philadelphia Geriatric Center, where I had the privilege to stay for a couple of months at the end of the 1980s. My main ambition regarding the ecology of aging has been to better link a person–environment interaction perspective with a life-span view of human development. Most recently, I see major new impulses toward better understanding the role of context for aging well. For example, new designs such as momentary ecological assessments and data linkage will add much to the ecology of aging at large and counteract the ongoing trend of decontextualizing aging processes and outcomes.

http://dx.doi.org/10.1891/0198-8794.38.17

BIOGRAPHICAL NOTES

As a student, I never planned to become a geropsychologist or a gerontologist, not to speak of an environmental gerontologist. The psychology of aging did not play a role at all in the psychology program of Heidelberg University at the end of the 1970s/beginning of the 1980s, when I completed my diploma in psychology. It is nevertheless true that I unexpectedly received the offer to start my professional life in a geropsychiatric research area at Heidelberg University and the Central Institute of Mental Health in Mannheim, Germany, an important partner institution of Heidelberg University. I accepted and gave it a try. However, I also told myself that this should be the beginning of the end of my aging research involvement. Thereafter, according to my professional anticipation, something "real important" in psychology should follow. However, things developed differently. I received the opportunity to work as a research associate with Margret M. Baltes (Margret) around the midst of the 1980s. My association with her completely changed my view on aging as a scientific matter. I realized that gero- and life-span psychologists are a "serious scientific species;" this has, of course, been the case already at the time in the United States and to some extent also in Germany, but it was simply, I must admit, not on my radar screen as a young psychologist.

Working with Margret brought the environment upfront in my emerging involvement in psychological aging. Margret's major conceptual research platform—social learning theory, was new to me at the time. I found it fascinating that there was empirical data on micro-level social interaction indicating that dependent behaviors in older adults are to a large extent produced by social contexts, particularly professional and informal care environments. Operating in this inspiring research atmosphere, I was also offered the opportunity to work together with Margret on a book chapter (Baltes & Wahl, 1987), published in Carstensen and Edelstein's *Handbook of Clinical Gerontology*. A large number of other joint publications followed over the years. Looking back, I feel that this 1987 chapter played a very important role for my "falling in love" with geropsychology and person–environmental aging perspectives, and resulted in the first international appearance of my name. Being a research associate and doctoral student of Margret also came with many opportunities for interacting with internationally well-established scholars visiting Berlin, that is, Margret's research unit as well as Paul B. Baltes' (Paul) research group at the Max-Planck Institute of Human Development. Scholars such as Margie Lachman, M. Powell Lawton (Powell), Carol Ryff, or Vern Bengtson (Vern), just a few names among many others, were several times around who opened my mind for fundamental issues related to behavioral and social aging.

As a consequence, in my internal struggle to define my own research interests, an interesting combination was created. On one hand, in my daily work with Margret's research on dependency in old age, it was highly sensible for the critical role of the social environment for aging processes and outcomes. It was quickly clear that I should also concentrate on my own dissertation work (published in Wahl, 1991, in *Psychology and Aging*) on this issue, although I strived to also collect direct data of older adults in nursing homes and in home health care as compared to our mostly observational data protocol previously used. Hence, I developed a semistructured interview based on psychological action theory and made an attempt to systematically reconstruct action-related cognitions and emotions directly after care-related behaviors in caregivers as well as in care receivers. Nevertheless, this approach was framed against contrasting institutionalized versus home settings and thus kept the consideration of the environmental part as I had learned it from Margret. On the other hand, I extended my understanding of "the environment" in two directions. First, the physical–spatial part of the environment, much focused conceptually and empirically by scholars such as Powell, still was not considered much in the psychology of aging. My plan was to address this research gap with my own work. Second, environmental thinking also needed reasoning in socio-structural and regional terms, and this opened my mind also for sociological and geographical views on aging.

What followed in 1988 was of high importance for my further academic development. Margret and Paul opened the doors for research visits to the Philadelphia Geriatric Center, Philadelphia, where Powell very successfully conducted his research nearly completely based on soft money, as well as the Andrus Gerontology Center in Los Angeles and Vern's research team, in particular. Hence, as a young scholar, I had direct contact with a giant in Environmental Gerontology (Powell) as well as with a giant in the social sciences of aging studies (Vern). Powell's influence was of high importance for my work until today and was driven by three elements: (a) his competence-environmental press theory and related conceptual elaborations, pointing to the increasing dependence on and profit from environmental characteristics as we age; (b) his rigor as an empirical researcher struggling to assess as optimally as possible the confounded nature of personal and environmental (P-E) processes; (c) his personality that combined in quite a unique way a critical attitude toward himself and others with personal warmth and generosity. In Vern's case, his clear-cut emphasis put on the role of theory for the understanding of aging was critical for me (indeed, the first edition of what later became *Handbook of Theories of Aging*, edited by Birren and Bengtson, was published in 1988). Honestly, however, I think that Vern's theory impulse which I received as a young scholar during my stay at end of the 1980s showed kind of a sleeper effect and I realized only later in full size the importance of theory in aging science. When I returned to Berlin, I did my duty and had my dissertation defense at the beginning of 1989. At the content level, my interest in the physical-spatial environments of aging had much increased and it was apparent that this should be a major pathway for my research in the next couple of years.

Besides Margret, a German colleague who was very influential on my views on person–environment aging perspectives, was Winfried Saup (Winfried) affiliated with the University of Augsburg. He was already engaged in Environmental Gerontology as the author of the first German textbook on the issue in 1993 (Saup, 1993; see also Wahl & Saup, 1994). I still vividly remember my several highly inspiring exchanges with Winfried, during our long walks in nature, on fundamental issues of person–environment transaction as people age and on the role of Environmental Gerontology in the gerontology enterprise at large. Sadly, I have to note that Winfried passed away in 2011 from cancer, at only 60 years of age. A major outcome resulting from my exchange with Winfried was my programmatic essay on an environmentally framed psychology of aging, which appeared in 1992 in the *Psychologische Rundschau*, the German Society of Psychology's official periodical (Wahl, 1992).

Afterwards, a dual life of sorts followed. Paul and the directorship of the Berlin Aging Study (BASE) offered me the position of the scientific coordinator of BASE, which I gladly accepted. In parallel, I furthered my interest in environmental geropsychology and gerontology and searched for an empirical paradigm which should fulfill three criteria: being inspiring in terms of learning about P-E relations, empirically not well researched, and practically important. This search brought me to an unexpected theme: age-related vision impairment. Losing one's sight late in life is a psychologically critical experience that predominantly impacts on the relation to the physical environment, whereas hearing loss mostly affects the relation to the social environment. However, not much was known at the time on how the nature of such P-E change due to vision impairment looks like and what kind of compensatory and optimizing strategies visually impaired older adults may use to counteract autonomy and wellbeing threats. My goal thus was to learn about adaptation in visually impaired older adults by explicitly taking the physical environment into consideration. Empirically, we assessed the living environment (particularly in-house, but also immediate surrounding) by means of a "walk-through" interview in addition to using established scales on coping, wellbeing, and depression. In terms of P-E interchange processes, we were interested in issues such as environmental hazards (e.g., light conditions, obstacles on floor, narrow pathways, bathing tubs), but also in how visually impaired older adults make use of the environment to remain as independent as possible (e.g., using frozen meals, using a tape recorder for cooking receipts, keeping order to always know where to find important things). My initial interest in age-related vision impairment quickly intensified and led to considerable research funding.

At the same time, after the completion of my BASE-related involvement in 1992, backed by my own funding money, I moved to Heidelberg University and its Institute of Gerontology chaired by Ursula Lehr. At Heidelberg, my age-related vision impairment research evolved into a full-blown research program, in which I headed for understanding psychological adaptation at the person level (e.g., coping and control-regulatory processes in dealing with vision loss), as well as the role of person–environmental interchange with emphasis on the physical–spatial environment. This resulted in different lines of publications. For example, I published the more environmental parts of research in an article in *The Gerontologist* (Wahl, Oswald, & Zimprich, 1999), while the more person-level parts appeared in the *Journal of Gerontology: Psychological Sciences* (Wahl, Schilling, Oswald, & Heyl, 1999). The messages coming from both of these research streams were that there is obvious loss in terms of increased "environmental docility" caused by the vision loss. At the same time, it was evident that older adults with vision loss adjust rather successfully using a range of creative compensatory strategies, and by these means, were able to maintain autonomy and wellbeing at least to a considerable extent. For me, this overall finding fitted well into and extended the picture that Powell had drawn in his landmark article on "the good life" in old age based on his Kleemeier Award lecture (Lawton, 1983). My vision research, later enriched by age-related hearing impairment, continues to run until present, although it increasingly turned to the person level (see for example Schilling et al., 2016, for our latest contribution in this area; see also below). It also brought in my long-standing collaborations with Frank Oswald (now at Goethe University Frankfurt) and with Amy Horowitz (now at Fordham University New York) and her research group, both starting at the beginning of the 1990s. My interest in person–environmental issues was also highly supported at the university level by the creation of a professorship position on social and ecological gerontology at the newly founded German Center for Research in Aging at Heidelberg University in 1997, the first of its kind in Germany.

Around the beginning of the new millennium, a series of publications in established formats significantly deepened my thoughts on and work in Environmental Gerontology. Warner Schaie invited me to contribute a chapter on Environmental Gerontology to the 5th edition of the *Handbook of the Psychology and Aging* (Wahl, 2001) and later also to edit a volume of the *Annual Review of Gerontology and Geriatrics* titled "Aging in Context: Socio-physical Environments," which I was very happy to do together with Rick Scheidt and Paul Windley (Wahl, Scheidt, & Windley, 2004). I myself had a chapter in this book coauthored by developmental and life-span psychologist Frieder Lang (University of Erlangen-Nuremberg), in which we made an attempt to systematically spell out the need to consider social and physical environments as closely intertwined, if not inseparable, environments of aging (Wahl & Lang, 2004, 2006). We did this in what we labeled the "Social-Physical Environments over Time" (SPOT) model; for me, such striving to consider both the social and physical environment was much inspired by what Lawton already had claimed much earlier (e.g., Lawton, 1982) as well as by my collaboration with Margret, but now new theoretical substance such as socio-emotional selectivity theory (e.g., Carstensen, 2006) was available. Other scholars of high relevance for my own thinking on person–environment issues at the time have been Laura Gitlin (e.g., contribution to *Encyclopedia of Gerontology*, Wahl & Gitlin, 2007), Gerald Weisman (*Forum* article in *The Gerontologist*: Wahl & Weisman, 2003), and Graham Rowles (see Oswald & Wahl, 2005 in volume edited by Rowles & Chaudhury, 2005), all visiting Heidelberg several times for research and conference occasions.

In parallel emerged an important European endeavor, that is, the ENABLE-AGE project and our collaboration (Frank and myself) with Susanne Iwarsson (Susanne) from Lund University, Sweden (see Chapter 7, From Occupational Therapy to Environmental Gerontology). In this project involving Germany, Hungary, Latvia, Sweden, and the UK and funded by the 5th Framework Program of the European Commission, we aimed to create a kind of an ideal data protocol for an Environmental Gerontology study in terms of the breadth of data collected, methods used, and conceptual grounding. We concentrated on very old (75–80 years and older) and living alone adults as a group particularly vulnerable for environmental demands. The data protocol contained an innovative person–environment fit index developed by Susanne's team based on her Housing Enabler Instrument (Iwarsson & Slaug, 2010), a range of newly constructed scales to assess meaning of home and coping with one's environments (e.g., housing-related control beliefs), as well as a large number of healthy aging-related outcomes, such as life satisfaction, affective wellbeing, and depressive mood. We were also able to implement a 1-year longitudinal component to transcend a sole cross-sectional design at least to some extent. Major findings of the ENABLE-AGE project were summarized in a special section in *The Gerontologist* in 2007 (opening paper: Iwarsson et al., 2007; an integration of all ENABLE-AGE findings is available in Iwarsson et al., 2016). The M. Powell Lawton Award of the Gerontological Society of America, which I received in 2009, was certainly only possible due to the outstanding collaboration and support offered by all of the individuals mentioned above and much backed by the ENABLE-AGE research.

We transformed the ENABLE-AGE study in Heidelberg to a new longitudinal project ("Lateline") with a strong focus on psychological adaptation in very old age, but with less emphasis put on the environmental component (e.g., Wettstein, Schilling, Reidick, & Wahl, 2015). An important background for this shift to the person level of aging was a new professorship position on psychological aging research installed at the Institute of Psychology at Heidelberg University which I received in 2006. Somewhat later, I started a new collaboration together with Manfred Diehl (Manfred) from Colorado State University on the role of subjective aging. In particular, we introduced a new concept, *awareness of age-related change* (Diehl & Wahl, 2010), and built (and continue to build) a full research program around the construct. Although views of aging always operate in societal contexts and are strongly driven by environmental dynamics, this research is highly person-centered and aims to further assessment devices of subjective aging and linkages between subjective aging and key endpoints such as health and wellbeing-related constructs (see also Diehl & Wahl, 2015).

Though, I never "left" the person–environmental view of aging and was happy to prepare chapters, for example, for the *Sage Handbook of Social Gerontology* (Wahl & Oswald, 2010), and more recently for the *Handbook of Theories of Aging* (Wahl & Oswald, 2016) together with Frank. I was also very happy to see my M. Powell Lawton lecture held in 2010 at GSA's Annual Scientific Meeting in a revised version together with Susanne and Frank as a Spotlight Article in *The Gerontologist* (Wahl, Iwarsson, & Oswald, 2012).

A new person–environment assessment approach now increasingly common and known as ambulatory assessment was used in a research project (project SenTra) together with Israeli geographer Noam Shoval (Hebrew University Jerusalem) based on GPS sensor tracking technology targeting out-of-home mobility of older adults with cognitive impairment (Wahl et al., 2013). Further, I recently completed a project (INNOVAGE) together with sport scientist Klaus Hauer (Bethanien Geriatric Center, Heidelberg) on the role of physical activity training in nursing homes environments, using the latest in accelerometry and sensor-tracking technology to assess training gain, as well as to characterize the daily ecology of living in long-term settings at large (Jansen, Claßen, Hauer, Diegelmann, & Wahl, 2014).

Finally, I also developed a strong interest in technology as a new and increasingly important environment of aging (e.g., Schulz et al., 2015). Most recently, I became interested in the issue of ecological validity and started to prepare together with Manfred a respective special section for *Research in Human Development* (Diehl & Wahl, n.d.). This is kind of a closing the circle experience, because Environmental Gerontology for me always has been, at the more general level, a striving toward better representation of daily ecologies, while considering aging persons and their environments in parallel, influencing each other in constant transaction.

CONCEPTUAL EVOLVEMENTS OVER TIME

As already indicated above, social learning theory has been important as an initial driving force to address the role of the socio-physical context for aging processes and outcomes, particularly dependent and independent behaviors. In all what I did afterwards in terms of theoretical referral and empirical research, this conceptual socialization I experienced during my working with Margret remained an important meta-view. Hence, whether I addressed the role of social partners including professionals or the role of various physical-spatial environments, a major issue for me always has been the consideration of its impact on dependency or independency of older adults operating in respective environments. That is, I assume that autonomy and mastery lie at the core of aging successfully, but can only be understood, when older adults are not seen as islands, but as closely interwoven with their environments.

Going further, my fundamental platform of theorizing aging as a behavioral scientist is that the pursuit of goals and actions important for an older person, and thus, quality of life in old age cannot be seen as an individualized outcome but also is triggered and shaped by facilitating or hindering environmental conditions. Therefore, I always had (and continue to have) problems with the commonly followed strategy to sample individuals in empirical research, but not situations in which these individuals are embedded in and transact with their environments. There is thus an ongoing paradox with which I've struggled until presently in what we do in empirical research: On one hand, a broad consensus within the aging research community exists that both personal and environmental characteristics contribute to aging well. On the other hand, the contribution of key elements of the immediate environment to aging well, including the home, public and community environments, and technology, remain largely overlooked in many of our key theories and projects, particularly longitudinal studies. Despite Lawton and Nahemow's (1973) conceptualization of aging well as involving both personal and environmental components, or more specifically a P-E transactional dynamic, and thus, P-E coconstruction (Valsiner, 1994; Youniss, 1987), the role of the environment has largely been neglected in gerontological research. For example, established reasoning on successful aging (Baltes & Baltes, 1990; Rowe & Kahn, 1998; Ryff, 1989) typically does not refer explicitly to environmental conditions, especially not to the physical–spatial part of the environment. This is all the more surprising, because as Lawton and Nahemow

(1973) convincingly argued more than four decades ago, that development in the late and most vulnerable phase of the adult human life span is particularly sensitive to the nature and character of P-E transactions.

It is worthwhile in this context to reflect upon fundamental concepts in the environmental psychology as well as developmental science literature. For me, the concepts of *transaction* and *co-construction* transport best what happens in human development seen as an open system (Overton, 2010). There is no one-way road and individuals are always shaping environments and being shaped at the same time by environments. Although this means conceptually that both processes are completely interwoven and hard, if not impossible, to separate, the concept of coconstruction assumes that life goals play a critical role in transactions. That is, it has been clear to me that older adults, even in highly vulnerable life circumstances, are not pawns of their environmental set-up; instead, they also invest in selecting suitable ecologies to act in.

Hence, my view of older adults always has been one of goal-directed individuals striving to remain "masters" of their per definition contextual lives. Environmental characteristics increasingly shape the process and outcome of such goal-direction as we age; at the same time, they also can help to cope with lost competencies by means of enabling (and not disabling) features. This may happen in the ideal case as naturally occurring and usable by the aging individual or may become the subject of designed environmental intervention (e.g., home modification). Hence, the environmental sphere is in my view a rather ambivalent force as part of aging, coming with inextricably interwoven elements of threat and reserve capacities for autonomy and wellbeing. The classic question of many older adults and particularly those with emerging functional and cognitive impairments "How long will I be able to stay at this place?" echoes such ambivalence quite directly. The strong desire to stay put becomes increasingly overshadowed by the fearful insight that enjoying the safety and wellness of one's living environment may find its limits in a hard to predict P-E constellation in the future that will no longer be acceptable (e.g., too risky and unsafe).

That said, my treatment of Environmental Gerontology, conceptually and empirically, has been and continues to be driven by two demands imposed on myself: (a) Although transaction and co-construction have been my most important theoretically driving concepts, I felt that there is no gold standard for how to take up such concepts at the empirical level. It has therefore been important for me to stay pragmatic in terms of what is empirically manageable and fruitful. (b) I strived to provide integrative suggestions that better link a P-E transaction of aging with key gerontology research perspectives, such as life-span developmental views and ideas on the role of cohort flow to understand aging.

Theoretical Treatment of P-E Transaction in Old Age That is Empirically Manageable and Fruitful

Objective Environments Matters in Old Age

For me, taking the "world out there" seriously is the platform of Environmental Gerontology. Key gerontological researchers have made classic contributions to understand the impact of objective environments and objective environmental transitions (e.g., Carp & Carp, 1984; Lawton, 1982, 1989; Lawton & Nahemow, 1973; see also Scheidt & Windley, 2006; Wahl, 2001). The ecology of aging perspective posits old age as a critical phase in the life course that is profoundly influenced by objective physical environments. According to Lawton (1982), the objective physical environment lies outside the skin, is inanimate and measurable. While there is consensus that the physical environment has the potential to impose significant constraints in late life, it may also enhance opportunities for aging well, as new housing solutions and new technologies support declining competencies. They may also enrich late-life development and thus contribute to successful aging trajectories. Based on Lewin's ecological equation, Lawton suggested an interaction term to account for the influence of person–environment interactions, that is, $B = f(P\ E\ P \times E)$. This interaction term suggests that because person-related competencies and needs manifest differently in different environments, they may lead to dissimilar outcomes. Lawton and Nahemow's (1973; see also Lawton, 1982) ecology theory of aging (ETA) continues to provide a broad, overarching framework that includes different types and levels of personal competence (e.g., sensory loss, physical mobility loss, cognitive decline) and characteristics of the objective environment (e.g., housing standards, neighborhood conditions, and public transport). A fundamental assumption of the ETA is that unique combinations of personal competence and environmental characteristics determine an individual's optimal level of functioning.

The idea to focus the transaction of rather objectively measurable person characteristics operating in rather objectively measureable environmental constellations may sound a bit strange for developmental science and geropsychology. However, I believe this focus is fundamental for the understanding of behavioral life-span development because of three primary reasons: First, it is the objective ecology in which psychological processes unfold. If an older adult with severe vision impairment lives in a housing situation which significantly constrains the person's remaining capabilities, then developmental reserve capacity and plasticity in terms of what is psychologically possible in life for this individual are under pressure. Second, the availability and use of objective action space may stimulate exploratory behaviors and the generation of new and possibly unexpected goals. Indeed, such exploratory behaviors may be seen as a form of training able to contribute to physical, social, and cognitive functioning maintenance and thus what has been coined *engagement* (Hertzog, Kramer, Wilson, & Lindenburger, 2008). Third, enabling objective P-E ecologies will likely provide a major facilitating platform for key late-life processes and outcomes such as life review, meaning making, and purpose of life reflections.

This reasoning has led to two consequences in our research program. On one hand, it has been important to provide additional data showing that environmental docility exists and leads to different everyday worlds of aging individuals. We found that severely visually impaired older adults living in objectively low P-E fit constellations do indeed have more constrained opportunities for the execution of autonomy, particularly in the domain of instrumental and thus more complex activities of daily living (IADL; Wahl et al., 1999). As we later presented in a systematic review paper, available research generally confirms a linkage among the objective environment, particularly the home environment, and disability-related outcomes (Wahl, Fänge, Oswald, Gitlin, & Iwarsson, 2009; see also Oswald & Wahl, 2004). On the other hand, it has been important to underscore, how older adults in specific life situations, such as age-related vision impairment, are coping with their specific P-E transactional demands in terms of goal engagement and disengagement. In this regard, we applied the life-span theory of control (now titled motivational theory of life-span development; Heckhausen, Wrosch, & Schulz, 2010) in order to better understand adaptational processes and outcomes. As we found with a generally framed as well as a vision-specific control strategy assessment instrument, older adults with vision loss overall invest more in secondary compensatory control strategies (SCC) to keep going and maintain wellbeing (e.g., Schilling et al., 2013, 2016; Wahl, Schilling & Becker, 2007). However, as we have also found in these studies, investment into SCC strongly depends on remaining IADL status. Only when surpassing a certain threshold of lowered IADL due to the vision impairment, increased use of SCC starts and is adaptive; too early use would lead to unnecessary undermining of still available action reserves. Inversely, as argued above, the IADL status of visually impaired older adults also is associated with the physical environment. Indeed, trends toward improvement in IADL functioning in more recent cohorts of older adults have been connected with contextual improvement, whereas ADL functioning more strongly depends on underlying disease processes (e.g., Feng et al., 2013; Parker & Thorslund, 2007). Hence, psychological adaptation in terms of goal engagement and goal disengagement always is embedded in given transactions with the objective environment coming with increased or decreased objective enabling or disabling P-E constellations.

Experiencing P-E Transactions Matters in Old Age

Although I regard objective constraints to development given in existing P-E constellations as fundamental in the driving processes of psychological adaptation, it is also clear that environmental constellations are subject to interpretations and evaluations. Living for a very long time at the same location, typically for older adults (quite often for several decades), seems to generate a rich portfolio of place-related meaning and bonding processes. Residential satisfaction in terms of global evaluations of home or geographic location is certainly important here (Pinquart & Burmedi, 2004). Interestingly and similar to the wellbeing paradox in general (Kunzmann, Little, & Smith, 2000), residential satisfaction remains high as people age, independent of changes at the person level (e.g., increasing functional impairment impacting on making use of one's environment) and characteristics of the environment such as a housing set-up with a number of environmental hazards. Thus, residential satisfaction may play an important protective role in making aging individuals resilient to fears of losing autonomy (staying put is a major indicator for many older adults of "still" being autonomous) and possibly a needed relocation in the not too distant future.

However, we (Frank and I) were more interested in processes of place attachment and identity (Neisser, 1988), emphasizing the transformation of "space" into "place" (Rowles & Watkins, 2003), and the better understanding how aging individuals form affective, cognitive, behavioral, and social bonds to their environment (Peace, 2005). This brought us to more qualitative work of how older adults experience feeling at home, resulting in five categories (Oswald & Wahl, 2005): (a) "Physical," focusing on the experience of housing conditions such as experience of the residential area and furnishing; (b) "Behavioral," related to the everyday behavior of the person at home and to ways of rearranging items in the home; (c) "Cognitive," representing biographical bonding to the home, such as the experience of familiarity and insideness; (d) "Emotional," expressing the experience of privacy, safety, pleasure, and stimulation; and (e) "Social," expressing relationships with fellow-lodgers, neighbors, or visitors. As we found in a study contrasting healthy older adults with older adults with severe vision impairment and older adults with mobility impairment, healthy participants were more appreciative of the physical location, access, and amenity aspects of the home. Both groups of functionally impaired participants emphasized the cognitive and biographical significance of the home. With respect to behavioral and social aspects, visually impaired older adults concentrated more on their social and cognitive sphere and less on behavioral and physical aspects of the home, while the meaning patterns for the mobility-impaired participants included behavioral aspects to a greater extent. About the same share of statements were made with regard to emotional themes in all three groups.

As I see it, these findings add important and differentiating facets to research on meaning making in later life as a major theme in developmental research. That is, older adults impose meaning on their environments, which in turn motivate them for action (e.g., "Jogging in this residential area is fun") or help them cope with lost functional capacities (e.g., "At home, I am feeling competent and fully functioning, although my eyesight is bad"). Hence, goal-engagement and goal-disengagement processes as spelled out in the motivational theory of life-span development (Heckhausen et al., 2010) not only are shaped by objective P-E constellations as argued above, but are also embedded in environment-related meaning structures and bonding processes (e.g., "This is my home which I will never leave"). In other words, goal-engagement or goal-disengagement processes in aging, particularly very old individuals, may be better understood, if environment-related meaning-making processes are also taken into consideration.

Integrative Efforts to Better Link Different Views on P-E Transactions With Gerontology Theorizing at Large[1]

Going for objective P-E constellations as well as the experiential component of aging in environments cries for integration, but most of the available frameworks previously proposed incorporated only one of these perspectives (e.g., ETA-focused objective environments). At the core of what Frank and I did in terms of integration has been the consideration of two processes, that is, P-E belonging and P-E agency (see Figure 2.1; Wahl et al., 2012; Wahl & Oswald, 2016). As we have suggested, processes associated with P-E belonging account for the experiential part of P-E transactions in terms of subjective evaluations and environmental representations at the cognitive and emotional levels.

While belonging oriented processes are environment-related meaning-making processes without goal direction, processes of agency include the full range of goal-directed behaviors related to environment, such as environment-related cognition and perceived control over the physical environment. They include reactive and proactive aspects of using, compensating, adapting, retrofitting, creating, and sustaining places, especially important in old age because of decreasing functional and cognitive capacity. Overall, the agency-belonging approach is predominantly seen as a meta-model able to reconcile the realm of key meaning-related environmental processes and classic theoretical-empirical work in the area (e.g., Peace, 2005; Rowles & Watkins, 2003; Rubinstein, 1989) with models anchored in the tradition of the ETA (Lawton, 1982; Lawton & Nahemow, 1973; Scheidt & Norris-Baker, 2004). However, we also broadened

[1]I strongly refer in this section to previous writings, particularly cooperative work done together with Frank Oswald.

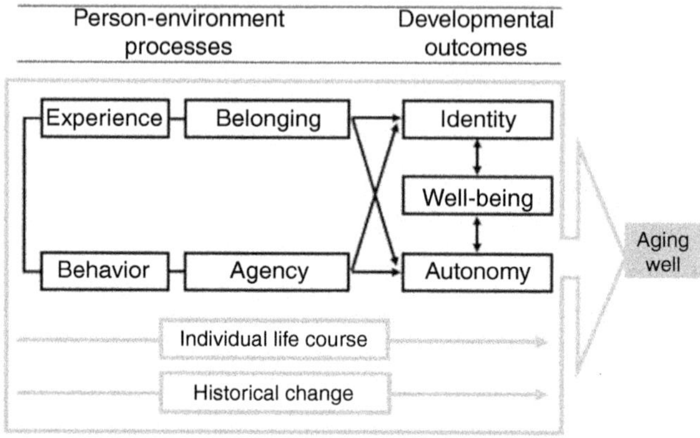

FIGURE 2.1 Toward a comprehensive model of P-E transaction in later life.
Source: Wahl and Oswald (2016, p. 629).

the agency component in that we considered control theory elements, that is, housing-related control beliefs (Oswald, Wahl, Schilling & Iwarsson, 2007). Finally, the model assumes that a range of outcomes needs consideration. P-E agency is expected to predominantly impact on autonomy, whereas P-E belonging plays an important role for personal identity issues. Wellbeing is another overarching endpoint to be considered.

The model so far has found its most profound empirical application in the ENABLE-AGE project. Overall, we found what we expected (e.g., Oswald, Wahl, Schilling, Nygren, 2007): Older adults living in better person–environment fit situations, assigning higher meaning to their housing, and having higher beliefs in that they are able to control their environments (not being pawns of their environments) also revealed higher cognitive and affective wellbeing, autonomy, and lowered depression (we did not consider identity related outcomes in ENABLE-AGE). Importantly, this pattern emerged in all countries involved in the ENABLE-AGE project; hence, we concluded that the covariance dynamics of environmental and personal constructs seemed to operate rather similarly across countries, although socio-economic level differences among countries obviously were pronounced.

Going further, contributing to a life-span developmental view of aging, processes of P-E *belonging* are expected to increase in importance as people enter old and particularly advanced old age, while the relevance of processes of P-E *agency* is expected to decrease. This would be in line with models of human development and aging (Erikson, 1950; Tornstam, 2005), but also with socio-emotional selectivity theory (e.g., Carstensen, 2006). Indeed, Wahl and Lang

(2004) have argued in their SPOT model that belonging and agency may similarly apply to the social and physical environments. That is, increasing belonging can be detected in more emotional closeness to selected places as well as selected social partners.

In terms of gerontology's important issue of the role of cohort flow, changes in aging individuals' relations with their physical environments may be seen as a frequently underrated important cohort effect. For example, one may argue that the impact of interaction with the environment on aging well has increased as new housing solutions for older adults, such as assisted living, retirement communities, or intergenerational arrangements, and new housing options for persons with dementia, have replaced traditional built environments. It may well be that future built-environment solutions for older adults may not only better support P-E agency-related processes (e.g., enhancing daily autonomy even among older adults with disabilities), but also nurture or even "provoke" new forms of belonging and respective outcomes. For example, the realm of "feeling at home" may increasingly extend to such new housing options and thus the exclusiveness of private housing as the key form of "Home" may significantly change. Going further, technology developments that were not available to the cohorts investigated empirically in Powell's research may considerably impact on future aging. For example, the Internet, the "automation" of everyday technology (e.g., teller machines, ticket machines, computer voice menus, car technology), and sensor- or GPS-based assistance have already changed the way older people interact with the environment (Charness & Boot, 2009; Schulz et al., 2015).

OUTLOOK

On one hand, it is obvious that notable bridges do already exist here and have for decades. A classic example is Bronfenbrenner's *bio-ecological model* now on stage since the end of the 1970s (Bronfenbrenner, 1979). This model expands on the concept of environment to include microsystems (activities and interaction patterns in immediate surroundings), mesosystems (connections among microsystems), exosystems (settings not containing the individual directly yet still affecting them), macrosystems (broader systems of culture, values, laws, customs), and chronosystems (life transitions). It focuses on the changing interrelationship among these layers of context in individuals over time and therefore has a direct linkage with human development in multilayered contexts. On the other hand, it is surprising that such long-time established bridges only found limited application so far in mainstream gerontology and its empirical programs. For example, with respect to theories of successful aging, P-E agency processes may have the potential to further develop the selective optimization with compensation (SOC) model inaugurated by Baltes and Baltes (1990). Home modification, relocation processes, and using a care robot (in the future) reflect important selection and compensatory strategies, beyond those typically included in the SOC model. At the same time, I argue that processes of P-E belonging are much underrepresented in currently dominant models of aging well. Also I strongly believe in the importance of an agency orientation and goal-directedness in older adults' daily P-E transactions, more experientially driven aging processes, hence P-E belonging oriented processes, seem to play an increasingly adaptive role when individuals move into advanced old age (Oswald & Konopik, 2015; Wahl & Lang, 2004; Wahl et al., 2012).

At the more empirical level, the recent strong trend toward event sampling and measurement in day-to-day ecologies (e.g., Ram & Gerstorf, 2009) may also benefit from a stronger P-E transactional perspective. Indeed, the ecology of aging view always made a strong claim to better consider concrete day-to-day behaviors in natural environments (Lawton & Nahemow, 1973; Wahl, 2001). For me, the "hype" toward ambulatory assessment that increasingly conquers the psychology of aging in key areas such as stress experience and coping, cognitive functioning, social relations, and physical activity in sense also may be seen as ecological gerontology "in dynamic action:" Understanding at the micro transactional level how older individuals' lives are embedded into contexts and daily co-constructional processes happen (Ram & Diehl, 2015). However, it seems also clear to me that ambulatory assessment approaches that may also shape Environmental Gerontology at large in the future need the consideration of meso-, exo-, macro-, and chrono-levels of contexts to grasp the complexity of human development.

In closing, I feel that taking contextual perspectives seriously in gerontology may bring a much stronger liaison among Environmental Gerontology and developmental science views and will deepen our views of what aging well may mean to older adults. I continue to enjoy operating both in the life span and still much person-centered psychology of aging as well as the Environmental Gerontology world, but best moments in my academic life happen when I stand on the bridge between those worlds, having a nice look on both at the same time.

REFERENCES

Baltes, M. M., & Wahl, H.-W. (1987). Dependency in aging. In L. L. Carstensen & B. A. Edelstein (Eds.), *Handbook of clinical gerontology* (pp. 204–221). New York, NY: Pergamon Press.

Baltes, P. B., & Baltes, M. M. (Eds.). (1990). *Successful aging: Perspectives from the behavioral sciences.* New York, NY: Cambridge University Press.

Birren, J. E., & Bengtson, V. L. (1988). Emergent theories of aging. New York: Springer Publishing.

Bronfenbrenner, U. (1979). *The ecology of human development. Experiments by nature and design*. Cambridge, MA: Harvard University Press.

Carp, F. M., & Carp, A. (1984). A complementary/congruence model of well-being or mental health for the community elderly. In I. Altman, M. P. Lawton, & J. F. Wohlwill (Eds.), *Human behavior and environment: Elderly people and the environment* (Vol. 7, pp. 279–336). New York, NY: Plenum Press.

Carstensen, L. L. (2006). The influence of a sense of time on human development. *Science, 312*(5782), 1913–1915.

Charness, N., & Boot, W. R. (2009). Aging and information technology use. Potential and barriers. *Current Directions in Psychological Science, 18*(5), 253–258.

Diehl, M., & Wahl, H.-W. (2010). Awareness of age-related change: Examination of a (mostly) unexplored concept. *The Journals of Gerontology Series B: Psychological Sciences and Social Sciences, 69*(2), 340–350.

Diehl, M., & Wahl, H.-W. (Eds.). (2015). Research on subjective aging: New developments and future directions. In *Annual Review of Gerontology and Geriatrics 2015*(Vol. 35). New York, NY: Springer Publishing.

Diehl, M., & Wahl, H.-W. (n.d.). Ecological validity and research on human development: Old and new challenges. *Research in Human Development*. [Manuscript in preparation.]

Erikson, E. H. (1950). *Childhood and society*. New York, NY: Norton & Company.

Feng, Q., Zhen, Z., Gu, D., Wu, B., Duncan, P. W., & Purser, J. L. (2013). Trends in ADL and IADL disability in community-dwelling older adults in Shanghai, China, 1998–2008. *Journal of Gerontology: Social and Psychological Sciences, 68*(3), 476–485.

Heckhausen, J., Wrosch, C., & Schulz, R. (2010). A motivational theory of life-span development. *Psychological Review, 117*(1), 32–60.

Hertzog, C., Kramer, A. F., Wilson, R. S., & Lindenburger, U. (2008). Enrichment effects on adult cognitive development: Can the functional capacity of older adults be preserved and enhanced? *Psychological Science in the Public Interest, 9*(1), 1–65.

Iwarsson, S., & Slaug, B. (2010). *The revised version of the Housing Enabler: An instrument for assessing and analysing accessibility problems in housing*. Nävlinge and Staffanstorp, Sweden: Veten & Skapen HB & Slaug Data Management.

Iwarsson, S., Löfqvist, C., Oswald, F., Slaug, B., Schmidt, S., Wahl, H.-W., et al. (2016). Synthesizing ENABLE-AGE research findings to suggest evidence-based home and health interventions. *Journal of Housing for the Elderly, 30*(3), 330–343.

Iwarsson, S., Wahl, H.-W., Nygren, C., Oswald, F., Sixsmith, A., Sixsmith, J., et al. (2007). Importance of the home environment for healthy aging: Conceptual and methodological background of the ENABLE-AGE Project. *The Gerontologist*, 47(1), 78–84.

Jansen, C.-P., Claßen, K., Hauer, K., Diegelmann, M., & Wahl, H.-W. (2014). Assessing the effect of a physical activity intervention in a nursing home ecology: a natural lab approach. *BMC Geriatrics, 14*(117), 1–12.

Kunzmann, U., Little, T. D., & Smith, J. (2000). Is age-related stability of subjective well-being a paradox? Cross-sectional and longitudinal evidence from the Berlin Aging Study. *Psychology and Aging, 15*(3), 511–526.

Lawton, M. P. (1982). Competence, environmental press, and the adaptation of older people. In M. P. Lawton, P. G. Windley, & T. O. Byerts (Eds.), *Aging and the environment* (pp. 33–59). New York, NY: Springer Publishing.

Lawton, M. P. (1983). Environment and other determinants of well-being in older people. *The Gerontologist, 23*(4), 349–357.

Lawton, M. P. (1989). Environmental proactivity in older people. In V. L. Bengtson & K. W. Schaie (Eds.), *The course of later life* (pp. 15–23). New York, NY: Springer Publishing.

Lawton, M. P., & Nahemow, L. (1973). Ecology and the aging process. In C. Eisdorfer & M. P. Lawton (Eds.), *The psychology of adult development and aging* (pp. 619–674). Washington, DC: American Psychological Association.

Neisser, U. (1988). Five kinds of self-knowledge. *Philosophical Psychology, 1*(1), 35–59.

Oswald, F., & Konopik, N. (2015). Bedeutung von außerhäuslichen Aktivitäten, Nachbarschaft und Stadtteilidentifikation für das Wohlbefinden im Alter. [Impact of out-of-home activities, neighborhood and urban-related identity on well-being in old age] *Zeitschrift für Gerontologie und Geriatrie, 48*, 401–407.

Oswald, F., & Wahl, H.-W. (2004). Housing and health in later life [special issue]. *Reviews on Environmental Health, 19*(3–4), 223–252. Retrieved from https://www.ncbi.nlm.nih.gov/pmc

Oswald, F., & Wahl, H.-W. (2005). Dimensions of the meaning of home in later life. In G. D. Rowles & H. Chaudhury (Eds.), *Home and identity in later life. International perspectives* (pp. 21–46). New York, NY: Springer Publishing.

Oswald, F., Wahl, H.-W., Schilling, O., & Iwarsson, S. (2007). Housing-related control beliefs and independence in activities of daily living in very old age. *Scandinavian Journal of Occupational Therapy, 14*(1), 33–43.

Oswald, F., Wahl, H.-W., Schilling, O., Nygren, C., Fänge, A., Sixsmith, A., et al. (2007). Relationships between housing and healthy aging in very old age. *The Gerontologist, 47*(1), 96–107.

Overton, W. F. (2010). Life-span development. Concepts and issues. In R. M. Lerner & W. F. Overton (Eds.), *The handbook of life-span development* (Vol. 1, pp. 1–29). New York, NY: Wiley.

Parker, M. G., & Thorslund M. (2007). Health trends in the elderly population: Getting better and getting worse. *The Gerontologist, 47*(2), 150–158.

Peace, S. M. (2005). *Environment and identity in later life.* Berkshire: Open University Press.

Pinquart, M., & Burmedi, D. (2004). Correlates of residential satisfaction in adulthood and old age: A meta-analysis. In H.-W. Wahl, R. Scheidt, & P. G. Windley (Eds.), *Annual Review of Gerontology and Geriatrics* (Volume 22, Focus on Aging in context: Socio-physical environments, pp. 195–222). New York, NY: Springer Publishing.

Ram, N., & Diehl, M. (2015). Multiple-time-scale design and analysis: Pushing toward real-time modeling of complex developmental processes. In M. Diehl, K. Hooker, & M. J. Sliwinski (Eds.), *Handbook of intraindividual variability across the life span* (pp. 308–323). New York, NY: Routledge/Taylor & Francis.

Ram, N., & Gerstorf, D. (2009). Time-structured and net intraindividual variability: Tools for examining the development of dynamic characteristics and processes. *Psychology and Aging, 24*(4), 778–791.

Rowe, J. W., & Kahn, R. L. (1998). *Successful aging.* New York, NY: Pantheon/Random House.

Rowles, G. D., & Watkins, J. F. (2003). History, habit, heart and hearth: On making spaces into places. In K. W. Schaie, H.-W. Wahl, H. Mollenkopf, & F. Oswald (Eds.), *Aging independently: Living arrangements and mobility* (pp. 77–98). New York, NY: Springer Publishing.

Rubinstein, R. L. (1989). The home environments of older people: A description of the psychosocial processes linking person to place. *Journal of Gerontology: Social Sciences, 44*(2), S45–S53.

Ryff, C. D. (1989). Beyond Ponce de Leon and life satisfaction: New directions in quest of successful ageing. *International Journal of Behavioral Development, 12*(1), 35–55. Retrieved from http://journals.sagepub.com

Saup, W. (1993). *Alter und Umwelt. Eine Einführung in die Ökologische Gerontologie* [Old age and the environment: An Introduction to ecological gerontology]. Stuttgart: Kohlhammer.

Scheidt, R. J., & Norris-Baker, C. (2004). The general ecological model revisited: Evolution, current status, and continuing challenges. In H.-W. Wahl, R. J. Scheidt, & P. G. Windley (Eds.), *Annual Review of Gerontology and Geriatrics* (Vol. 22, pp. 34–58). New York, NY: Springer Publishing.

Scheidt, R. J., & Windley, P. G. (2006). Environmental gerontology: progress in the post-Lawton era. In J. E. Birren & K. W. Schaie (Eds.), *Handbook of the psychology of aging* (6th ed., pp. 105–125). Amsterdam: Elsevier.

Schilling, O. K., Wahl, H.-W., Boerner, K., Horowitz, A., Reinhardt, J. P., Cimarolli, V. R., et al. (2016). Developmental regulation with progressive visual loss: Use of control strategies and affective well-being. *Developmental Psychology*, *52*(4), 679–694.

Schilling, O. K., Wahl, H.-W., Boerner, K., Reinhardt, J. P., Brennan-Ing, M., & Horowitz, A. (2013). Change in psychological control in visually impaired older adults over 2 years: Role of functional ability and depressed mood. *The Journals of Gerontology Series B: Psychological Sciences and Social Sciences*, *68*(5), 750–761.

Schulz, R., Wahl, H.-W., Matthews, J. T., de Vito Dabbs, A., Beach, S. R., & Czaja, S. J. (2015). Advancing the aging and technology agenda in gerontology. *The Gerontologist*, *55*(5), 724–734.

Tornstam, L. (2005). *Gerotranscendence. A developmental theory of positive aging.* New York, NY: Springer Publishing.

Valsiner, J. (1994). Irreversibility of time and the construction of historical developmental psychology. *Mind, Culture, and Activity, 1*(1–2), 25–42.

Wahl, H.-W. (1991). Dependency in the elderly from an interactional point of view: Verbal and observational data. *Psychology and Aging*, *6*(2), 238–246. Retrieved from https://www.ncbi.nlm.nih.gov/pubmed

Wahl, H.-W. (1992). Ökologische Perspektiven in der Gerontopsychologie: ein Blick in die vergangenen drei Jahrzehnte und in die Zukunft [Ecological perspectives in geropsychology: A view into the recent three decades and into the future]. *Psychologische Rundschau*, *43*, 232–248.

Wahl, H.-W. (2001). Environmental influences on aging and behavior. In J. E. Birren & K. W. Schaie (Eds.), *Handbook of the psychology of aging* (5th ed., pp. 215–237). San Diego, CA: Academic Press.

Wahl, H.-W., Fänge, A., Oswald, F., Gitlin, L. N., & Iwarsson, S. (2009). The home environment and disability-related outcomes in aging individuals: What is the empirical evidence? *The Gerontologist*, *49*(3), 355–367.

Wahl, H.-W., & Gitlin, L. N. (2007). Environmental gerontology. In J. E. Birren (Ed.), *Encyclopedia of gerontology: Age, aging, and the aged* (2nd ed., pp. 494–501). Oxford: Elsevier.

Wahl, H.-W., Iwarsson, S., & Oswald, F. (2012). Aging well and the environment: Toward an integrative model and research agenda for the future. *The Gerontologist*, *52*(3), 306–316.

Wahl, H.-W., & Lang, F. (2004). Aging in context across the adult life course: Integrating physical and social environmental research perspectives. In H.-W. Wahl, R. Scheidt, & P. Windley (Eds.), *Annual Review of Gerontology and Geriatrics* (Vol. 23, pp. 1–33). New York, NY: Springer Publishing.

Wahl, H.-W., & Lang, F. (2006). Psychological aging: A contextual view. In P. M. Conn (Ed.), *Handbook of models for human aging* (pp. 881–895). Amsterdam: Elsevier.

Wahl, H.-W., & Oswald, F. (2010). Environmental perspectives on aging. In D. Dannefer & C. Phillipson (Eds.), *The SAGE handbook of social gerontology* (pp. 111–124). London, UK: Sage.

Wahl, H.-W., Oswald, F., & Zimprich, D. (1999). Everyday competence in visually impaired older adults: A case for person-environment perspectives. *The Gerontologist*, *39*(2), 140–149.

Wahl, H.-W., & Oswald, F. (2016). Theories of environmental gerontology: Old and new avenues for ecological views of aging. In V. L. Bengtson & R. A. Settersten (Eds.), *Handbook of theories of aging* (3rd ed., pp. 621–641). New York, NY: Springer Publishing.

Wahl, H.-W., & Saup, W. (1994). Ökologische Gerontologie: mehr als die Docility-Hypothese? [Ecological gerontology: More than the docility hypothesis]. *Zeitschrift für Gerontologie*, *27*, 347–454.

Wahl, H.-W., Scheidt, R., & Windley, P. (Eds.). (2004). Aging in context: Socio-physical environments. *Annual Review of Gerontology and Geriatrics* (Vol. 23). New York, NY: Springer Publishing.

Wahl, H.-W., Schilling, O., & Becker, S. (2007). Age-related macular degeneration and change in psychological control: Role of time since diagnosis and functional ability. *Journal of Gerontology: Psychological Sciences*, *62*(2), P90–P97.

Wahl, H.-W., Schilling, O., Oswald, F., & Heyl, V. (1999). Psychosocial consequences of age-related visual impairment: Comparison with mobility-impaired older adults and long-term outcome. *Journal of Gerontology: Psychological Sciences*, *54*(5), P304–P316.

Wettstein, M., Schilling, O. K., Reidick, O., & Wahl, H.-W. (2015). Four-year stability, change, and multidirectionality of well-being in very-old age. *Psychology and Aging*, *30*(3), 500–516.

Wahl, H.-W., & Weisman, J. (2003). Environmental gerontology at the beginning of the new millennium: Reflections on its historical, empirical, and theoretical development. *The Gerontologist*, *43*(5), 616–627.

Wahl, H.-W., Wettstein, M., Shoval, N., Oswald, F., Kaspar, R., Issacson, M., et al. (2013). Interplay of cognitive and motivational resources for out-of-home behavior in a sample of cognitively heterogeneous older adults: Findings of the SenTra project. *The Journals of Gerontology Series B: Psychological Sciences and Social Sciences*, *68*(5), 691–702.

Youniss, J. (1987). Social construction and moral development: Update and expansion of an idea. In W. M. Kurtines & J. L. Gewirtz (Eds.), *Moral development through social interaction* (pp. 131–148). New York, NY: John Wiley.

CHAPTER 3

Being There

Personal Reflection on a Quest for Understanding the Meaning of Place in Environmental Gerontology

Graham D. Rowles

ABSTRACT

This autoethnography essay provides a life course perspective on a career-long exploration of the meaning of place and its connection with the early years of Environmental Gerontology. I trace the evolution of a cumulative perspective in three phases, corresponding to sojourns at Clark University, West Virginia University, and the University of Kentucky. At Clark University, in-depth ethnographic study of five older adults in a run-down inner city neighborhood revealed four modalities of environmental experience: action, orientation, feeling, and fantasy. Elaboration on this research at West Virginia University, based on a 3-year study of older adults in a rural Appalachian community, resulted in the theme of insideness, as manifest in physical, social, and autobiographical expressions of affinity with place. At the University of Kentucky, explorations of the notion of being in place and development of a longitudinal life course perspective on this construct further deepened my understanding of the meaning of place. Moving forward it is important to pursue more sophisticated qualitative methodologies, consider diverse populations, incorporate greater consideration of the influence of technological change, and develop more refined grounded theory in the quest for deeper understanding of the meaning of place for older adults.

http://dx.doi.org/10.1891/0198-8794.38.39

BIOGRAPHICAL NOTES

I was born in 1946. I have resided in at least 23 different places since a "home birth" in the warm and loving family embrace of an upstairs room at grandma's house in Carshalton, Surrey, on the outskirts of London, England. The majority of moves were made during the first three decades of my life. This does not include a period during adolescence when, as the son of a naval officer who was posted to a new base or ship every couple of years, I would travel to boarding school at the beginning of a term and return to a different residence at its end. When I was 24, I relocated to the United States with sojourns in Worcester, Massachusetts (three locations), Morgantown, West Virginia (two locations), and Lexington, Kentucky, before moving to my current residence in Georgetown, Kentucky. Each location involved adaptation to an entirely new environment.

Being shaped by different places is interwoven with my professional career. It reflects a blending of personal and professional life—components of being an environmental gerontologist I cannot separate. Second, it generated a life-long inclination to not move, to put down roots and achieve the sense of meaning and belonging to a place that was denied me as a child. Finally, early experience of repeated separation has fueled a 40-year quest to unravel the meaning of place.

In this essay, I use autoethnography to trace a life-course perspective on the meaning of place and its connection with the birth and early years of Environmental Gerontology. There are many different perspectives on autoethnography (Anderson, 2006; Chang, 2008; Jones, Adams, & Ellis, 2013). My focus is on interweaving three elements in an autoethnography that is ethnographic in its methodological focus, contextual in its interpretative orientation, and autobiographical in its perspective (Chang, 2008, p. 48). The story is framed in three phases, corresponding to research at three different institutions. Each provides the historical backdrop for a deepening understanding of the meaning of place in Environmental Gerontology and its relevance and potential contributions to an aging society.

IN THE BEGINNING (1970–1976)

Expansion from a personal to a professional interest in person-environment relationships began in graduate school at Clark University where I found myself in the midst of scholars in geography and psychology who were forging links between the two disciplines during the foundational years of environmental psychology (Rowles, 1988). Geographer Anne Buttimer introduced me to phenomenology, to the work of Paul Vidal de la Blache on regional *genre de vie*, and to classic French scholars' Maximillien Sorre and Paul-Henri Chombart de Lauwe's ideas on social space (Buttimer, 1969). Saul Cohen, a geographer, at this time working with Clark psychologists Seymour Wapner and Bernard Kaplan on developing an organismic developmental person-environment transactional model (Wapner, Kaplan, & Cohen, 1973), nurtured an interest in expanding beyond a stimulus-response behaviorist perspective on Kurt Lewin's fundamental B=f(P.E) ecological equation. I also had the good fortune to share my doctoral experience with David Seamon, Gary Moore, Roger Hart, and Michael Godkin who went on to make significant contributions to the fledgling field (Buttimer & Seamon, 1980; Godkin, 1980; Hart, 1979, 1997; Moore & Gollege, 1976; Seamon, 1979; Seamon & Maugerauer, 2012).

Interest in the lived experience of older adults, prompted me to reach out to scholars who shared my interest in aging and environment. Sandra Howell at MIT engaged me as local field director for a major national study of special housing for the elderly and enthusiastically embraced my fledgling ideas, providing unwavering intellectual and emotional support as I tried to employ the perspective of humanistic geography to understand older adults' experience of their environment. Perhaps the most important intellectual influence was luminary M. Powell Lawton. I wrote him a short letter enclosing a rambling 30-page dissertation proposal and requesting feedback. He responded almost immediately with a three-page single-spaced letter providing detailed comments including a suggestion that we meet. I drove the 270 miles from Worcester, MA, to Philadelphia, PA. The result was a lengthy luncheon and Powell's mentorship for the rest of his life.

This fortuitous confluence of people and ideas resulted in a doctoral dissertation that questioned prevailing views of aging and environment in an in-depth ethnographic study of five older adults living in a run-down inner city neighborhood in New England (Rowles, 1978a, 1978b). The study involved participant observation in the neighborhood (immediately adjacent to my home), more than two dozen in-depth interviews, most of them tape-recorded, with each participant over a period of several months, and event analysis (monitoring and discussion of specific events in the participants' lives as they occurred). Interpreting the data involved more than "having insight" or waiting for inspiration (Rowles, 1978b). It entailed synthesizing notes from my participant observation journal. This was complemented by systematic listening and relistening to my tape-recorded interviews and tape recordings of less formal exchanges with each participant (to detect nuances that were overlooked during the actual interactions). In addition, it involved reading and rereading the transcripts of the interviews to identify key themes. Although I was unaware of this at the time, this involved an inductive process very similar to the constant comparative analysis approach advocated in grounded theory—progression through a sequence of open, axial and selective coding to organize the data into a series of themes (Corbin & Strauss, 1990). As my ideas began to take shape, I shared them with the participants to gain feedback and assess the degree to which they felt I had authentically captured their experience. Numerous refinements resulted from these "member checking" conversations. I discovered that these older adults' lived experience of their environment was far more complex than the limiting stereotype of a progressively closing life space prevalent at the time. Four modalities of environmental experience were revealed.

The first was *action*, the physical use of space. This occurred on three levels: *immediate action*, defined by physiological capability, and illustrated in 83-year-old Marie Dion's reduced ability to reach for a high shelf or crouch to hem a skirt; *everyday activity*, the participants' routine daily and weekly patterns of travel to the grocery store, church, and to visit friends that was increasingly restricted by mobility limitations; and *occasional trips*, paradoxically, an increased propensity to make long-distance trips to vacation or visit distant family members (during one 6-month period, Marie visited her son in Indiana, her birthplace in Quebec, and a daughter in Florida).

Action was grounded in *orientation*, the cognitive differentiation of space (Figure 3.1). A *personal schema* provided bodily orientation, the propensity to distinguish front from back, up from down, left from right, and to maintain

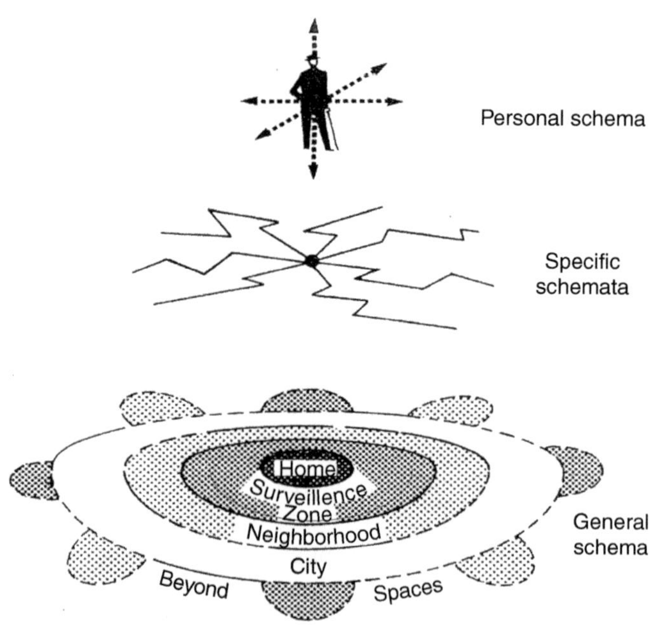

FIGURE 3.1 Dimensions of orientation.
Source: Rowles (1978a).

balance. Awareness of routes walked on a regular basis provided *specific schemata* that guided the participants in tracing familiar pathways. Sixty-eight-year-old Stanislav Linsky's day was defined by a routine of trudging from bar to bar within the neighborhood tracing the same pathway at the same time each day. The familiarity of repetition enabled him to traverse his neighborhood without conscious thought. Cognitive awareness of familiar routes was embedded in a *general schema,* an implicit array of "mental maps" of the places of their life—knowledge the participants carried around in their head (much of it subconscious) that was evoked as needed to visualize, navigate and frame an understanding of the world. Each participant had intimate taken-for-granted awareness of the configuration of their home. They were also strongly oriented within their surveillance zone (space within the visual field of their dwelling). General schemas were progressively less detailed and more fragmentary as they moved from the neighborhood to the scale of the city. The exception, was detailed awareness and integration of selected locations far away, "beyond spaces" they had frequented and remembered from visits to relatives or for vacations.

Third, places of the participants' lives were suffused with emotion. Such *feelings* ranged from *immediate* visceral reactions to particular neighborhood locations to *permanent* expressions of the aura of the neighborhood developed over a lifetime. Particularly important were *personal* locations where key events had transpired. The excitement evoked by a now demolished hall where Marie had danced in a red velvet dress provoked a reaction every time we passed the site, and the leaning Dion Square street sign with the emblazoned gold star was a constant emotional reminder of her son and her gold star mother status. Some locations evoked *shared* feelings. A rueful sense of loss of the supportive social ambiance of the neighborhood during the 1940s, when neighbor would help neighbor, was shared and sustained by the participants who had mutually witnessed the neighborhood become progressively more run down and alienating.

A fourth and final modality was *fantasy* (vicarious immersion in locations displaced in space and/or time). Each participant could, in their minds eye, transport themselves back to the environments of their past, places where they had lived previously or visited. They could resurrect and vicariously re-engage in the neighborhood as it had been. They could also project themselves across space to contemporary although geographically displaced environments. Sixty-nine-year-old Raymond could visualize his daughter's garden in Arkansas as he recalled visits to her home. He could imagine what his son in the Air Force would be doing in Tokyo as he glanced at a clock on his mantle telling the time in Japan. Fantasy involved vicarious engagement in environments displaced in space and time spanning each participant's entire life history.

Viewing simultaneous systematic changes in the four modalities as the participants had aged led to a *hypothesis of changing emphasis*. I hypothesized that limitations in action with advancing age were accompanied by an increase in fantasy as physical and mobility limitations necessitated increased vicarious experience. This change was accompanied by changes in orientation, including increased emphasis on the home, surveillance zone and proximate environments, and by intensification of feelings for selected treasured spaces, for example, the home and locations where memorable life events transpired. Relocation to West Virginia University provided an opportunity to build on this initial conceptualization.

PROBING DEEPER (1976–1985)

At West Virginia University, I was embraced by the department of psychology, the cradle of a life-span developmental perspective. Although luminaries K. Warner Schaie and Paul Baltes had departed, their inspiration remained. Nancy Datan and young scholars, including Laura Carstensen, quickly socialized me to the value of this focus. My new Appalachian home also nurtured an interest in rural environments and the meaning of place on a community rather than solely individual level. Would what was discovered in an inner city neighborhood apply in a rural context? I reached out for help from leaders in rural aging. The ideas of Raymond Coward at the University of Florida, John Krout at Ithaca College, and Rick Scheidt at Kansas State University became increasingly relevant as I began to study growing old in "Colton," a community of 403 people located in the heart of Appalachia. Three years of experiential fieldwork (Rowles, 1978b), funded by the National Institute on Aging (AG 00862), and once again involving a combination of participant observation, repeated in-depth interviewing and event analyses, resulted the theme of "insideness" as an element in the meaning of place (Rowles, 1980).

Again, the stereotypes were misleading. The 15 rural older adult participants were far more satisfied with their *genre de vie* than the literature on rural poverty, inadequate housing, social isolation and poor access to health care and social services would suggest. These older adults viewed themselves as "insiders" in a Colton milieu of historically grounded existential meaning as an integral part of their culture and identity. Elements of my initial conceptualization were reinforced. Regular patterns in daily and weekly use of community space (action) generated the rhythm and routine of a *physical insideness*—intimate and taken-for-granted proprioceptive familiarity with the configuration of home and community space. The importance of the surveillance zone was reinforced and distance decay in participant knowledge, affinity and meaning of zones of space moving away from the residence was confirmed (orientation) (Rowles, 1981, 1983a). Life-long residence and enduring relationships with age peers created a *social insideness* manifest in a "society of the old" paralleling the social and historical meaning of the neighborhood I had discovered in urban New England (feeling). Finally, detailed personal histories of remembered events and the places where they had transpired generated the temporal and biographical depth of an *autobiographical insideness* which was an essential component of the meaning of Colton to its life-long residents (Rowles, 1983b). The meaning of place derived from a melding of location and identity.

During fieldwork in Colton, it became apparent that some elderly residents were literally "between worlds" as they experienced the tensions of a multiyear process of gradual separation from the community and relocation to live outside Appalachia (Rowles, 1983c). With increasing difficulty in maintaining their home and failing health and self-care abilities, an annual exodus to spend Christmas with children became an absence of weeks, then months and eventually permanent relocation. I found myself focusing on the role of time in conditioning the meaning of place and with issues of severance from familiar place and the process of creating or recreating meaning in a new location. Once again, my own relocating, this time to Lexington, Kentucky, provided the opportunity and stimulus for deeper exploration.

WIDENING HORIZONS (1985–PRESENT)

Moving to the University of Kentucky provided exposure to new colleagues including anthropologist Nancy Schoenberg who increased my awareness of the role of culture in filtering lived experience, and John Watkins who nurtured an interest in a life-course perspective. The move to Kentucky was also accompanied by gravitation toward another discipline. A 1988 invitation to present at an American Occupational Therapy Foundation conference at Pingree Park in Colorado provided an introduction to occupational science. I found myself developing professional identification with occupational scientists who encouraged me to share an emerging perspective on *being in place* and contemplate practical implications of this perspective (Rowles, 1991). Affinity with occupational science provided inspiration for reframing the role of habit, ritual, and routine in shaping the meaning of place (Rowles, 2000; Rowles & Watkins, 2003). The theoretical work of Susanne Iwarsson and Malcolm Cutchin also widened my horizons: Iwarsson through her expansion of the ecological equation to embrace activity within a more holistic conceptualization of P-E-A transactions (Iwarsson, 2003); and Cutchin through his introduction of *place integration,* an action-based perspective grounded in the pragmatism of John Dewey, that revealed how, over time, commitment to place intensifies through a dynamic situation-defined transaction of person and place (Cutchin, 1997, 2003, 2004; Cutchin, Owen & Chang, 2003).[1] Both of these perspectives contributed to transcending the simple dualism of person and environment and moving toward understanding the meaning of place as a dynamic, situation-defined, transactional fusion of person, environment, and activity/action.

Since the 1990s, a series of invitations to spend time overseas have resulted in collaborations with scholars promoting the newly minted phrase "Environmental Gerontology" to characterize their work. Clare Wenger in Bangor, Wales; Habib Chaudhury in Vancouver, Canada; Miriam Bernard in Keele, England; Rose Gilroy in Newcastle, England; Frank Oswald and Hans-Werner Wahl in Heidelberg, Germany; and Tom Scharf and Kieran Walsh in Galway, Ireland, all made contributions to increasing the sophistication of my perspective.

Sometimes it takes a career to fully internalize the obvious, that no space or location has inherent meaning, that all meanings of place are attributed; they are created and sustained by the individual, albeit, frequently colored and reinforced by shared experience with others. Being in place is partially "received" in response to circumstance and context. It is also partially volitionally generated through our agency. Most important, being in place is an elemental component of being in the world. I now believe that the quest for being in place, and specifically, achieving a sense of home and at-oneness in our environment, is a fundamental underlying motivation of life itself and that this imperative permeates our lives (Walsh, Rowles, & Scharf, 2014). When I was young, there was a reason for my sense of alienation from place during an itinerant childhood. Each person has an inherent need for being at home and at each phase of our life course we adjust to change through the lens of this imperative. Each time we relocate, we go through a process of making and remaking home and reinventing meaning in place (Rowles, 2008).

This process is represented in Figure 3.2. Linking back to my original conceptualization, each place of residence has meaning based on use (action), awareness (orientation), and emotion (feeling and fantasy). Each move involves transferring artifacts, familiar ways of using space, memories, and meanings to the new environment. Each new place of residence, offers fresh opportunities—a fireplace or a sun porch that was not in our former home, as well as a new set of neighbors, and new constraints such as previously unencountered barriers (perhaps the need to negotiate more stairs). Within this context of transferred past and new opportunities we create a new sense of being in place. Generally,

[1]Ironically, many years earlier I had directed Malcolm's doctoral dissertation in Geography on this topic, little knowing how, subsequently, his scholarship would so strongly influence my own views.

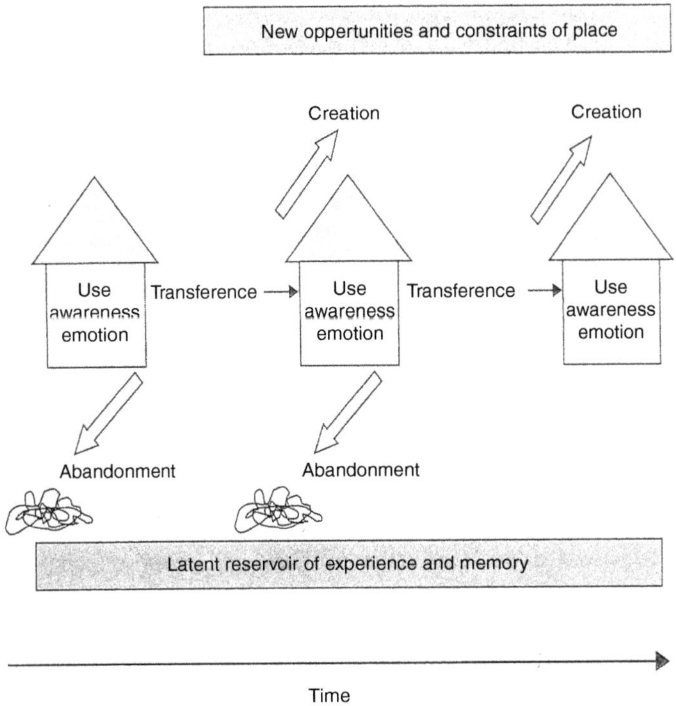

FIGURE 3.2 Making and remaking home.
Source: Rowles and Bernard (2013).

this also involves abandonment as we throw some things out, make adjustments in our social network, and filter memory as details of the places of our past fade from memory or are reconstituted as part of a new being in place. We abandon the detritus of our past. But this past is never completely forgotten. There always remains a latent reservoir of experience and memories that can be resurrected and used in recreating place and meaning. And so the process continues as we sequentially make and remake place, each time abandoning part of our past and each time creating a present that embraces elements of that past within the context of new possibilities.

I have recently become more interested in the role of human agency in this process. In childhood we move at the whim of our parents; making and retaining a sense of being in place is often highly constrained and in some ways beyond our control, as it was in my life. I had no choice about moving or about the environment in which I would find myself. Reflecting Lawton's and Simon environmental docility hypothesis, I could merely react (Lawton

& Simon, 1968). This reactivity reflected reluctance to be separated from place, torn away from home. As we grow older and gain more control, reacting to the decisions of others is gradually replaced by environmental proactivity (Lawton, 1989, 1990). Moving into middle age, we exert increasing personal influence on shaping place and its meaning. Especially as we move toward retirement, those who are fortunate enough to have the resources, have the very real possibility of consciously shaping environments in ways that nurture being in place. I am engaging in this process in striving to make my current residence a place of at-oneness.

As we progressed through a series of "homes," my wife and I gradually developed preferences (and dislikes) in envisioning the place where we want to spend our old age. We are deliberately making "home" in our current residence. There is the study with its custom fitted wrap-around walnut desk and abundant bookshelves. The walls are adorned with photographs and artwork accumulated over our lifetimes. There is a back porch where we sit during summer evenings. There is the pond we installed that upon reviewing old family photographs I discovered has been a prominent feature in most of the places I have lived. There are the iris flowerbeds that link me back to my grandfather's garden. We are creating a "homeplace" where our children can visit. In sum, we are seeking a sense of being in place that represents the best of our previous homes and experiences we have accumulated. My wife is an integral part of this process. There are spaces for craftwork and pursuing her interests in genealogy and, outside, the herb garden she enjoys cultivating.

There is, of course, an inevitable looming challenge. We grow old. Eventually my quest to understand the meaning of place to older adults will move into a new phase as at first I anticipate and then experience the increased dependency of frailty and reluctant return to the reactivity of my childhood. Although the tension between reactivity and proactivity will always provide an underlying motif, over the coming years it is likely I will once more return to the point where, consistent with the environmental docility hypothesis, what happens to me becomes increasingly beyond my control.

GROWING OLD (2016-20__?)

"We shall not cease from exploration, and the end of all our exploring will be to arrive where we started and know the place for the first time." T. S. Eliot

In August of 2016, I turned 70. Understanding the meaning of place in old age is becoming lived experience. In the prologue to my doctoral dissertation, completed in 1976, I wrote:

> When I grow old, I will experience what it is like to be elderly. Until then I can only speculate and seek to understand from the outside; for experiential awareness is personal and ultimately incommunicable. As Simone de Beauvoir notes ". . . there is one form of experience that belongs only to those who are old—that of old age itself" (Rowles, 1978a, p. xviii).

Now I am here. Perhaps I can understand. Autobiography now becomes relevant as I attempt to gain deeper understanding from critical self-examination. I am not alone in this endeavor; age peer colleagues whose journeys have been part of the intellectual convoy of my life and who are still alive remain to share their insight. The legacies of Tom Byerts, Sandra Howell, Powell Lawton, Lucille Nahemow, Paul Windley, and other Environmental Gerontology pioneers, through the legacy of their writing, still shape my thinking from beyond their graves. New colleagues and doctoral students remain invaluable in critiquing my perspective.

As I begin to personalize changes and concerns I used to glibly discuss in my "Aging and Environment" course, the issues become very real. It is late at night and I am tired: *Do I have the energy to climb these stairs to turn off the light of the tropical fish tank on the landing? How long will it be before I can't get out of this bathtub?* In the coming years, I will doubtless divine the answers to some of these questions and gain progressively deeper insight into the meaning of place in old age from lived experience. I am fortunate: How many scholars are in a field that empowers them, indeed demands that they harness such a unique opportunity?

REFLECTING AND PROJECTING

In the interim, I can summarize what I have learned to date and identify priority directions for future exploration. I am fairly sure that understanding the meaning of place in old age involves: accepting the lived experience of the individual as a legitimate focus in gerontology; embracing vicarious environmental engagement; using the lens of the life course; recognizing a universal imperative for "being in place"; seeking to understand processes of making and remaking place in response to personal and environmental change; and probing the tension between proactivity and reactivity in framing the meaning of place.

Placing this experience within the larger context of Environmental Gerontology, where should we be probing for deeper insight? From a methodological stance, it is important to focus on research aimed at revealing the essence of the lived experience of place by harnessing the full array of sources that offer qualitative insight, including literary interpretation and poetry, deep narrative interviews, oral histories of place, reflective focus groups and study panels, and participatory action research—all approaches that give voice and opportunity to older adults to express what may be taken-for-granted and difficult to articulate.

Triangulation, and the simultaneous use of multiple methods and measures provided by an ethnographic approach will be essential (Mertens & Hesse-Biber, 2012). There is a need for increased concern with employing member checking to assess the validity and trustworthiness of our insights from the perspective of the lived experience of participants (Birt, Scott, Cavers, Campbell & Walter, 2016). Indeed, this should become standard practice. There is also rich potential, on a more fundamental paradigmatic level, to adopt new lenses in the very framing of research on the meaning of place. For example, the philosophy and practice of appreciative inquiry facilitates liberation from the constraints of exclusively problem-focused research (Reed, 2007). The perspective of autoethnography, as employed in this essay, enables us to legitimately harness the rich reservoir of our own lived experience in ways that transcend the preciousness and narcissism that sometimes pervades autobiographical work (Chang, 2008; Jones, Adams, & Ellis, 2013).

From a substantive perspective, inquiry must embrace more diverse populations. In contrast with previous generations, fewer older adults now experience their old age in traditional nuclear-family-oriented middle-class suburban settings that have been the dominant source of insight to date. It is important to focus on persons growing old as part of contemporary family structures and living arrangements. What is the meaning of place to people who grow old alone (de Medeiros, Rubinstein & Doyle, 2013; Rubinstein & de Medeiros, 2005)? How is place experienced by older members of the LGBTQ community? How do older adults of different ethnicities and from different cultures, especially non-Western cultures, attribute meaning to place? What about nomadic societies and populations whose engagement with environment is less domicentric? While notions of home and belonging give us a warm and fuzzy feeling inside, not all people are able to enjoy this level of being in place. Are people experiencing social exclusion and alienation from place trapped by circumstances that preclude them from making or remaking place as a source of meaning (O'Shea, Walsh, & Scharf, 2012; Phillipson & Smith, 2005)? Is the imperative for being in place as universal as I have suggested?

Environmental gerontology will also need to become sensitive to changing technologies. Radical expansion of capabilities and modalities for experiencing place in an increasingly digital universe of the World Wide Web and Facebook, Skype, and social media that facilitates real-time participation in geographically displaced environments, is fundamentally altering process of engagement. How will this translate into our ability to imbue places with meaning? Does technology now allow us to transcend memory, imagination, and vicarious immersion in place by enabling new forms of "being there?" In the context of such changes, does our need for "being-in place" become less important? Is there currently, or can we anticipate, a fundamental shift in the meaning of place for individuals and groups? Is there the potential for a world in which place will no longer matter? Is a universal malady of placelessness on the horizon (Relph, 1976)? I think not. On the other hand, in the context of changing perspectives on people's relationships with place, we can anticipate potential contributions from additional disciplines beyond those that have traditionally been the focus of Environmental Gerontology. Engineering, computer science and communications, for example, are already joining the family of disciplines (geography, psychology, sociology, and architecture) that have nurtured Environmental Gerontology. As perspectives on the meaning of place become more sophisticated, ever more disciplines may be embraced in its investigation.

More sophisticated experientially grounded theory and conceptualizations that embrace transformations of place are becoming essential. Wahl and Oswald's framework of person-environment processes in later life integrates themes of behavior, experience, belonging (manifest in residential satisfaction, place attachment, and meaning of home), and agency (manifest in housing-related control beliefs, environmental docility and proactivity, and person-environment fit) in predicting interwoven developmental outcomes of identity, wellbeing, and autonomy (Wahl & Oswald, 2010). Stephen Golant's important insights on *residential normalcy* as an underlying motif in understanding older adults relationship with place provides a parallel and highly complementary perspective to the theme of being in place (Golant, 2011, 2015). There is need for broader and deeper emphasis on the social meanings of place at multiple scales from home to community, including the social places of both private and public life. For example, Gardner (2011), building on original ideas developed by Oldenburg (1989, 2000), has explored the distinction among first (home), second (work), and third places (key sites of public life such as café's, post offices, parks, and main streets). The idea of third places as sources of meaning resurrects the theme of "behavior settings," locations that nurture common activities and hold shared meanings regardless of the participants present at any one time (Barker, 1968; Barker & Barker, 1961). Thang and Kaplan (2013) are also providing fresh insight in their work on intergenerational strategies for building relational spaces and places. Creating meaningful shared spaces is becoming critical in a world where globalization has increased tension and the need for the sharing of place by multiple populations that can no longer ignore each other's presence. It is no longer viable to remain cocooned in our own little portion of space, oblivious to a larger relational world. The ultimate aspiration of an enlightened Environmental Gerontology is the design of dwelling places and communities that bring us together rather than render us asunder.

Finally, there is a need for Environmental Gerontology to more directly translate insight into practical interventions and public policy (Rowles & Bernard, 2013). The signs here are encouraging. A flood of research on the meaning of home is enabling us to build residential environments that facilitate identity and belonging (Oswald & Wahl, 2013; Rowles & Chaudhury, 2005). On a larger scale, exponential growth, in less than a decade, of concern with creating aging friendly and livable communities, initially stimulated by the World Health Organization (2007), and by the AARP Public Policy Institute (2000), represents an international movement that continues to gain momentum (Scharlach & Lehning, 2016). Communities throughout the world are now seeking to create environments supportive of people of all ages and that foster competence, place identification, inclusion, and belonging. The ageing friendly communities movement provides an opportunity for environmental gerontologists to inform practice by translating what has been learned into sensitive and inclusive environmental design, culturally informed community planning, and even human services initiatives that routinely acknowledge the importance of the meaning of place.

EPILOGUE

The end of this story is murky, for it is still to be written. If it were possible to draft a communique from beyond the grave, I hope I would be able to write: *"I died in 20_ _. The setting was equivalent to where I was born—far from a hospital and free from invasive technology. My final hours, as were my first, were embraced in the quiet and nurturing warmth of family. There was the at-oneness with place I had strived to understand and attain throughout my life. My physical capability was maximized I remained oriented and aware in familiar surroundings. This place was emotionally significant to me; it providing cues and resources that enabled me to reminisce, savor, reflect on, and integrate the places and events of my life within a sense of being in the world I was about to leave that made me whole."* It is a task of Environmental Gerontology to make this possible.

REFERENCES

AARP Public Policy Institute. (2000). *Livable communities: An evaluation guide*. Washington, DC: AARP Public Policy Institute.

Anderson, L. (2006). Analytical autoethnography. *Journal of Contemporary Ethnography*, 35(4), 373–395.

Barker, R. G. (1968). *Ecological psychology*. Palo Alto, CA: Stanford University Press.

Barker, R. G., & Barker, L. S. (1961). The psychological ecology of old people in Midwest, Kansas and Yoredale, Yorkshire. *The Journal of Gerontology*, 16(2), 144–149.

Birt, L., Scott, S., Cavers, D., Campbell, C., & Walter, F. (2016). Member checking: A tool to enhance trustworthiness or merely a nod to validation. *Qualitative Health Research*, *26*(13), 1802–1811.

Buttimer, A. (1969). Social space in interdisciplinary perspective. *Geographical Review*, *59*(3), 417–426.

Buttimer, A., & Seamon, D. (Eds.). (1980). *The human experience of space and place*. London, UK: Croom Helm.

Chang, H. (2008). *Autoethnography as method*. Walnut Creek, CA: Left Cast Press.

Corbin, J., & Strauss, A. (1990). Grounded theory research: Procedures, canons and evaluative criteria. *Qualitative Sociology*, *13*(1), 3–21.

Cutchin, M. P. (1997). Physician retention in rural communities. *Health and Place*, *3*(1), 25–41.

Cutchin, M. P. (2003). The process of mediated aging in place: A theoretically and empirically based model. *Social Science and Medicine*, *57*(6), 1077–1090.

Cutchin, M. P. (2004). Using Deweyan philosophy to rename and reframe adaptation to environment. *American Journal of Occupational Therapy*, *58*(3), 303–312.

Cutchin, M. P., Owen, S. V., & Chang, P-F. J. (2003). Becoming 'at home" in assisted living residences: Exploring place integration processes. *Journals of Gerontology: Social Sciences*, *58*(4), S234–S243.

de Medeiros, K., Rubenstein, K., & Doyle, P. (2013). A place of one's own: Reinterpreting the meaning of home among childless older women. In G. D. Rowles & M. Bernard (Eds.), *Environmental gerontology: Making meaningful places in old age* (pp. 79–104). New York, NY: Springer Publishing.

Gardner, P. J. (2011). Natural neighborhood networks—important social networks in the lives of older adults in place. *Journal of Aging Studies*, *25*(3), 263–271.

Godkin, M. A. (1980). Identity and place: Clinical applications based on notions of rootedness and uprootedness. In A. Buttimer & D, Seamon (Eds.), *The human experience of space and place* (pp. 73–85). London, UK: Croom Helm.

Golant, S. M. (2011). The quest for residential normalcy by older adults: Relocation but one pathway. *Journal of Aging Studies*, *25*(3), 193–205.

Golant, S. M. (2015). *Aging in the right place*. Towson, MD: Health Professions Press.

Hart, R. A. (1979). *Children's experience of place*. New York, NY: Irvington.

Hart, R. A. (1997). *Children's participation: The theory and practice of involving young citizens in community development and environmental care*. New York, NY: Earthscan.

Iwarsson, S. (2003). Assessing the fit between older people and their physical home environments: An occupational therapy research perspective. In H-W. Wahl, R. J. Scheidt & P. G. Windley (Eds.), *Annual Review of Gerontology and Geriatrics*, *22*, 85–109.

Jones, S. H., Adams, T. E., & Ellis, C. (Eds.). (2013). *Handbook of autoethnography*. New York, NY: Left Coast Press.

Lawton, M. P. (1989). Behavior-relevant ecological factors. In K. W. Schaie & C. Schooler. (Eds.), *Social structure and the psychological aging process* (pp. 57–78). New Jersey: Erlbaum.

Lawton, M. P. (1990). Residential environment and self-directedness among older people. *American Psychologist, 45*(5), 638–640.

Lawton, M. P., & Simon, B. (1968). The ecology of social relationships in housing for the elderly. *The Gerontologist, 8*, 108–115.

Mertens, D. M., & Hesse-Biber, S. (2012). Triangulation and mixed methods research: Provocative positions. *Journal of Mixed Methods Research*, 6(2), 75–79.

Moore, G. T., & Golledge, R. G. (1976). *Environmental knowing: Theories, research and methods*. Pennsylvania.: Dowden, Hutchinson & Ross.

O'Shea, E., Walsh, K., & Scharf, T. (2012). Exploring community perceptions of the relationship between age and social exclusion in rural areas. *Quality in Ageing and Older Adults, 13*(1), 16–26.

Oldenburg, R. (1989). *The great good place: Cafes, coffee shops, community centers, beauty parlors, general stores, bars, hangouts, and how they get you through the day*. New York, NY: Paragon House.

Oldenburg, R. (2000). *Celebrating the third place: Inspiring stories about the "great good places" at the heart of our communities*. New York, NY: Marlowe & Company.

Oswald, F., & Wahl, H-W. (2013). Creating and sustaining homelike places in residential environments. In G. D. Rowles & M. Bernard (Eds.), *Environmental gerontology: Making meaningful places in old age* (pp. 53–75). New York, NY: Springer Publishing.

Phillipson, C., & Smith, A. (2005). *Extending working life: A review of the research literature* (Vol. 299). Corporate Document Services for the Department for Work and Pensions, Department for Work and Pensions and University of Leeds, UK.

Reed, J. (2007). *Appreciative inquiry: Research for change*. Thousand Oaks, CA: Sage Publications.

Relph, E. (1976). *Place and placelessness*. London, UK: Pion.

Rowles, G. D. (1978a). *Prisoners of space? Exploring the geographical experience of older people*. Boulder, CO: Westview Press.

Rowles, G. D. (1978b). Reflections on experiential fieldwork. In D. Ley & M. Samuels (Eds.), *Humanistic geography: Prospects and problems* (pp. 173–193). New York, NY: John Wiley.

Rowles, G. D. (1980). Growing old inside: Aging and attachment to place in an Appalachian community. In N. Datan & N. Lohmann (Eds.). *Transitions of Aging* (pp. 153–170). New York, NY: Academic Press.

Rowles, G. D. (1981). The surveillance zone as meaningful space for the aged. *The Gerontologist, 21*(3), 304–311.

Rowles, G. D. (1983a). Geographical dimensions of social support in rural Appalachia. In G. D. Rowles & R. Ohta (Eds.), *Aging and milieu: Environmental perspectives on growing old* (pp. 111–130). New York, NY: Academic Press.

Rowles, G. D. (1983b). Place and personal identity in old age: Observations from Appalachia. *Journal of Environmental Psychology, 3*, 299–313.

Rowles, G. D. (1983c). Between worlds: A relocation dilemma for the Appalachian elderly. *International Journal of Aging and Human Development, 17*(4), 301–314.

Rowles, G. D. (1988). The grand fiction of a personal odyssey. *Journal of Environmental Psychology*, *7*(4), 357–365.

Rowles, G. D. (1991). Beyond performance: Being in place as a component of occupational therapy. *American Journal of Occupational Therapy*, *45*(3), 265–271.

Rowles, G. D. (2000). Habituation and being in place. *Occupational Therapy Journal of Research*, *20*, S52–S67. [Special Supplement].

Rowles, G. D. (2008). Place in occupational science: A life course perspective on the role of environmental context in the quest for meaning. *Journal of Occupational Science*, *15*(3), 127–135.

Rowles, G. D., & Bernard, M. (Eds.). (2013). *Environmental gerontology: Making meaningful places in old age*. New York, NY: Springer Publishing Company.

Rowles, G. D., & Chaudhury, H. (2005). *Home and identity in late life: International perspectives*. New York, NY: Springer Publishing.

Rowles, G. D., & Watkins, J. F. (2003). History, habit, heart and hearth: On making spaces into places. In K. W. Schaie, H-W. Wahl, H. Mollenkopf & F. Oswald (Eds.), *Aging independently: living arrangements and mobility* (pp. 77–96). New York, NY: Springer Publishing.

Rubenstein, R. L., & de Mederios, K. (2005). Home, self and identity. In G. D. Rowles & H. Chaudhury (Eds.), *Home and identity in later life: International perspectives* (pp. 47–62). New York, NY: Springer Publishing.

Scharlach, A., & Lehning, A. (2016). *Creating aging-friendly communities*. Oxford, UK: Oxford University Press.

Seamon, D. (1979). *A geography of the lifeworld: Movement, rest and encounter*. London, UK: St.Martin's Press.

Seamon, D., & Maugerauer, R. (Eds.). (2012). *Dwelling, place and environment: Towards a phenomenology of person and world*. Dordrecht: Martinus Nijhoff Publishers.

Thang, L. L., & Kaplan, M. S. (2013). Intergenerational pathways for building relational spaces and places. In G. D. Rowles & M. Bernard. (Eds.). *Environmental gerontology: Making meaningful places in old age* (pp. 225–251). New York, NY: Springer Publishing Company.

Wahl, H-W., & Oswald, F. (2010). Environmental perspectives on aging. In D. Dannifer & C. Phillipson (Eds.), *International handbook of social gerontology* (pp. 111–124). London, UK: Sage.

Walsh, K., Rowles, G. D., & Scharf, T. (2014). Constructing home over the life course: Toward a model of at-oneness. *Proceedings of the 67th Annual Scientific Meeting of the Gerontological Society of America*. Washington, DC: District of Columbia.

Wapner, S., Kaplan B., & Cohen, S. B. (1973). An organismic-developmental perspective for understanding transactions of men and environments. *Environment and Behavior*, *5*(3), 255–289.

World Health Organization. (2007). *Global age-friendly cities: A guide*. Retrieved from http://www.who.int/ageing/publications/Global_age_friendly_cities_Guide_English.pdf

CHAPTER 4

Intellectual Origins of Residential Normalcy Theory

Stephen M. Golant

ABSTRACT

My award-winning paper designed to advance Environmental Gerontology theory proposed that older persons achieve residential normalcy when they are in their residential comfort and residential mastery zones. They then experience pleasurable, hassle-free, and memorable emotional experiences and feel both competent and in control of their everyday environments. However, when older persons fail to achieve residential normalcy, they initiate adaptive behaviors designed to manage or eliminate their discrepant individual and environmental circumstances. To understand both my motivations and abilities to construct this theory, I engage in an academic life review to identify those factors that most influenced my intellectual development. This exercise reveals that several critical and serendipitous interactions with universities, departments, organizations, faculty members, mentors, and colleagues motivated and channeled my research and writing on older people and their residential and care environments. It also emphasizes how throughout my career, a wealth of theoretical and empirical research by other academics both stimulated and reinforced my Environmental Gerontology focus.

Validation

In 2012, I received the Richard M. Kalish award for my paper: "The Quest for Residential Normalcy by Older Adults: Relocation but one Pathway." The

http://dx.doi.org/10.1891/0198-8794.38.57

Gerontological Society of America (GSA) presents this award to papers that make insightful and innovative contributions to aging and life development in the behavioral and social sciences. This was an especially meaningful honor because it affirmed that my professional peers recognized the value of my work.

In this and subsequent papers (Golant, 2011a, 2011b, 2015a, 2015b, 2015c), I advanced a theoretical model proposing that older persons achieve *residential normalcy* when they appraise their residential settings as congruent or fitting with their needs and goals. This happens when they report having two sets of overall favorable or positive emotional experiences or feelings that I labeled, *residential comfort* and *residential mastery* experiences. When these outcomes occur (Golant, 2011b, p. 193):

> Older people experience overall pleasurable, hassle-free, and memorable feelings that have relevance to them; and they feel both competent and in control—that is, they do not have to behave in personally objectionable ways or to unduly surrender mastery of their lives or environments to others.

I further theorized that when older people unfavorably appraise their residential circumstances, they do not passively sit back and accept their unfortunate fates. Rather, their residential incongruence may be short-lived because they initiate adaptive behaviors designed to manage or eliminate their negative experiences to regain their residential normalcy (Golant 2011b, 2015c).

I will examine my residential normalcy theory in more detail later in this chapter and show how its constructs and relationships were influenced by the literature I read earlier in my academic career. First, however, I will identify those events, places, and persons in my biography that contributed to my strong academic ties with Environmental Gerontology and in so many unanticipated ways influenced the derivation of my residential normalcy theory. Writing this life review was a rewarding but also a challenging exercise because it was often difficult to reconstruct the detailed pathways of my past professional life.

A Geographer at the University of Toronto

My undergraduate education at the University of Toronto (1964–1968) had little to do with either Environmental Gerontology or aging. I majored in geography and was especially interested in courses that focused on the internal social and economic structure of urban areas. In retrospect, however, this urban emphasis was to influence—however unpredictably—my later research on the residential locations, migration patterns, and travel behaviors of older urban adults (Golant, 1987). The only hint of my eventual focus on the environments of older people was my early intrigue with the environmental (climatic) determinism of the controversial Ellsworth Huntington (1922).

My professors were top-notch. I benefited from recently hired faculty who received their PhDs in geography from the University of Chicago, mentored by the internationally renowned urban geographer, Professor Brian Berry. They included Larry Bourne, James Simmons, and Alan Baker, who were on the cutting edge of urban geography research. Consistently, my BA honor's paper was an empirical investigation of the journey-to-work behaviors of urban residents.

I entered the master's program in urban and regional planning (then a separate department) at the University of Toronto, but disenchanted with its narrow disciplinary focus, I left after about 1 month. I returned sheepishly to the Department of Geography that fortunately admitted me as an MA graduate student (1968–1969). Herein occurred one of the first of several serendipitous events in my career. I was offered a research assistant position with Professor Ian Burton, then also a young PhD from the University of Chicago, but who had studied under the internationally renowned Professor Gilbert White, with a very different geographic focus on natural resources and environmental hazards. He immediately introduced me to research that focused on how to predict human responses to natural hazards. I became familiar with the semantic differential research of Osgood, Suci, and Tannenbaum's (1957) and the theoretical and applied research of Richard Lazarus (1966) that investigated how people appraise and cope with stressful events. This led to my first published refereed paper that examined the connotative meaning of natural hazards, based on responses from a convenience sample of university students (Golant & Burton, 1970). Little did I know how this research experience would frame my Environmental Gerontology interests many decades later.

This environmental focus, however, was short-lived. Under the mentorship of Professor James Simmons, my MA thesis was consistent with a spatial science geographic paradigm and I focused on the urban travel and migration behaviors of an urban population. Very importantly, however, Simmons was willing to accept a thesis that did not report on empirical research. I produced a purely theoretical analysis of how human spatial movements could be interpreted as adjustment processes by individuals in response to their stressful events (Golant, 1971). I revisited the psychological constructs of Lazarus (1966) and immersed myself in the living systems' theoretical frameworks of James Miller (1978) and Von Bertalanffy (1968). I was early enamored with theory construction.

Newly Born Gerontologist at the University of Washington (Seattle)

In 1969, I was accepted into the PhD program of the Department of Geography, University of Washington, to study under Dr. Richard Morrill, a nationally renowned social geographer who also viewed the discipline as a spatial/quantitative science with interests in medical geography, transportation, population movements, and residential distributions.

Early on in this graduate program, a second serendipitous event profoundly influenced my career path. As a teaching assistant administering a tutorial session for a large undergraduate introductory geography class, I required the students to write a paper on any topic of human geography. One student produced a well-written paper focused on the transportation problems of older people. Fascinated, I checked out her sources—low and behold, undergrad plagiarizes several sections of a paper written by Professor James Birren (1970) in *Psychology Today*. I still passed her. She at least had the good sense to borrow the insights of a prominent scholar.

Birren's paper substantially channeled my reading and research focus during the rest of my PhD program. I contacted my College Dean's office and asked about faculty who knew about gerontology. Remember, this was 1970 and gerontology as an inquiry was only in its embryonic stage. This resulted in a very productive intellectual relationship with Professor Arthur Farber, a social worker. At first, he was reluctant to be on my PhD committee, warning me that he was not a researcher. That was fine with me for I did not lack for research counsel. What he offered me was even more valuable—a guided tour of the literature on social gerontology.

As I was deliberating on what I should do for my PhD dissertation, I benefited from a third serendipitous event. On a return visit to the University of Toronto, Professor James Simmons (my former urban geography mentor) informed me about a new data source, a recently completed urban transportation survey—the Metropolitan Toronto Area Region Transportation Study. What he thought would interest me was that the urban residents who reported on their auto, transit, and pedestrian travel behaviors were distinguished by their chronological age. The analysis of this rich data resulted in my PhD dissertation focused on the residential location and transportation patterns of older Toronto residents. Although this was a conventional spatial analysis, unlike other comparable geographic studies, it innovatively recognized older persons as a distinctive population group. However, it lacked any environmental focus, which was only to come later.

The University of Chicago Connection

After completing my PhD in 1972, I received an invite from Professor Brian Berry to join the Department of Geography at the University of Chicago as an assistant professor. This was my fourth and career-changing serendipitous event. Remember that all my University of Toronto mentors reigned from here. Here, I was surrounded by renowned faculty, each a recognized expert in their respective specialties. As a bonus accompanying this appointment, my dissertation was published in the celebrated University of Chicago, Department of Geography Research Paper series (Golant, 1972).

My invitation in 1974 to hold a joint assistant professor position with the Committee on Human Development (part of the Department of Psychology, University of Chicago) was a critically important fifth serendipitous event. It was then one of the most respected centers on aging research in the world. I do not remember how I actually connected, but I forged extraordinarily rewarding academic relationships with new colleagues that included Professors Bernice Neugarten, Morton Lieberman, Mike Czikszentmihalyi, Bert Cohler, Gunhild Hagestad, and Robert Havighurst.

A sixth serendipitous event occurred 2 years later. Professor Bernice Neugarten invited me to participate as a principal investigator in a Program Project Grant, titled "Adult Lives and Patterns of Aging in an Urban Setting." The project consisted of four independent component studies having in common their concern with the patterns of social and psychological adaptation of an older urban population. No doubt, Neugarten and her colleagues were intrigued with an urban geographer interested in older people.

I proposed a study, "Community Ecology and the Adaptation of Older Persons" that focused on the subjective environmental experiences of a sample of age 60 and older people in Evanston, Illinois (a Chicago suburb), relying on survey research methodology. Under the tutelage of Bernice Neugarten, I learned painfully how to write a research grant and it was funded for 3 years (1976–1979) by the National Institute on Aging (NIA-PHFS P01 AG00123).

Achieving the goals of this empirical analysis was made immensely easier because of the highly talented graduate students that the University of Chicago typically attracted. Two played important roles as research assistants in my study and deserve special mention: the late Allan McCutcheon who assisted on the survey construction and computer analysis and Rosemary McCaslin who served as field director for the social service data collected for the study. Allan later became director of the University of Nebraska-Lincoln (UNL) Gallup Research Center and chair of UNL's survey research program. Rosemary became professor of social work at California State University at San Bernardino. I coauthored publications from my Evanston study with both (Golant & McCaslin, 1979; Golant & McCutcheon, 1980).

I reported the results of my research in my book, *A Place to Grow Old, The Meaning of Environment in Old Age* (Golant, 1984). It unfortunately took me more time to complete than I expected and Columbia University Press published it only after I left the University of Chicago (1980) to assume an associate professor position at the University of Florida in its Department of Geography. I wrote a short sentence in this book that was to be my intellectual companion throughout my career: "It is better, more enjoyable, easier, and less adaptationally costly to grow old in some places than in others" (Golant, 1984, p. 2).

My research program at the University of Chicago marked the beginning of a life-long focus on the subjective environments of older people. I did not know it at the time, but I was morphing into an environmental gerontologist. I was to become focused on how the everyday residential and care arrangements occupied by older adults influenced the quality of their lives and how successfully they adapted to the vagaries of getting old.

Initially, however, because I was intellectually raised and trained as a geographer, I felt like an interloping outsider to this Environmental Gerontology paradigm. My discipline attachments were strong and positively reinforced by my faculty position at a leading U.S. geography department. When I transitioned to the Department of Geography at the University of Florida in 1980, I soon assumed the department chair mantle which further nurtured my geography identity. Furthermore, a dedicated group of geographers in the 1980s and early 1990s were still acknowledging their interests in aging and old age (Golant, Rowles, & Meyer, 1989). And in 1990, I received a 2-year grant from the National Science Foundation (Geography section) to study the effects of aging-in-place on the housing quality of U.S. elderly (SES-8922053).

These disciplinary ties were to weaken substantially later in the 1990s and through to the present. I felt more estranged from geography as a field of study, felt intellectually more at home attending the GSA annual conference, identified more with journals published by gerontologists, and the scholars who I looked to for inspiration were all outside of geography (e.g., Powell Lawton, Jon Pynoos, Rick Scheidt, Rudolf Moos, Victor Regnier, and Jay Gubrium).

In Retrospect

A fortuitous combination of supportive universities, departments, organizations (GSA), mentors, and colleagues unquestionably influenced my current focus on Environmental Gerontology. However, it would be unfair to ignore the wealth of theoretical and research writings during the 1970s, 1980s, and early 1990s that fueled my interests and initially played an especially important role in my University of Chicago "community ecology" study. Disciplinary branches in geography, gerontology, sociology, planning, architecture, and psychology variously focused on how everyday environments interacted with and influenced human behavior (Campbell, Converse, & Rodgers, 1976; French, Rodgers, & Cobb, 1974; Ittelson, 1973; Lazarus & Folkman, 1984; Mehrabian, 1980; Michelson, 1976; Osgood et al., 1957; Perin, 1970; Proshansky, Ittelson, & Rivlin, 1970; Rapoport, 1977; Rowles, 1978; Saarinen, 1976; Stokols, 1978; Wapner, Cohen,

& Kaplan, 1976). In gerontology, of course, Powell Lawton's pioneering conceptual and empirical work dominated (Lawton, 1977; Lawton, 1983; Lawton & Kleban, 1971; Lawton & Nahemow, 1973). But also influential were the works of so many other researchers interested in aging issues, including Byerts (1975), Howell (1983), Kahana (1982), Pastalan and Carson (1970), and Scheidt and Windley (1985).

In retrospect, this literature helped frame the theoretical constructs and relationships found in my residential normalcy formulation. In the remainder of this chapter, I elaborate on these intellectual connections.

Intellectual Origins of Residential Normalcy Theory: Revisiting the Literature in My Past

What was original about the residential normalcy theory was not its distinctive constructs, several of which (but not all) I shamelessly borrowed from the theoretical formulations of others. Rather, what differentiated my contribution was its ability to show how these well-established parts operated together in specified ways and holistically explained how older people reacted and adapted to their everyday environments to achieve their needs and goals (Figure 4.1). Explanations for the successful functioning of complex living systems have long recognized that the whole is greater than the sum of its parts (Miller, 1978; Von Bertalanffy, 1968).

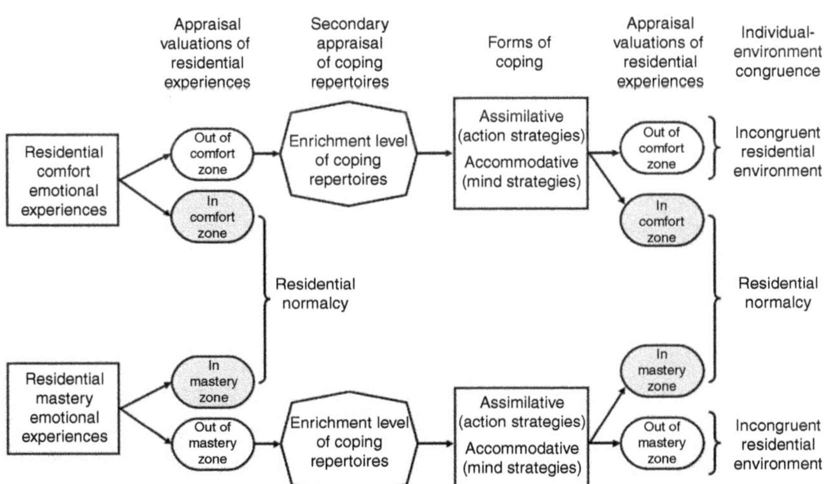

FIGURE 4.1 Theoretical model of residential normalcy.
Source: Golant (2015c).

Rejecting Residential Satisfaction as an Indicator of Individual–Environment Congruence

I was unhappy with the preponderance of housing quality assessments that relied on "residential satisfaction" as a subjective indicator of well-being. Such empirical treatments implicitly assumed that environmental congruence was a unidimensional construct. My distrust for such scaling approaches developed after I became familiar with Neugarten, Havighurst, and Tobin's (1961) empirical validation of "life satisfaction" as a multidimensional construct.

This helps explain why I relied on the multidimensional scales of Osgood et al. (1957) and Mehrabian and Russell (1974) when I formulated the residential normalcy construct. I had used both these sets of scales when I earlier studied the meanings of natural hazards and the subjective experiences of older people (Golant, 1984; Golant & Burton, 1970). Particularly valuable was Mehrabian and Russell's emotional response framework. It argued that when people (of all ages) interact with their everyday environments, they have a limited set of three basic and relatively orthogonal emotional reactions—pleasure, arousal, and dominance. In their words, the "evidence shows that [these] emotional (affective, connotative, feeling) reactions represent the common core of human response to all types of environments" (Mehrabian & Russell, 1974, p. 10).

To conceptualize residential normalcy, my model incorporated two of these orthogonal sets of emotional experiences—pleasure and mastery/control (dominance). This resulted in four possible sets of emotional outcomes: in comfort zone/in mastery zone; in comfort zone/out of mastery zone; out of comfort zone/in mastery zone; and out of comfort zone/out of mastery zone.

I believed that the formulation of residential normalcy as a multidimensional construct offered a more accurate representation of how older individuals subjectively appraised their places of residence. The literature often showed that the housing arrangements of older persons had spilt personalities. On the one hand, when in their *residential comfort zone*, older persons felt emotionally attached to their dwellings and possessions, enjoyed rewarding relationships with their friends or families, felt a sense of belonging with their communities, or enjoyed living in their culturally rich cities. However, on the other hand, when out of their *residential mastery zones*, they felt stressed because they had difficulty maintaining their independent households or paying for their dwellings, they continually worried about falling or had difficulty getting to their grocery stores. Clearly, these two sets of feelings could be operating independently at the same time.

I incorporated the third emotional reaction dimension of arousal as my "salience" construct. I argued that older people weighted their emotional experiences by how central or salient they were to their goals and needs (Lazarus, 1991). As an example, the older widow could feel *out of her residential comfort zone* because she had few nearby friends, disliked her neighbors, and felt her house was physically unattractive. She could also feel *out of her residential mastery zone* because she recently lost her driver's license and had difficulty reaching her doctor. But she could also believe that all these experiences were relatively unimportant or lacked salience in her overall residential assessment (Golant, 2015a). Rather, what mattered most to her was the very important loving social relationship she had with a daughter living close-by (a major source of *pleasurable* feelings) and the tasks she was able to accomplish with her help (buttressing her feelings of *competence and being in control*).

Coping or Adaptive Processes

The empirical research on how individuals coped with natural hazards and made migration decisions had emphasized that we should not construe their negative environmental appraisals as static outcomes. When individuals felt threatened with the imminent flooding of their houses, they usually took actions to get out of danger. Similarly, when individuals appraised their places of residence as incompatible with their way of life, they moved elsewhere (Rossi, 1955; Wolpert, 1966).

There was also considerable theoretical support to argue that when confronted with stressful circumstances, individuals take corrective actions. Lazarus and Folkman's (1984, p. 179) cognitive-relational theory argued that the coping actions of individuals served the overriding function of "managing or altering the problem with the environment causing distress." Several human development and Environmental Gerontology formulations similarly emphasized that older individuals initiate action-oriented adaptive processes—exercise agency—to achieve their personal goals and rectify their incongruent environments. Baltes and Baltes (1990), for example, argued that when older persons confronted age-related declines or losses, they initiated three types of adaptive regulatory processes—selection, optimization, and compensation—to achieve their developmental goals. For Scheidt and Windley (1985, p. 245), the underpinnings of an ecology of aging was "the adaptation of individuals to demands posed by the interaction of the environmental and intrapersonal changes that accompany aging." And for Lawton (1989), "older adults are increasingly proactive in seeking the kinds of social environments that allow them to avoid negative affect and conflict and which permit sufficient intellectual and emotional stimulation" (Magai, 2001, p. 404). These theoretical treatments were the basis for my residential normalcy theory arguing that older people are motivated to initiate coping actions when they feel *out of their residential comfort* and/or *mastery zones*.

Consequently, the theorized emotional experience outcomes of residential comfort and residential mastery were not necessarily fixed or permanent end states, but rather were often in flux. Individual–environmental congruence or incongruence was always being established and reestablished because older people's personal attributes (e.g., their self-perceptions, motivations, and capabilities), their objectively defined physical and social environments, and their subjective environmental experiences were continually changing (Golant, 2003).

Consequently, over the course of their aging lives, older people may experience many new "residential normals" and these may be very different from their pasts.

> They do not necessarily replace lost activities, reestablish the integrity of a past residential setting, or maintain the continuity of their past lives or environments. They end up in residential or care settings and conducting activities different from their pasts. (Golant, 2015c, p. 79)

Dual Process Coping Framework

The residential normalcy theory incorporated the dual process coping framework of Brandtstadter and Greve (1994) that distinguished between *assimilative* and *accommodative* adaptive strategies. The assimilative mode referred to external-directed action efforts and activities whereby older individuals attempt to prevent, correct, or modify the offensive or discrepant aspects of their environments. In contrast, the accommodative mode referred to inner-directed mind strategies whereby older individuals rationalized or denied their problems. Consequently, they changed, downgraded or de-emphasized their expectations or aspirations, devalued their existing goals or plans, or less harshly judged their lives or environments to make them more consistent with their current individual and environmental realities. Individuals rely on these mind adaptive strategies when they lack viable assimilative coping options or appraise them as overly taxing or stressful, when they judge their goals or needs as less salient to achieve, or when they lack strong self-efficacy beliefs.

I was early aware of these theoretical distinctions. Lazarus (1966) had distinguished between "problem-focused" (or "direct-action" coping) and "defensive reappraisals" when he accounted for how individuals responded to threatening situations like natural disasters. Other researchers had also distinguished these dual coping processes to explain their empirical findings. In the 1970s, the authors of a large survey research study offered an intriguing explanation for why low-income persons were more satisfied with their housing than higher income persons, even though the latter group occupied housing that was "better" by most objective indicators (Campbell et al., 1976). They argued that unlike wealthy individuals who often had higher but unfulfilled expectations, low-income persons did not aspire or expect to occupy high quality housing. Consequently, the perceived gap between the reality of their housing status and their expectations was often going to be smaller than for wealthier individuals. This resulted in the greater residential satisfaction of low-income individuals and explained their lack of motivation to move to alternative places.

Fried (2000) also concluded that the emotionally and symbolically charged attachments that older people formed with their residential settings despite their severe inadequacies could be pathological and destructive (Fried, 2000). He argued that these coping responses revealed their "submission to decline and decompensation" (Fried, 2000, p. 198). He concluded that such attachments become "dysfunctional when adaptation to new growth opportunities or possibilities of greater gratification in personal or community life are renounced" (Fried, 2000, p. 202). Similarly, Peterson, Maier, and Seligman (1993) speak of the hopelessness of longtime housing occupants in denial because they have become habituated to the less desirable features of their dwellings. Such interpretations also accounted for why older people were aging in place despite occupying residential environments that by objective standards were not congruent with their observable needs or goals (Golant, 2008).

Coping Produces Unexpected Outcomes

Most of the literature also theorized that the initiation of assimilative adaptive processes resulted in positive outcomes. Oswald, Schilling, Wahl, and Gang (2002, pp. 283–284), for example, reasonably concluded that when older people move, it is to pursue "individual interests and [to] enhance personal development as well as to overcome environmental restrictions or 'environmental press.'" Much earlier, Kahana and Kahana (1983, p. 206) argued that "Environmental change may also be a positive experience, if it is interpreted as a pathway toward personal control" and hope for improving one's future in later life...and an increase in "person–environment fit." And for home modification advocates, physical changes to the dwelling are interpreted as a means to alleviate current individual–environment mismatches that could increase the risk of falling (Pynoos, Liebig, Overton, & Calvert, 1997).

But my former Committee on Human Development colleagues had shown that the coping actions of older persons do not always produce positive outcomes. They had studied frail older people transitioning from their homes to nursing homes because they had difficulties maintaining their independent households. However, the residential moves of these old—often made involuntarily—did not necessarily result in their occupancy of positively experienced environments. Lieberman and Tobin (1983), for example, found that although these older adults occupied settings that were more secure and helped them to cope with their limitations, these places were very incompatible with their earlier "home" environments (Golant, 2015c). Consequently, after they relocated to their new institutional settings, a significant percentage experienced poor emotional outcomes.

This is why in my residential normalcy theory I argued that even as older people cope successfully with one set of incongruent environmental features, their adaptive responses may unintentionally produce new undesirable residential experiences and they still end up in discordant environments. For example, when frail older people move to assisted living developments because they require help to live independently, they again feel in their residential mastery zones because they no longer have to worry about accomplishing their instrumental activities of daily living (e.g., shopping, housework, or preparing meals). However, if they have difficulty establishing emotionally rewarding friendships or hate the smallness of their accommodations, they will newly feel out of their residential comfort zones (Golant, 2015c).

Explaining Why Some Older People Cope Better

Most Environmental Gerontology theories argue that because the older population is comprised of heterogeneous group of individuals, they interact differently with their everyday environments. Lawton's environmental docility hypothesis, for example, proposes that older persons who are more physically impaired are more likely to have their behaviors explained by the attributes of their residential settings (Lawton & Nahemow, 1973). Similarly, Kahana's congruence model argues that optimal environments must be congruent with individual preferences (Kahana, 1982).

The residential normalcy theory also recognized the importance of these individual–environment interactions, but not as antecedents of older people's residential assessments. Rather, the focus was on how older individuals differently coped with their incongruent residential environments, what Lazarus (1966) referred to as secondary appraisal processes. The theory argued that older individuals with more efficacious and viable coping opportunities (who I characterized as having *more enriched coping repertoires*) also had resilient personalities, made their own decisions, and had access to resource-rich environments offering potential solutions. Unlike the other constructs and relationships of my residential normalcy theory, these relationships were based on my more recent readings by Aldwin and Igarashi (2012), Skodol (2010), and Wild, Wiles, and Allen (2013).

Going Forward

Environmental gerontologists typically focus on the physical and social attributes of older people's residential and care environments. I believe the next "big thing" will be the formal inclusion of the "technological" environment, subsumed under labels such as smart technologies, gerontechnology, ambient assisted technology, telehealth, and telemedicine (Schulz et al., 2014). We are entering an era of omnipresent wireless devices implanted in our bodies or swallowable, attached to our wearable clothing, inserted in portable devices such as smart phones, in the walls, floors, ceilings, beds, appliances, furniture, and infrastructure of our residential and care settings, and embedded in robots with human qualities. They will record a wealth of data about the physical and mental health conditions, cognitive and sensory performance, mobility, social connectedness, and everyday social and leisure activities of older individuals. They will also monitor the health and functioning of their built environments including their appliances and building's infrastructure to detect threats such as allergens, toxins, air pollutants, dampness, water leaks, mold, bacterial infections, and extreme temperatures. They will communicate this information to older persons, their families, and their clinicians who can intervene to prevent, manage, or treat bad outcomes.

These new information and communication technologies hold tremendous promise as strategies that can optimize the health, activities, and social functioning of an aging population. However, we require far more information about how older persons will react to having these devices introduced into their homes.

Consequently, I have constructed a new theoretical model identifying the factors that will influence their acceptance behaviors (Golant, 2017). It recognizes that how older individuals appraise their unmet needs for assistance will be a motivating factor and that their adoption behaviors will also depend on how they process information about the efficaciousness and usability of these technological alternatives and their possible unintended consequences. Furthermore, the model will recognize that however favorable their appraisals, older persons may reject these technological solutions, considering them as less desirable than traditional family care giving and assistive device alternatives.

REFERENCES

Aldwin, C., & Igarashi, H. (2012). An ecological model of resilience in late life. In B. Hayslip & G. C. Smith (Eds.), *Annual review of gerontology and geriatrics* (pp. 115–130). New York, NY: Springer Publishing.

Baltes, P. B., & Baltes, M. M. (1990). Psychological perspectives on successful aging: A model of selective optimization with compensation. In P. B. Baltes & M. M. Baltes (Eds.), *Successful aging: Perspectives from the behavioral sciences* (pp. 1–34). New York, NY: Cambridge University Press.

Birren, J. E. (1970). Abuse of urban aged. *Psychology Today*, *3*(10), 37–38.

Brandtstadter, J., & Greve, W. (1994). The aging self: Stabilizing and protective processes. *Developmental Review*, *14*(1), 42–80.

Byerts, T. O. (1975). Symposium: The city: A viable environment for the elderly? Phase I. *The Gerontologist*, *15*(1), 13–46.

Campbell, A., Converse, P. G., & Rodgers, W. (1976). *The quality of American life*. New York, NY: Russell Sage.

French, J. R. P., Rodgers, W., & Cobb, S. (1974). Adjustment as person-environment fit. In G. V. Coelho, D. A. Hamburg & J. E. Adams (Eds.), *Coping and adaptation* (pp. 316–333). New York, NY: Basic Books.

Fried, M. (2000). Continuities and discontinuities of place. *Journal of Environmental Psychology*, *20*(3), 193–205.

Golant, S. M. (1971). Adjustment process in a system: A behavioral model of human movement. *Geographical Analysis*, *3*(3), 203–220.

Golant, S. M. (1972). *The residential location and spatial behavior of the elderly: A Canadian example*. Chicago, IL: University of Chicago, Department of Geography Monograph Series.

Golant, S. M. (1984). *A place to grow old: The meaning of environment in old age*. New York, NY: Columbia University Press.

Golant, S. M. (1987). Residential moves by elderly persons to U.S. Central cities, suburbs, and rural areas. *Journal of Gerontology*, *42*(5), 534–539.

Golant, S. M. (2003). Conceptualizing time and space in environmental gerontology: A pair of old issues deserving new thought. *The Gerontologist*, *43*(5), 638–648.

Golant, S. M. (2008). Commentary: Irrational exuberance for the aging in place of vulnerable low-income older homeowners. *Journal of Aging and Social Policy*, *20*(4), 379–397.

Golant, S. M. (2011a). The changing residential environments of older people. In R. H. Binstock & L. K. George (Eds.), *Handbook of aging and the social sciences* (7th ed., pp. 207–220). New York, NY: Academic Press.

Golant, S. M. (2011b). The quest for residential normalcy by older adults: Relocation but one pathway. *Journal of Aging Studies*, *25*(3), 193–205.

Golant, S. M. (2015a). *Aging in the right place*. Baltimore, MD: Health Professions Press.

Golant, S. M. (2015b). Residential normalcy and the aging in place behaviors of older Americans. *Progress In Geography*, *34*(2), 1535–1557.

Golant, S. M. (2015c). Residential normalcy and the enriched coping repertoires of successfully aging older adults. *The Gerontologist*, *55*(1), 70–82.

Golant, S. M. (2017). A theoretical model to explain the smart technology adoption behaviors of elder consumers. *Journal of Aging Studies*, *42*, 56–73.

Golant, S. M., & Burton, I. (1970). A semantic differential experiment in the interpretation and grouping of environmental hazards. *Geographical Analysis*, *2*(2), 120–134.

Golant, S. M., & McCaslin, R. (1979). A functional classification of services for older people. *Journal of Gerontological Social Work*, *1*(3), 187–209.

Golant, S. M., & McCutcheon, A. L. (1980). Objective quality of life indicators and the external validity of community research findings. *Social Indicators Research*, *7*(1–4), 207–235.

Golant, S. M., Rowles, G. D., & Meyer, J. W. (1989). Aging and the aged. In G. Gaile & C. Willmott (Eds.), *Geography in America* (pp. 451–466). New York, NY: Merrill Pub. Co.

Howell, S. (1983). The meaning of place in old age. In G. D. Rowles & R. J. Ohta (Eds.), *Aging and milieu* (pp. 97–107). New York, NY: Academic Press.

Huntington, E. (1922). *Civilization and climate*: New Haven, CT: Yale University Press.

Ittelson, W. H. (1973). Environment perception and contemporary perceptual theory. *Environment and cognition*, 1–19.

Kahana, E. (1982). A congruence model of person-environment interaction. In P. G. Windley, M. P. Lawton & T. O. Byerts (Eds.), *Aging and the environment: Theoretical approaches* (pp. 97–121). New York, NY: Springer Publishing.

Kahana, E., & Kahana, B. (1983). Environmental continuity, futurity, and adaptation of the aged. In G. Rowles & R. J. Ohta (Eds.), *Aging and milieu* (pp. 205–228). New York, NY: Academic Press.

Lawton, M. P. (1977). The impact of the environment on aging and behavior. In J. E. Birren & K. W. Schaie (Eds.), *Handbook of the psychology of aging* (pp. 276–301). New York, NY: Van Nostrand Reinhold.

Lawton, M. P. (1983). Environment and other determinants of well-being in older people. *The Gerontologist*, *23*(4), 349–357.

Lawton, M. P. (1989). Environmental proactivity and affect in older people. In S. Spacapan & S. Oskamp (Eds.), *The social psychology of aging* (pp. 135–163). Newbury Park, CA: Sage.

Lawton, M. P., & Kleban, M. H. (1971). The aged resident of the inner city. *The Gerontologist*, *11*(4), 277–283.

Lawton, M. P., & Nahemow, L. (1973). Ecology and the aging process. In C. Eisdorfer & M. P. Lawton (Eds.), *The psychology of adult development and aging* (pp. 619–674). Washington, DC: American Psychological Association.

Lazarus, R. S. (1966). *Psychological stress and the coping process*. New York, NY: McGraw-Hill.

Lazarus, R. S. (1991). Cognition and motivation in emotion. *American Psychologist*, *46*(4), 352–367.

Lazarus, R. S., & Folkman, S. (1984). *Stress, appraisal, and coping*. New York, NY: Springer Publishing.

Lieberman, M. A., & Tobin, S. S. (1983). *The experience of old age: Stress, coping and survival*. New York, NY: Basic Books.

Magai, C. (2001). Emotions over the life span. In J. E. Birren & K. W. Schaie (Eds.), *Handbook for psychology and aging* (5th ed., pp. 399–426). San Diego, CA: Academic Press.

Mehrabian, A. (1980). *Basic dimensions for a general psychological theory: Implications for personality, social, environmental, and developmental studies*. Massachusetts: Oelgeschlager, Gunn & Hain, Publishers, Inc.

Mehrabian, A., & Russell, J. A. (1974). *An approach to environmental psychology*. Cambridge: MIT Press.

Michelson, W. (1976). *Man and his urban environment: A sociological approach*. Reading, MA: Addison-Wesley.

Miller, J. G. (1978). *Living systems*. New York, NY: McGraw-Hill.

Neugarten, B. L., Havighurst, R. J., & Tobin, S. S. (1961). The measurement of life satisfaction. *Journal of Gerontology*, *16*, 134–143.

Osgood, C. E., Suci, G. J., & Tannenbaum, P. H. (1957). *The measurement of meaning*. Champaign, IL: University of Illinois Press.

Oswald, F., Schilling, O., Wahl, H-W., & Gang, K. (2002). Trouble in paradise? Reasons to relocate and objective environmental changes among well-off older adults. *Journal of Environmental Psychology*, *22*(3), 273–288.

Pastalan, L. A., & Carson, D. H. (1970). *Spatial behavior of older people*. Ann Arbor, MI: University of Michigan Ann Arbor.

Perin, C. (1970). *With man in mind*. Cambridge, Mass: Massachusetts Institute of Technology Press.

Peterson, C., Maier, S. F., & Seligman, M. E. P. (1993). *Learned helplessness a theory for the age of personal control*. New York, NY: Oxford University Press.

Proshansky, H. M., Ittelson, W. H., & Rivlin, L. G. (1970). *Environmental psychology: Man and his physical setting*. New York, NY: Holt.

Pynoos, J., Liebig, P., Overton, J., & Calvert, E. (1997). The delivery of home modification and repair services. In S. Lanspery & J. Hyde (Eds.), *Staying put: Adapting the places instead of the people* (pp. 171–192). New York, NY: Baywood Publishing Co.

Rapoport, A. (1977). *Human aspects of urban form: Towards a man-environment approach to urban form and design*. New York, NY: Pergamon Press.

Rossi, P. H. (1955). *Why families move*. Glencoe, IL: Free Press.

Rowles, G. D. (1978). *Prisoners of space?: Exploring the geographical experience of older people*. Boulder, CO: Westview Press.

Saarinen, T. F. (1976). *Environmental planning: Perception and behavior*. Boston, MA: Houghton Mifflin.

Scheidt, R. J., & Windley, P. G. (1985). The ecology of aging. In K. W. Schaie & J. E. Birren (Eds.), *Handbook of the psychology of aging* (2nd ed., pp. 245–258). New York, NY: Van Nostrand Reinhold.

Schulz, R., Wahl, H-W., Matthews, J. T., De Vito Dabbs, A., Beach, S. R., & Czaja, S. J. (2014). Advancing the aging and technology agenda in gerontology. *The Gerontologist*, *00*(00), 1–11.

Skodol, A. (2010). The resilient personality. In J. W. Reich, A. J. Zautra & J. S. Hall (Eds.), *Handbook of adult resilience* (pp. 112–125). New York, NY: Guilford Press.

Stokols, D. (1978). Environmental psychology. *Annual Review of Psychology*, *29*(1), 253–295.

Von Bertalanffy, L. (1968). *General system theory: Foundations, development, applications*. New York, NY: G. Braziller.

Wapner, S., Cohen, S., & Kaplan, B. (1976). *Experiencing the environment*. London, UK: Plenum Press.

Wild, K., Wiles, J. L., & Allen, R. E. S. (2013). Resilience: Thoughts on the value of the concept for critical gerontology. *Ageing & Society*, *33*(1), 137–158.

Wolpert, J. (1966). Migration as an adjustment to environmental stress. *Journal of Social Issues*, *22*(4), 92–102.

CHAPTER 5

Personal Biography and the Development of Gerontological Environmental Theory

Robert L. Rubinstein

ABSTRACT

This chapter summarizes career, research, and environmental ideas of Robert Rubinstein, a cultural anthropologist. Starting with ethnographic fieldwork in Vanuatu in the 1970s, it presents his work undertaken at the Philadelphia Geriatric Center and more recently at the University of Maryland Baltimore County (UMBC) in the following decades, focusing on ideas concerning aging and the environment and on numerous collaborations with colleagues.

BIOGRAPHICAL NOTES

My work in Environmental Gerontology came about without preintention. I originally did not know much about gerontology (I hope I know more by now) and had intended to be a more or less standard cultural anthropologist. But, coming out of graduate school, there were few academic jobs and I applied for an opening at the Philadelphia Geriatric Center (PGC) and was hired for what was initially a year-long position. It was my work interviewing older informants in their own homes that directed me compellingly to the home environment as an area of interest. I did not have to dig. This is what people talked to me about and it was obvious that home life was quite important to the persons I interviewed, many of whom lived alone. I will say more about this below.

http://dx.doi.org/10.1891/0198-8794.38.73

GRADUATE SCHOOL ORIENTATIONS

When I was in graduate school, studying cultural anthropology, I learned about the numerous theoretical approaches to the collection and analysis of field data, some of which are quite distinct from contemporary theoretical approaches. Among those that interested me the most at the time were (a) cultural ecology, or the analysis of the interrelationship among ecology, cultural meaning, ritual and social life. This approach is best typified by Roy Rappaport's classic book, *Pigs for the Ancestors* (Rappaport, 1968), which analyzed caloric intake, human versus pig populations, and how they were all intertwined in a larger regional ritual system that regulated war and peace in a small area of Papua New Guinea. Other prominent approaches which interested me were (b) structuralism or a culturally situated pan-human construction of important binary oppositions among cultural categories that meaningfully underlined social life as well as social exchange, marriage, and mythology found in distinctive societies, an approach fostered by Claude Levi-Strauss (1966) and other scholars. The perspective of structuralism seems to no longer be a focus of anthropological research and was superseded by work from a post-structural perspective. And, (c) symbolic anthropology, or the study of key cultural symbols in particular societies and how such symbols dominated or reduced the meaning systems of local societies (Turner, 1966). While few persons are still symbolic anthropologists in any sense, I still find myself attracted to this approach and a good deal of my current work in adult day services in fact relates to the intersection of Alzheimer's disease and semiotics. However, symbolic anthropology did not fully take into action elements such as social action, power, and inequality. Finally (d) the work of Clifford Geertz (1973), including his notion of ethnography as text and his methodological emphasis on "thick description," showed the way for anthropologists to better use and understand the act of interpretation by the field worker as part of their methodological tool-kit to explain findings and as the goal of research and social explanation. The focus on interpretation of meaning is critical and it is one of the most important methodological tools that are generally missing from mainstream gerontology.

What I did not realize at the time (the 1970s) was that I would find in these approaches a central focus on place and environment as key crosscutting themes. For example, in some of the work of Levi-Strauss and his colleagues, the binary opposition between center and periphery in a village or setting became an important cultural way of symbolically classifying culturally identified space and social practice in a village or encampment which was inhabited by specific group of people in various parts of the world.

DISSERTATION WORK

When it came to do my own doctoral dissertation work, I spent more than a year on the island of Malo (Na Tamambo) in Vanuatu (formerly the New Hebrides) in the southwestern Pacific Ocean. Malo is a small island and had about 2,000 inhabitants, who were horticulturalists living primarily on yams and taro, who raised coconuts to make copra for cash, raised cattle to feed attenders at weddings and other large events, and also raised pigs, which were used in interpersonal and intergroup exchange payments. Malo was well known in the region historically for the use of both male and intersex pigs as objects of wealth. Male and intersex pigs were graded in value based on the growth of a tooth toward a full circle. This was a very valuable symbol and commodity. Traditional culture was based, for men, on the killing of larger number of male and intersex tusked pigs necessary for rising in grade in the local pig-killing system or *Sumbuea;* at the time of my visit this system was nearly moribund with very few practitioners remaining.

There, some of the cultural themes or key symbols that also emerged in research concerned notions of place; land; connections to land; movement among lands; the metaphor of "walking"; history as represented in and on the land and its features; personal, land-based biography; and attachment to place. Some of these ideas, for example the notion of place, have become important notions in contemporary Environmental Gerontology and environmental psychology, but I never learned to view them through the lenses of these disciplines until much later. Rather, to me, they were manifestations of a meaningful cultural system shared to some degree by the people of Malo and I could see them in operation in our own society. One thing I also found out on Malo was that the phenomenology of the person was somewhat distinctive from that of the West. On Malo, the cultural boundary of the body did not always end at the skin, but rather continued, especially for men, into the land that was their patrimony. That is to say, men and their land were part of one another, closely aligned and largely inseparable. By land, I mean relatively small parcels of named territory that were associated with the senior male's patrilineal ancestors and patrilineal descent group, that formed the territory for patrilineally and patrilaterally related groups of men and in-married women. The close association, identity coherence, and inseparability of men and their lands led me to wonder about the connection between person and object, a theme I was to take up in my work in gerontology later on. Each piece of named land was marked with specific, meaningful features that included stone constructions, mostly formerly used for pig killing, significant trees, and a number of other historically important features, knowledge of which was passed down to children.

From my graduate work and my initial fieldwork in the Pacific grew the significance of two concepts. First, the notion of data gathering, especially gathering subjective, person-centered knowledge, through ethnographic fieldwork and cultural interpretation loomed as significant. Second, the idea of culture itself became highly significant. When I was on Malo for my dissertation work, it was very hard to tell if this small island constituted a single socially integrated society in the Durkheimian sense, or if it was a collection of distinctive individuals and opposing groups, somewhat linked, and sometimes not linked, by history, identity, kinship and affinal ties, and exchange. There were many cross-cutting groupings, factions, and distinctive individuals among this small population. Where one lived, how one was politically oriented, how one was temporally oriented (to the past or to the future), gender, social status, education level, income, social networks, all these elements both brought people together and pulled them apart. There were profound political disputes, which at times made the island unworkable as a single entity. Factions sometimes made fun of one another behind their backs. A minority of Maloese were members of a political movement that looked toward both political independence with the hope of bringing aspects of the past (called *kastom*) back into the present together with traditionalists from other islands in the then-New Hebrides. The majority of Maloese were affiliated with more modernist political movements, which were pushing toward independent nation status (the New Hebrides was a colony of both France and Great Britain, which caused a great deal of confusion, evidenced in two school systems, two currency systems and a separate currency for postage stamps, which were printed in both English and French). The Malo social system seemed to be held together because persons had both affinal and kinship relations with one another, found attachment to their lands as a significant aspect of social identity, and there was little economic or class ranking; a class system had not yet developed (to my knowledge, this has since happened, with co-occurring income, class inequality, and more movement to and away from the island).

In reality, I never really stopped to consider the processes by which culture itself, which was then thought of as a system of sometimes shared meanings and interpretations, could in fact exist on the level of the individual specifically. I could not really figure this out although I spent a good deal of time pondering it. This understanding had to wait until my first work in gerontology at the PGC, a period which, through my research interviews, showed me how older adults in the United States could be thought of as inhabiting a singular cultural world that for the most part was found in individuals. This was especially true in my initial work in the United States with older men who lived alone (see below), who created a miniaturized and subjectively significant culture of one in their own homes. These were points that were made much earlier in the 20th century by the great ethnographer-linguist, Edward Sapir, who emphasized the individual level as the ultimate locus of culture and also by A.I. Hallowell (1954), whose work on *The Self in its Behavioral Environment* proved influential.

I also never stopped to consider how individuals on Malo, primarily men who owned land and were descendants of patrilineal ancestors who lived on the land for generations, could be thought of as acting together as person, place, and object, in some ways as phenemonologically inseparable. A question I raised was: How could a person (who, in my thinking, assumed ontological primacy) project themselves into objects, places, or even behavioral routines and personalize or possess them? Were these psychoanalytic types of projections, some form of psychoanalytic "object relations," or were they thoroughly cultural and therefore part of the cultural constitution of the person? Ultimately, I landed on the cultural side of this question and attributed such "projections" as part of the Western cultural constructs of autonomy and individualism, or more properly possessive individualism. On Malo, people were attached significantly to place through patrimony and through transaction (that is, women attached to land via marriage exchanges and payments) and were in some ways socially larger than the entity encased by their skin.

Some years after returning from my initial trip to Vanuatu, I managed to read Bourdieu's book, *An Outline of a Theory of Practice* (Bourdieu, 1990), which had been translated from French into English. There, I found the term *habitus*, which had been previously known in anthropology from the work of Marcel Mauss. The concept habitus was used by Bourdieu to overcome preexisting problems with developing a perspective on person and the social environment, among other relationships, which linked both subjective and objective approaches to the person in a single conceptualization. How are subjective perceptions and objective constructions aligned? Although the definition of habitus is not easy to comprehend, it essentially means a system of social structures along with structuring personal dispositions that together are oriented to practical outcomes in the world. Based on social and cultural habits developed by individuals alone and as group members, habitus represents embodied and psychological dispositions that shape and are shaped by larger social attitudes and affect how individuals react to social categories and beings around them. Habitus, a structuring element of living, is determined by factors such as socio-economic status (SES), family, social relations, religion, education, ethnicity, and many others. As such, habitus produced a "model of" the world that again shapes and is shaped by orienting structural features, also to be conceived as a model for the world, as Geertz might say. Orientation to places and to the environment are some of the features that are reproduced both over time and over and again by this orienting structure. Essentially, as some say, habitus reproduces a person's place in the larger social structure.

KEY THEMES AND GERONTOLOGY

This leads to several important elements that ultimately concern the relations of older persons and the environment. It shows the significance of person-environment relations that are *more than just* the result of, for example, a press-competence perspective, as Lawton, Kahana, and others have developed in gerontology. Or more than (even as Bourdieu was later to attend to), aspects of social distinction and social class that identify, socially reproduce, and variously divide and unify people. The habitus approach shows how social identities are formed beyond the biophysical, both subjectively and objectively, through structuring and its effects on individual citizens. Considering a gerontological press-competence approach in the context of habits thus shows a way of combining press and competence as experienced by the person-as-organism into the larger context of social life, the social world, and as individuals with identities in a larger meaningful cultural context.

In 1981, Powell Lawton, at the PGC, hired me to conduct a one-year grant-funded study of older men living alone in the Philadelphia-area and he also encouraged me to write National Institutes of Health (NIH) research about older adults. I managed to stretch the funds for the grant out to more than 1 year and was luckily still employed by the time my first NIH grant was funded. This NIH research was called "The meaning and function of 'home' for the elderly," a 3-year study of aging and the environment in the Philadelphia region.

These two early studies on older men living alone and the meaning of home to older adults in many ways let me see important aspects of older Americans' relationships with home and local environments. In the study of old men living alone, I interviewed 47 men age 65 and over, usually each once a week for 5 consecutive weeks, about their life histories, residential and family histories and the life they experienced in their home environments, their attachments, activities, social networks, family relations and most importantly, critical cultural-personal themes, or organized areas of personal meaning, which they found to be central in their lives. The results were written in the book, *Singular Paths* (Rubinstein, 1984). I was also influenced by the work of anthropologists Clark and Anderson and by the work of Sharon Kaufman, who discussed the term *theme* as one way older adults have to organize personal meaning and biographical experience. She also showed how a theme functioned to construct or shape a self that seemed ageless, since a theme can itself be adapted as a continuous framework to fit many biographical changes that might occur over time. Biographical disconnection and rebuilding lives after tragedy or unexpected events occurred was later treated by Gay Becker.

In the NIH-supported study on the meaning and function of home, I was able to ethnographically follow nine older adults, making weekly visits to their homes for periods of 5 months to 2 years. In the second part of the study, I was able to interview more than 50 older adults in their own homes and collected lifetime residential histories from them, which ranged from one residence to dozens and, along with this, an account of who lived with them, what they were doing at the time, and whatever information about lingering emotional attachment to former and present-day residences that I could elicit. Results were written in a series of papers (Lawton & Rubinstein, 2000; Rubinstein & Lawton, 1997).

KEY CONCEPTS

From these two projects emerged a number of concepts that would prove crucial in my own understanding of the attachment and allocation of meaning by older adults to their homes: the biographical approach, the culture of living alone, miniaturization, and the notion of a personal meaning system. I have written about these concepts in various places, focusing primarily on the biographical approach and the personal meaning system. Studies of miniaturization have been limited and I can only recall one conference paper in which I discussed it in much detail, but I think it is worthy of expansion (Rubinstein, 1987, 1989a, 1989b, 1990).

The Biographical Approach

In these two early studies, I visited informants in their own homes in a wide range of neighborhoods, ranging from the truly deplorable and dangerous to the elite. By a stroke of luck, I approached interviewing so that, after initially collecting background and demographic information about each informant, I asked them to tell the story of their lives in whatever way they wanted. Later, I collaborated with Mark Luborsky in utilizing the life-history approach, a staple in anthropology, which we refined for work with older adults, in other research studies. With Helen Black, I later collaborated on studies of chronic, life-long poverty and several other topics using as central the life-history method. It was our feeling that we really could not know much about a person until we had some picture of what their lives had been like and had some context for understanding what they were telling us.

In the two studies I am discussing here, most informants interpreted this request to tell a life story as a chance to construct a story that was fairly coherent, edited or scripted (things were often left out), often emotional, and that led retrospectively to the present day. Not all were chronologically oriented, although most were; some were thematic, some chaotic, some topical in nature (e.g., family and kin first, then work, then schooling). Nevertheless, informants were in some sense giving the history of their lives, which was constructed by them *in the present day* as an explanation of events of the present day and how the informant got to be where she or he was right now. Thus, they were using the events of the past as malleable raw material to construct a story about the present day. Their stories were not "the truth" in any absolute sense (a point which seemed to be beyond the comprehension of some of the grant reviewers we had), but rather was a story about identity in the present made up of material that occurred in the past and was selected for the telling to illustrate an informant's identity at the present time. Often, the life story was told with reference to key possessions that were located in the home and could be shown as illustrations of the things the informant was speaking about—a souvenir from a vacation, family photos ("my generations" as one informant put it), artwork, a piece of furniture, medicine bottles, and similar items became elements to back up the story that was being constructed and told. And the story that was being told was a story of one's personal identity: who that person found herself to be at the present time and how they got there. In the intimacy of an interview undertaken in the home environment, the story of present-day identity occurred in dialogue with the home environment and its objects. Thus the home and objects and representations in the home became inherently tied up in the story of one's present-day identity as constructed biographically.

The biographical approach has been critical to my work over the years and it has almost always been utilized in a manner, which incorporates the built and in-filled environment as a central player in the story.

The Culture of Living Alone

In these two studies, I interviewed many people who lived alone, and I came to the conclusions that living alone shaped a particular orientation to time, place, and action. This meant that for some informants, behavioral routines became objectivized, that the routine itself became an object of consciousness for the person, part of phenomenological intentionality, part of a daily or weekly or other temporal round that was subjectively singled out as an important event in the person's life. One man I interviewed made it his routine to pay his utility bills at the utility office, instead of just mailing the check in from the corner post box, so that he could spend the better part of the day travelling by city bus to the utility office, having lunch out, and returning home by bus for the next set of scheduled activities. In this lifestyle, having routines not only filled in time and structured that day, they forced the person to get up, washed, dressed, and engage with others. Again, the routine seemed more important subjectively than just a meaningless activity. Some spoke about activities with a capital A. "Its my Activity," one man said about a certain routine. In this way, the home acted as a staging area for personal projects as well as a node in a conscious map of both time and space. This may seem somewhat trivial, but on further consideration, I felt this required an active presence and a conscious cultural construction of daily life, part of personal identity, using the home as a central place. It was indeed not trivial for the persons involved. In further thought about this over the years, I believe that the cultural construct of autonomy, an important marker of cultural personhood in America, was being constructed through such small-scale routines both when living alone and when living with others. To be sure, regular routines valorize work, an important concept in American life, and especially for retirees. Recall that in the earliest days of gerontology, people spoke about later life as a set of "role less roles." Further, in households in which more than one person lives, cultural autonomy can be validated by reference to other peoples' acknowledgments of one's social and personal identities. While living alone, it is sometimes incumbent on the solo dweller to undertake such forms of validation.

Miniaturization

Some of the persons I interviewed in the early projects were frail or infirm. This required them to make important choices about the use of space in the home and in some cases led to what I called miniaturization. Parts of the home were closed off and the active world became quite miniaturized. One man I interviewed reduced his space to a desk, on which he put his phone and important papers, where he could sit and read, and from which he could see his television. Pathways to the bathroom, kitchen, and bedroom were traced by absence of dust on the floor. He was quite ill, used oxygen at times, and could not do much cleaning. His niece, his closet relative, occasionally came by to clean for him. His space had indeed become miniaturized. I once referred to this as the miniaturization of satisfaction: everything of necessity was close by and at-hand. But it certainly incorporates a sense of spatial miniaturization in life. In a related sense, the miniaturization was also one of time as the man was well aware of the limited amount of lifetime he probably had left. This sense of finitude could be muted by the time invested in reading, which was his major activity. Spatially, his was an adaptation to press by his remaining spatial competence, but it permitted him to continue as a citizen and as a person with an active social identity. It also permitted him to engage with those things that were personally meaningful to him and through which he defined himself, still.

The Personal Meaning System

I found that each informant had a system of personal meaning that was often tied to and represented by the home environment and the objects within the home. I called this the personal meaning system. The discovery, so to speak, of this, was not anything I consciously did, and I would say most of what I did with informants was to listen as carefully as I could. Through listening, the appearance of an interconnected system of key meanings, principles, events, relationship, and activities became quite clear. This system of meaning was more than biographical themes. It consisted of a variety of meaning-referents and meaning-contexts and related to many activities, decisions, types of affect, activities, and understandings.

I found appreciating the personal meaning system to be foundational for understanding any decision or event in the life of that person at the present time. This is why the biographical approach to understanding the lives of older adults is so very necessary. To understand an event or decision made by an individual, it needs to be placed in the larger context of personal meaning in order to be understood by observers. Research on aging, without appreciating the various sources of meaning for any person, and how meaning might be organized through themes, activities, beliefs, reminiscence, events, chronology, affect, and connections, seems entirely futile to me. For example, how can one understand the spiritual or religious beliefs of another person, or their economic circumstances, or their social relations, or their health without having a larger cultural and personal context, is a question that gerontology has failed to face and has led to what I believe is a current crisis in gerontology. And this process of meaning making and interpretation is continuous for most people, I believe. It does not stop. It is often dialogic, a process in which people nut over meaning with both oneself and with others over time.

I found the personal meaning system to be bound up into the present-day constructed life story; the story provided the backdrop for the meaning system. And the constructed life story was intimately tied to and represented in the home environment and its objects and subjectively defined significances.

Another great advantage in working at the PGC at the time, besides the support I received from my many colleagues over the years, was the ability to become familiar in a first-hand way with Dr. Powell Lawton's work. For example, his work on press and competence and person and environmental fit was well known in gerontology and really provided a map for environmentally sensitive design that was able to deal with physical and cognitive decrements experienced by older adults. To my knowledge, the Weiss Institute of PGC was the first research-based environment (designed by Dr. Lawton) specifically designed for persons with Alzheimer's disease and related disorders. As originally envisioned, rooms were situated around a central courtyard; the effect of this, in contrast to the long hospital-like corridors featured in traditional and pervasive designs, was to bring people out of their rooms and into social connection with one another in the central courtyard, where meals and activities occurred. One of the few things that we know is beneficial to persons with dementia is social interaction, which is cognitively stimulating. This was now designed into the living environment.

However, to me, as an anthropologist with an interest in culture, there was always a problem with press-competence approaches to environmental fit. These approaches were largely biocognitive in nature and were filtered through abilities as measured in activities of daily living and instrumental activities of daily living (ADLs and IADLs). They thus matched physical abilities, for example the ability to go up and down stairs, or cognitive abilities, for example being properly able to keep a checkbook, to some sort of environmental fit and the related need for supportive environments and other forms of external help. While press-competence has very significant implications for environmental design (in fact, Lawton and Nahemow's [1973] model might be the most important theoretical construction to come out of gerontology), they in no way accounted for the meaning of what was being pressed and who was having competence for what reason. One might argue, most positively, that the most important aspect of press-competence approaches was to maximize autonomy for the older adult through environmental manipulation and design and this is indeed the case. However, one must realize that autonomy is a Western, cultural construct; it is not "natural" or part of nature, as many biopsychologically oriented gerontologists seem to believe. Autonomy is also relational, relative, and contextual. However, a biopsychological approach to autonomy, there was no accounting for two important things. First, press-competence in no way dealt with the sense of loss that was likely to accompany decrements in abilities, even with supportive environments, nor did it deal with for the meaning of any loss of autonomy that could not be prosthetically treated. Second, there was no accounting for the personal meaning of the activities that could remain, or those that departed, or that had to be environmentally supported. That is to say, loss, change, and adaptation were not a part of or fully integrated into theories of press competence. In contrast to what has been said as part of the successful aging paradigm, that gerontology and the public presentation of aging had traditionally focused on loss and decline, press-competence approaches were perhaps unduly optimistic about what could be done to help people. This brings us to another idea that came from early work on the home environment. Interviewing individual older adults helped me to understand that there is ultimately nothing more basic or more foundational than individual subjectivity; there is no deeper level. Therefore it is very difficult to apply a generic theory, such as press competence, to a group, but almost all environmental design is done for groups and what is more the membership of these groups changes all the time as people move away or die and new people arrive, both residents and staff. This has been a problem in long-term care in settings in which the health characteristics of residents have become worse over time, but there is not much that can be done to alter the build environment. More recently, some of our research has been undertaken in assisted living settings and nursing homes where wheelchairs often overwhelm the setting and render elevators and corridors dysfunctional because of the press of people in wheelchairs. Sometimes, meals are now scheduled in two seatings to accommodate the flow of people onto elevators in an efficient fashion.

Let me give one example concerning press competence. The inability to climb stairs would be a fairly easy environmental fix through ramps or elevators. Consider, though, an older woman whom I interviewed in Philadelphia. She lived in a typical small row house in a poor neighborhood and her washer and dryer were in the basement of her house. She described to me at some length the elaborate procedure she had developed, because of her inability to be up and down stairs effectively, to do her wash. She described to me how she packed small amounts of dirty clothes and placed them into pillowcases and then shoved them down the stairs into the basement. She then sat on the top step and gradually moved down the steps, one at a time, in a manner in which she felt was both safe and efficient. When she got to the bottom, she was able to stand up and gradually do her wash. She sat on a chair in the basement while the washing and drying were being done. When the wash was dry, she folded the clothes and placed them neatly into the pillow cases again, and moved them up the stairs one step at a time and one step above where she sat as she moved upwards, step by step, sitting, moving the clothes up, and moving herself one step at a time one step below the pillowcases filled with laundry. I remember clearly her telling me about this procedure. She seemed to be very proud about how cleverly she felt she handled this problem. It would not have been possible for her to install a ramp or an elevator in this small house nor was she financially of means. There was no room to move the washer and dryer upstairs. Alternative solutions were finding someone to come to her house to do her laundry for her or moving, also probably not very easy given her income level. However, it is quite clear that it would be far easier for her to find some other way of doing her laundry and that the environmental press of this task barely matched her competence level. Yet this elaborate procedure had some important meaning for her, perhaps a manifestation of the pioneer spirit, a representation of cleverness and competence, a remaining ability to manipulate and use her body in a creative way, the ability to take care of herself yet, the value of work, and an accomplishment of some sort, an element of self-esteem. Eventually, she would surely need to move to some place in which life was easier, but for the time being she seemed satisfied with her arrangement.

So, this was the difference between a press-competence approach and a personal-meaning approach. She was gradually, over time, entering the zone of maximal press as defined by Lawton and Nahemow. It was the case that she was in the process of losing the autonomy that was key in her life, but the procedure she developed was in fact a positive statement of autonomy on her part. There was much about herself she retained in the meaning content of her washday procedure. And all this meaning content was contained in the zone between remaining competence and expanding press. Yet press-competence theories, being strangely acultural, do not account for the meaning content. Yet everything human is cultural. This is a conundrum.

CURRENT DAY APPROACHES

Above, I mentioned some of the theoretical perspectives that were important in anthropology at the earliest portion of my career, these approaches have by now been superseded at the present time by a number of new concerns that include perspectives that are more explicitly political, including topics such and biopolitics and knowledge/power, associated with the work of Foucault; globalization; suffering; poverty; status and income inequality; dispossession; minority status (of various sorts); a concern with the effects of neoliberalism; health inequality; and many other approaches from a critical perspective. In contrast, gerontology has retained its extremely conservative methodological and substantive perspective and an increasingly pervasive focus on quantitative methodologies as a "fix" of some kind in place of social, cultural, and personal knowledge. It is the case that my continuing work still utilizes some of the early theoretical approaches that I mentioned above including the biographical approach and the centrality of a personal meaning system for understanding the subjectivity of older adults and events in their lives. For example, in a recent study, I and Kate de Medeiros, with our research group (Kim DeMichele, Susan Hannum, Sarah Canham and others) interviewed (a) about 140 older women who had no children and the relationship of childlessness to generativity and (b) small comparison groups of older women with children also with an eye toward forms of generative action. However, the built environment and the meaning of home did not play a prominent role in this project. Nevertheless, most of the research work with which I've been involved in the past decade has been in long-term care, specifically assisted living settings, nursing homes, and other long-term care and continuum of care settings. With J. Kevin Eckert, Leslie Morgan, Ann Christine Frankowski,

John Schumacher, and many others, we undertook projects that examined transitions in long-term care, stigma in long-term care and local definitions of autonomy in assisted living. Interestingly, we found out several important things regarding environmental relations in long-term care. Perhaps most pressing and of greatest concern is the pervasive presence of stigma in these built environments. In one multilevel care campus we studied, which had independent living, assisted living and a Dementia Care Unit (DCU), we found that both non-DCU residents and even some family members labeled the DCU as "the dark side" and stigmatized the residents. It was the last place anybody wanted to be and the residents were seen as pitiable, as to be avoided (people stopped visiting once you entered there) and as "less than" human, somehow. Now, because most press-competence theories are cultural, there was never a theoretical consideration that creating environments to support the deeply cognitively impaired, might bring about stigmatization. We discovered that stigma comes to long-term care settings just the way it does to anyplace else: through the front door. People, including both residents and their family members bring with them all the biases and stigmatizations that are part of everyday life, but diffused and less pointed in the larger community. The problem is that negative social, cultural, cognitive, and physical attributes of people become heightened through the act of relative comparison in the multilevel setting, so that people who are in independent living, for example, often know that it is a matter of time before they enter the DCU via assisted living. They are moving on a culturally downward trajectory and are becoming locally devalued and those remaining outside the DCU have greatly heightened sensibilities of what the future will bring them and a more thoroughgoing social critique of the negative attributes of those "others." It seems to be that the amelioration of generic press was never anticipated to bring such negative labeling, in part because the perspective taken was of person-as-organism, not person-as-cultural entity living in a meaningful cultural context. It seems that the only solution to this problem in existing environments is a program of massive training and education to eradicate stigma, but such may be unlikely given the cognitive status of residents and the biases already built in to family members and, yes, even care workers. Another project we will be starting soon will examine the pervasiveness of lying to residents with Alzheimer's disease and related disorders by staff members and others in assisted living. Is this good or bad. Does it matter? Even though there are clinical protocols for eliminating lying to the cognitively impaired, our research has found this practice to be widespread. Sometimes, the lying is environmental in nature, when residents are lied to, in order to get them to change rooms.

As I mentioned above, the recent refocus in anthropological topics and theory is essentially about power and about politics. A lot of the early studies I undertook were from the "inside," examining emic constructions. I have turned more to structural and regulatory factors in micro-politics of long-term care settings; this was one of the goals of the project on autonomy in assisted living, a 4-year study that examined how autonomy was managed in five assisted living settings and three DCUs. We are currently writing an account of the multiple forces that shape the governance of autonomy in the assisted living settings, using a modified or more culturalized press-competence approach.

ACKNOWLEDGMENTS

Research projects discussed in this chapter were supported over the last 30-some years by the National Institute of Aging, the National Science Foundation, and several private foundations. They are too numerous to list in specifics, but I want to acknowledge them and my extreme gratitude to these organizations for their support of my research and that of my colleagues.

REFERENCES

Bourdieu, P. (1990). *An outline of a theory of practice.* Stanford, CA: Stanford University Press.

Geertz, C. (1973). *The interpretation of cultures*. New York, NY: Basic Books.

Hallowel, A. I. (1954). The self in its behavioral environment. In A. I. Hallowell (Ed.), *Culture and experience* (pp. 75–110). Philadelphia, PA: University of Pennsylvania Press.

Lawton, M. P., & Nahemow, L. (1973). Ecology and the aging process. In C. Eisdorfer & M. P. Lawton (Eds.), *The psychology of adult development and aging* (pp. 619–674). Washington, DC: American Psychological Association.

Lawton, M. P., & Rubinstein, R. L. (2000). *Alzheimer's disease and related disorders: Strategies in care and research.* New York, NY: Springer Publishing.

Levi-Strauss, C. (1966). *The savage mind.* Chicago, IL: University of Chicago Press.

Rappaport, R. (1968). *Pigs for the ancestors.* Ann Arbor, MI: University of Michigan Press.

Rubinstein, R. L. (1984). *Singular paths: Old men living alone.* New York, NY: Columbia University Press.

Rubinstein, R. L. (1987). The significance of personal objects to older people. *Journal of Aging Studies*, *1*(3), 225–238,

Rubinstein, R. L. (1989a). The home environments of older people: A description of psychosocial processes linking person to place. *The Journal of Gerontology: Social Sciences*, *44*(2), S45–S53.

Rubinstein, R. L. (1989b). Themes in the meaning of caregiving. *Journal of Aging Studies, 3*(2), 119–138.

Rubinstein, R. L. (1990). The environmental representation of personal themes by older people. *Journal of Aging Studies, 41*, 131–147.

Rubinstein, R. L., & Lawton, M. P. (1997). *Depression in long term and residential care.* New York, NY: Springer Publishing.

Turner, V. (1966). *The forest of symbols.* Ithaca, NY: Cornell University Press.

CHAPTER 6

Reflections on a Professional Journey to Making Home Life Better for Older Adults and Families

Laura N. Gitlin

ABSTRACT

In this essay, I assume the stance of a "reflective practitioner," critically examining my research practices and trajectory to gain insight as to how I have engaged in and possibly impacted Environmental Gerontology. I first examine the "what" (description of what has been done), then examine the "so what" (factors contributing to success [or not] and key achievements), and finally, the "now what" (logical next steps or vision for future endeavors). I characterize my stance towards Environmental Gerontology as a consumer or "user" of its concepts and principles. My research focus is on employing key environmental constructs to develop and evaluate biopsychosocial environmental interventions to improve the "good life" or quality of life of older adults and family caregivers. I have considered the socio-physical environment from varied roles: as cause of behavioral or psychological outcomes; as moderator of outcomes, as mediator of outcomes, as an outcome itself, or as the context in which behavioral, cognitive, and affective processes unfold. I suggest that modifying physical and social environments results in clinically meaningful benefits to older adults and caregivers; and that understandings from Environmental Gerontology may advance the science of implementing interventions in real-world community, clinical, and service settings.

http://dx.doi.org/10.1891/0198-8794.38.89

A REFLECTIVE RESEARCH PRACTITIONER

Without doubt, writing this essay has been challenging and filled with uncertainty as to whether I was wasting my time or that of others. It was daunting for several reasons. First, it is humbling to write a reflective essay—in doing so, one feels a strong obligation to get it right—to uncover important lessons about one's own particularities, to accurately portray and historically locate one's professional life course, and to identify nuggets of a career pathway involving Environmental Gerontology that make it a worthwhile read for others. It is not clear to me that I have accomplished this.

Second, it is challenging to balance the telling of personal life choices, circumstances, and events that shape career decision making with scholarly reflection that can contribute to new knowledge and understandings of how a field such as Environmental Gerontology advances, or at least how it has influenced one's research career, and in turn been explored and possibly impacted through one's own research endeavors.

Third, it is hard to believe that I am "senior" and have contributed sufficiently to warrant an autobiographical telling! I have previously read with great admiration the professional/personal narratives of luminaries in Environmental Gerontology who have served as my intellectual guideposts (Birren & Schroots, 2000). Frankly, I do not quite feel there yet nor equal to the groundbreaking contributions of the founders and previous and current developers of the field.

Finally, writing this essay was hard work—it tests one's ability to be self-critical and insightful and to dig deep to identify and define personal events that others may find useful for explicating the field. Consideration must be given to how what one chose to study was shaped by time and place and how one's personal reflections are/were/may be fraught with known and unknown biases. Further, recognition must be given to the limitations imposed by the particular historic juncture in which one matures as a researcher as well as the point in time in one's life course in which one engages in a self-reflection of this nature. Thus, this has been an imposing assignment. I must thank the Editors for their patience, encouragement, and strong belief in the project's potential historical and sociological import—a strong motivator for pursuing this type of essay.

In writing this essay, I assumed the stance of a "reflective practitioner," defined by Schön (1983) as the ". . . capacity to reflect on action so as to engage in a process of continuous learning." In this regard, the purpose here is to critically examine one's own research practices to gain new "developmental insights" (Bolton, 2010). In a reflexive analysis of research as a form of practice, the investigator examines his or her own perspectives and as they emerge within a socio-political and historical juncture, to evaluate not only how one has been influenced, but how in turn one has influenced advancement of new knowledge generated from one's own research practices. While there are various methodologies for reflection to uncover the essence of practice, I adopt here a simplified approach by first examining the "what" (e.g., description of what has been done), then examining the "so what" (e.g., factors contributing to success (or not) and key achievements) and finally, the "now what" (e.g., the logical next steps or the vision for future endeavors) (Driscoll & Teh, 2001; Laverdure, 2017).

More specifically, I start my reflections by offering the big picture or my stance toward Environmental Gerontology and the principles from this field guiding my research from start to present (the what). I then move on to a chronological telling of key influential life events, followed by an interpretative recap of significant research findings, and what might be viewed as contributory to the field (the so what) with conclusions as to what may be next steps for me and the field (what next).

THE BIG PICTURE

In reflecting backwards, I would have to conclude that I have worked within similar conceptual frameworks over the past 30 years, although refinements of course and branching out to involve emergent theoretical work and a wide array of evolving environmental and gerontological constructs occurred along the way. However, there does not appear to have been big pivots or major course corrections with regard to the core set of operating principles, thematic stances and perspectives I assumed and operationalized in my research pursuits. This reveal through this reflective essay, was actually surprising to me.

Stance Toward Environmental Gerontology

I would characterize my stance toward Environmental Gerontology as a consumer or "user" of its concepts and principles. My main focus has been to actively employ key environmental constructs for the purpose of intervening in people's lives. That has been and is, a persistent passion—from start to present—to intercede, to impact directly and to transform the daily life challenges of older adults and their families where they live at home. The purpose has been and is—to put it simply—to make life better by enhancing/realigning person capabilities, goals, and preferences with environmental conditions (social and physical) at home. This has taken the form of collaborating with diverse interprofessional teams to develop, evaluate, and implement (and more recently on a wide scale) over 15 different home-based interventions designed to address the cognitive, physical, and/or emotional consequences and challenges imposed by chronic conditions including but not limited to physical frailty, dementia, depression, caregiving, and other comorbidities.

Applying Environmental Gerontology to the intervention context facilitates an evaluation of the potential explanatory and predictive benefits and limitations of its principles. In application, constructs and propositions can be validated, and their meanings extended and/or bounded. Thus, intervention research represents an important strategy for theoretical verification (or not) and in this way I hope to have advanced and be advancing the field.

Overall, my intervention work is hung together by two broad, overarching conceptual frameworks developed principally by M. Powell Lawton. The first has been Lawton and Nahemow's (1973) foundational "competence environmental press" model. Although it has alluded measurement and specificity, it has provided an overarching structure for broadly understanding home interactions and types of adjustments that can be made and for whom to improve quality of life.

The second is Lawton's (1983) articulation of "quality of life" as the "Good Life," a multifactorial construct composed of four highly interactive quadrants: behavioral competence, objective environment, psychological wellbeing, and perceived quality of life, each of which in turn is composed of specific domains that have conceptual and measurement properties. One focus of my work has been to identify which quadrant(s) and specific domain(s) within are amenable to modification, the benefits and limits of making change, and how adaptations in one quadrant and domain may affect others. For example, realigning an older adult's functional capacity with home environmental objective conditions to enable persons to carry out preferred and valued activities results in greater behavioral competence and perceived quality of life. However, this realignment may not directly affect other quadrants and/or domains such as improving depressive symptoms (a domain within psychological wellbeing). Further, each quadrant and its domains can be a target, mediator, moderator, or outcome of intervention.

Both mega-constructs taken together offer a big picture of a person's "self" as the intersection of multiple considerations involving objective and subjective conditions including the physical and social environment. From this perspective, a logical and key conclusion is that quality of life or the "good life," cannot be reduced to a simple health or medical state; rather it reflects the interplay of multiple considerations including, but not limited to function, preferences, personal goals, perceived wellbeing, and objective environmental conditions (e.g., housing, finances, social capital); in turn, these considerations fluctuate as people age and experience age-associated and chronic disease impositions and deteriorating or improving environmental conditions.

This broad conceptualization suggests the potential power of multicomponent and multimodal interventions that simultaneously impact manifold quadrants and domains to realign or obtain the just-right person-environment fit to solve a quality of life challenge. Furthermore, Several important points can be derived from these conceptualizations. First, the models (the Good Life in particular) reinforce the notion that individuals are more than their health. As a wide array of factors inform quality of life, what is perceived as a good life for one person will differ for another (Lawton, 1991). Second, it follows then that individual preferences and perceptions are important to take into account with person-directed and person-centered approaches possibly being the most effective when the goal is for quality of life improvements. Third, the concept of "tailoring" to the unique constellation of factors (quadrants and domains) and taking into account what is of salience to older adults becomes important methodologically. Finally, of interest is to understand how targeting one quadrant and/or set of domains affect outcomes in other areas to understand the full impact of any one intervention. These conceptualizations and principles underlie my intervention work.

Thematic Threads

Diving deeper, I would identify five key related thematic threads that have been woven throughout my intervention research endeavors. These can be characterized as: (a) the audacious attempt to move health care away from a strictly medical model to a more balanced bio-psycho-social-environmental paradigm, considering home as central to wellbeing, particularly in old age; (b) examining, understanding and intervening in behavior(s) within the environmental (physical and social) context(s) or life space (the home) of older adults to basically make life better; (c) understanding adaptive psychosocial-environmental processes and family involvement in chronic illness management from which to design better and more targeted interventions; (d) involving a team perspective, particularly interprofessional and community members as collaborators who reflect environmental stakeholders in intervention delivery; and (e) engaging in theoretically based, action-oriented research geared toward initially adjusting person-environment gaps to improve everyday life to more recently addressing gaps between research, practice and policy environments shaping health-care delivery.

Emerging Variables of Interest

Over the course of my research endeavors, key person-centered constructs of great interest and that I have contributed to advancing can be located within the Good Life Model (see Figure 6.1). These include in the behavioral competence sector of the Good Life model, the construct of control (e.g., primary and secondary orientations; Gitlin, Hauck, Dennis, & Schulz, 2007), readiness to change (e.g., to adopt new behavioral and environmental strategies; Gitlin & Rose, 2016), efficacy (e.g., mastery of caregiving strategies also involving environmental

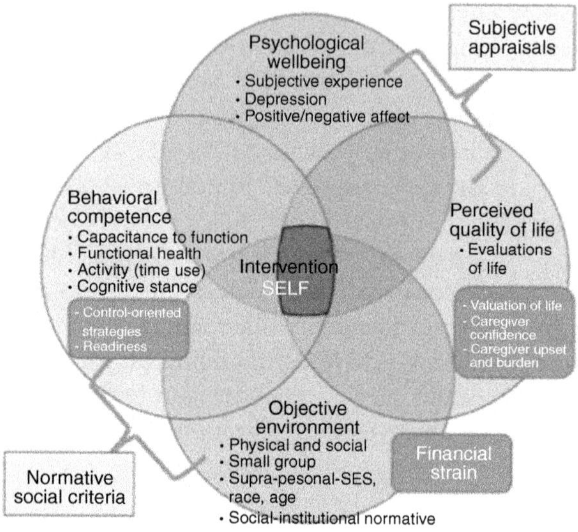

FIGURE 6.1 Adapted model of M. Powell Lawton's 1983 Good Life Model.
Note: Dark grey boxes reflect newly emerging constructs of interest; Light grey boxes and intersection (intervention/self) reflect Lawton's implications)

modifications; Gitlin, Winter, Dennis, Hodgson, & Hauck, 2010a), cognitive functioning (e.g., linking cognitive changes to enactment of everyday activities of living in the home environment; Gitlin, Hodgson, Jutkowitz, & Pizzi, 2010); and strategy use (e.g., simplification of interactions with environments through task performance; Gitlin, Winter, et al., 2002); in the perceived quality of life quadrant, my focus has been on valuation of life (e.g., appraisal of various factors in consideration of whether life is worth living; Gitlin et al., 2017), and behavioral activation (Gitlin et al., 2013).

On the environmental side of the equation, my interest has been on the role of physical features including assistive devices (Gitlin, 1995), as well as sociocultural elements of home environments and the extent of and limits to their modifications to support everyday functioning (Gitlin, 2003) and the somewhat illusive but powerful P-E fit construct (Iwarsson, 2004; Iwarsson, Horstmann, Carlsson, Oswald, & Wahl, 2009). Furthermore, of critical interest are the correlates of different levels and types of competencies/chronic issues with environmental conditions (Swenor et al., 2016; Wahl, Fänge, Oswald, Gitlin, & Iwarsson, 2009; Wahl, Oswald, Schilling, & Iwarsson, 2009). To this end, the environment has served in my research as backdrop for and/or as a form of intervention, as well as outcome (e.g., increasing home safety, wayfinding, functionality, decreasing disorientation, physical-care burdens).

More recently, my focus has been enlarged to include the role of technology (e.g., online platforms for family caregivers) as part of the home living environment (Kales et al., 2016); and for delivery of interventions; and understanding the environmental context for implementing evidence-based programs (Gitlin & Czaja, 2016). As to the latter, I would argue that Environmental Gerontology is implicitly reflected in the rise of implementation science which seeks to identify and understand contextual factors (e.g., the physical, organizational and cultural) supporting or deterring knowledge transfer. When implementing evidence-based programs in the real world, it is the environment that takes center stage and is key to considerations of adoption, scalability of evidence, and success (Wahl & Gitlin, n.d.).

Putting It All Together

These themes and core constructs are expressed throughout my research and publications and guide how I think about and view aging processes. While this consistency in focus may make it appear that my professional pathway has been steady, unswerving, logical, or purposively constructed, this is furthest from the truth nor how I have experienced my research trajectory. As Dr. Lawton definitively declared: ". . . my intellectual biography that discerns a grand and organized plan should be immediately revised. It is full of caprice and coincidence" (Lawton, 2000). His comment humbly applies to my research trajectory as well.

One could perhaps also impose a sequential, linear research pipeline to understand my intellectual development that reflects progression from discovery (e.g., describing home environments and use of assistive devices and home modifications by older adults; Gitlin, 1995) to explanatory (e.g., examining correlates of wellbeing including relationships between quality of life and social and physical environmental features; Choi, Budhathoki, & Gitlin, n.d.), to predictive (e.g., testing effectiveness of interventions involving environmental modification, Gitlin, Winter, Dennis, Hodgson, & Hauck, 2010b). Yet in real life, movement from discovery to explanation and prediction type research questions is an entirely iterative process and that is how I have practiced research.

IN SEARCH OF MAKING LIFE BETTER

How and why my interests have persistently been localized to these two broad frameworks and five key themes and variables, reflect a combination of personal conditions, historical/societal influences, personal agency, chance (accidental opportunities), and afforded privileges. In thinking about the contextual (bio-psycho-social-environmental) factors impacting my professional stance and entry into Environmental Gerontology, I would have to say that there have been four notable influential phases that have unfolded chronologically.

Typically, the questions and problems researchers seek to answer and solve are deeply embedded in personal life situations, and that is the case for me as well. Thus, the first important influential juncture on my research development was having grown up within a family struggling with significant chronic and life-threatening illnesses, initially that of my brother and then in combination with my father. My early life to adulthood was consumed with long hospital visits, separations from parents and brother, and daily fear of suffering and death. There were no "normal" life activities, only emergencies, which meant living in a state of liminality and differentness, and the acute sense of the fragility and ephemeralness of life. Small and "normal" aspects of daily life were inconsequential, giving me what I have come to realize an advantage of living life on the perimeter, being able to see the big picture, and not being consumed with small stuff. Travel early on became a form of escape and as such, I took every opportunity to leave (and still do!), to find and understand dissimilar worlds, cultures, places, people and how they have lived and adopted to different living conditions and adversities. Thus, I sought early on and continuously, exposures to differentness and as such, travel was and continues to be an important energizing vehicle for such exploration. I was and continue to be in search of how to make life better.

Not surprisingly, in college, I gravitated to learning about and understanding chronicity and familial adaptation, and was concerned early on with the interconnectedness of social, psychological, and biological processes that shaped health, wellbeing, and daily living. I sought interdisciplinary insights as I bored easily and found any one perspective or discipline limiting or one-sided in its lens and explanations. I tended to gravitate to social and psychological explanations in part influenced by my exposure to psychology through my father, a clinical psychologist and who along with my mother taught me early on to understand people's behavior not just through psychological frameworks but through the context in which behaviors occur and larger socio-economic and historical conditions. A little known fact is that I was a dance major until my goal of becoming professional was thwarted by a serious back injury. At that time, dance provided an important avenue for expression and a way to change space and meaning through placement of body—this background has partially influenced a later secondary interest in understanding how movement patterns at home can be detected (e.g., sensors) and serve as an indicator of functionality.

A second highly influential juncture was my exposure to exceptional mentors as an undergraduate major in anthropology and social psychology at Temple University in Philadelphia, Pennsylvania. I had the honor and great fortune to be mentored by anthropologists who offered qualitative analytic tools, theoretical grounding in ways to understand culture and the environmental contexts in which daily life choices are made and in different ways based on socio-economic and cultural considerations. I also worked with economists who provided guidance in economic principles and relationships to daily life choices. Finally, my mentor in social psychology (Dr. Robert Kleiner) introduced me to Kurt Lewin's force field, life space and foundational formula of behavior as a function of person and environmental interactions [B=F(P × E)], as well as action research principles and direct experience with data collection and analytics.

From these experiences, I was hooked on applied research, social psychological principles and the P × E formula. I consequently pursued a doctorate in sociology at Purdue University, as that department also included anthropology and the cross fertilization of ideas concerning sociological constructs and cultural manifestations remained important to me. At that time I became an avid reader/follower of Michael Foucault's work and his "archeological" deconstruction of science and medical practice. His complex understandings of scientific discourse as grounded in epistemological assumptions of particular historical junctures, offered the larger sociological-historical geography for P × E interventions; his constructs, writings also reinforced the role of reflection for understanding why certain variables become of interest and certain methodologies prevail. I remained as well concerned with the dynamics of power and studied in depth the work of Karl Marx, as well as modern philosophers such as Pierre Bourdieu, complimented of course by the classics of Weber, Durkheim, and Levi-Strauss among others. Within this context perhaps it is a bit more understandable why my dissertation involved a socio-historical-political analysis of the rise of psychiatry as a profession and its consequent role in shaping our understandings of "insanity" "depression" and other forms of mental illness.

Despite a highly theoretical dissertation, I still preferred the practical, and the action-oriented approach of intervention science. Nevertheless, I did not want to lose sight of theoretical underpinnings of my interests and thus felt it was important to be involved with philosophical traditions. I also rejected a strictly clinical pull and singular focus on psychology as well as health services research which all presented as possible higher degree options. At that time there was no formal training in gerontological programs and, as such, I had little to no exposure to the work under construction in the field. Upon receiving my PhD, I remained a bit adrift in terms of career goals. I rejected strictly academic positions as being too removed from clinical and everyday realities of individuals with disabilities. Instead, I sought applied settings in which I could utilize my research skills to enhance programming, particularly for individuals with social, physical, financial, emotional distresses. Hence, I worked a bit with troubled youth and in low-income and poorly resourced educational environments, providing tutoring and program evaluation. Although there was some modest immediate gratification, I felt I could and should do more, and I was not fully satisfied.

The third major and perhaps most important influence on my intellectual development was accepting a position at this time at the Philadelphia Geriatric Center as a research coordinator for Dr. M. P. Lawton which lasted from 1982 to 1986. This was the hallmark of my research career, my first true solid research position in which I worked on an NIH-funded clinical trial examining the physical and affective benefits of physical exercise in the well elderly. This career-altering serendipitous opportunity planted me squarely into Environmental Gerontology through Dr. Lawton's and Elaine Brody's visionary work. I delved into readings and learning about gerontology and immediately felt at home with Dr. Lawton's competence-environmental press framework as an outgrowth of Lewin's formula; and this perspective, as I have indicated earlier, has continued to form the broad conceptual backdrop to my intervention research. I remember one time sitting around the library conference table with about 15 other researchers as Dr. Lawton sketched out his thoughts on a small blackboard as to what constitutes his vision of the "good life," which he then formally presented as part of the Kleemeier Award offered to him by the Gerontological Society of America. I was also highly influenced by Dr. Lawton's reflective stance toward science—he always questioned his assumptions, made course corrections, and expanded upon and refined his influential theories, constructs, and measures. He never stood still intellectually and fought against reifying and freezing his work—he sought continuous improvement—a true scientist. Furthermore, his maxim that knowledge should be useful and in application to support the "good life" of older adults, formed my professional moral fabric moving forward.

As old age is a critical phase in the life course in which the socio-physical environment is perhaps the most profoundly and acutely impactful, I began to view gerontology as an excellent forum for examining the persistent issues I was passionate about—chronicity, self-management, adaptation, and the role of the physical and social environment. I was extremely energized by this 5-year apprenticeship with Dr. Lawton, one of the most brilliant and amazing scientists I have met, and thus began my foray into Environmental Gerontology.

The fourth influential juncture concerning my intellectual development was my employment in the Department of Occupational Therapy and the College of Health Professions at Thomas Jefferson University, initially as research coordinator and then advancing to founder and director of the Center for Applied Research in Aging. Occupational therapists are uniquely trained in P-E constellations and integrating cognitive, social, psychological, and functional profiles with objective environmental conditions to derive the just-right-fit to reduce decline or changes in competencies. As such, I purposely accepted a position within that department which afforded the opportunity to examine in greater depth and with clinical collaborators, P-E challenges. Teaching in and working with occupational therapists and then directing a research center on aging involving other disciplines, kept me connected to clinical realities and ways to operationalize P-E fit concepts in practice and research for over 24 years.

In this context, initially my focus was on "proving" that the lives of older adults with any type of chronic condition (frailty, depression, dementia, care giving) could be improved by enhancing their control over everyday exigencies through behavioral and environmental modifications. Also, I insisted on developing interventions that were not just person-centered but person-directed (environmental pro-activity hypothesis). This has involved approaches to enabling older adults with decision-making capacity to help identify and prioritize areas of daily life they wish to improve or address through intervention; and for those with cognitive functional challenges who are most vulnerable to environmental docility, ways to elicit capacity, intrinsic interests, and increase participation. Concomitantly, I was interested in the methodological challenges and nuances of conducting research in homes which had hitherto not been explicated (Gitlin, 2003). At that time, nursing homes were the preferred site for study and I had been informed by many that the home was too complex, and an uncontrolled environment that alluded measurement. Yet, as home is where people age and want to age, and is imbued with important meanings (Rubinstein, 1989), it became and continues to be my central environmental space for research.

At that time, I also explored with others the limits, meanings, and consequences of home by working with individuals who were homeless as well as examining housing in low-income and low-resourced countries. These afforded opportunities to explode what was the same (e.g., lack of adequate housing stock for older adults with a range of needs) and what was different (e.g., the hidden cultural biases of assumptions and measurements of home); and in turn heightened awareness of the boundedness of my/our research questions—how such questions are located in a historical moment reflecting socio-cultural trends, and in response to specific value propositions of scientists and policy stakeholders.

After over 24 productive years with wonderful teams including my occupational therapy colleagues (Drs. Corcoran, Piersol, Vause Earland among others), colleagues from other disciplines and my extremely supportive dean (Dr. Erdmann), I found myself itching to advance my science in ways that was not possible to achieve at an academic health science center in which the primary focus is on teaching and producing clinicians. As such, I decided to leave for a research-intensive university, Johns Hopkins University, but my compromise was to purposively locate myself in the School of Nursing and School of Medicine, to remain close to the real world context of intervening in the health and wellbeing of older adults and instruction in how to do so. With the full encouragement and support of deans and colleagues at Hopkins for whom I am most grateful, I developed the Center for Innovative Care in Aging (Center) to advance the science of behavioral intervention research. Now 6½-years-old, the Center serves as a focal point in the School of Nursing and at Hopkins at-large as well as nationally and internationally, for the conduct of behavioral intervention research as well as for preparing the next generation of scientists in this area by mentoring faculty and students through our various activities (Summer Research Institute on intervention research, monthly seminar series [the "Issue is. . ."] in which core faculty lead high level discussions examining key issues in intervention research, and working groups on behavioral interventions, role of engagement/activity]. Through this Center and my programs of research, I continue to explore the benefits and limits of the environment in making life better for diverse older adults and their families. Also, given the infrastructure and resources, I have been able to accelerate my attempts at scaling up and implementing our proven approaches in the United States and worldwide.

In summary, the confluence of familial context (imbued of course with specific values, beliefs, and practices and socio-economic standing affording opportunities), early and continuous exposure to and working with applied and action-oriented amazing researchers, delving into different disciplinary theories and cultures along with continuous travel, involvement with Dr. Lawton, followed by application of environmental gerontological principles in collaboration with occupational therapists and other health and human service professionals, have all been crucial, strategic stepping stones, factors in my intellectual evolution and entry to and dance within Environmental Gerontology. Perhaps most importantly, although it appears as though I mention this as a footnote, I could not be dancing within the field without the continuous support and grounding of my amazing husband, Eduardo, and two incredible sons, Eric and Keith, who keep me balanced, real and focused. They have provided the environment in which I have been able to flourish.

KEY SUCCESSES

I would summarize my key contribution to the field as applying a social-environmental framework to improving the health and wellbeing of older adults and their caregivers. This has involved using a person-centered/person-directed, tailored and multicomponent approach, attending to persons' needs and capacities, their social and physical living environments and their interactions, by which to effectively promote effective adaptational strategies to address daily challenges (e.g., functional decline, lack of meaningful activity, caregiving) of older adults and their families. These challenges are not typically addressed in health care and social services; and when unattended, lead to rapid decline, hospitalizations, nursing home placement, and mortality. Overall, our intervention approaches have yielded new ways of thinking about health and wellbeing and supporting older adults and families challenged by cognitive and/or physical changes that involves consideration and involvement of the home environment in ways hitherto not systematically considered. These findings can be encapsulated by three, simple broad maxims: small is big; engagement as the pill/ prescription; and care for the caregiver.

Small Is Big

The various interventions I have developed with my teams show foremost that small changes result in big benefits; that is, small behavioral (simplification or modification of the way a task is performed) and home environmental adaptations (e.g., use of assistive devices, removal of clutter, home modifications, and home repairs), yield BIG positive changes in the lives of older adults and families. Outcomes from different trials and with older adults with different cognitive and functional challenges have included reductions in hospitalizations, functional dependencies, mortality, depression, behavioral symptoms, and burden. Providing older adults with different strategies involving the home environment enhances control over the immediate life space and facilitates engagement in valued activities.

An exemplar is the Advancing Better Living for Elders (ABLE) clinical trial (funded by the National Institute on Aging) involving 319 older adults (≥70) living at home with physical difficulties. In up to six sessions, occupational therapists identify participants' own daily functional concerns and priorities (versus what health professionals view as problematic) and provide task modification strategies, positive primary and secondary control-oriented strategies, home modifications and assistive devices, and home safety whereas a physical therapist provides fall recovery techniques and balance exercise all designed to be linked to and help older adults achieve their self-identified daily functional goals (Gitlin, Winter, Dennis, Corcoran, Schinfeld, et al., 2006). This person-directed/ person-centered program resulted in reduced functional difficulties, near falls (behavioral competence of the Good Life), and fear of falling, and improvements in self-efficacy (psychological wellbeing of the Good Life), and perceived quality of life. ABLE also resulted in a 9% mortality reduction compared to usual care controls and 21% reduction for those previously hospitalized by 12 months. Survivorship benefits endured up to 3 years (Gitlin et al., 2009).

This approach has informed development of other powerful interventions including ABLE's extension to include a nursing component to address pain, depressive symptoms, and medication management (Szanton, Leff, Wolff, Roberts, & Gitlin, 2016). Applying a similar approach to persons with dementia, we have shown that helping families communicate effectively, set up simplified daily routines and modify the home environment can result in reducing functional dependence and behavioral symptoms in persons with dementia, and in caregivers, their upset and burden (Gitlin et al., 2010a, 2010b).

Engagement As Pill/Prescription

Our interventions also highlight the significance of helping older adults reengage within their environment by being able to assume/resume activities/tasks that are most meaningful to them. Activities may include but are not limited to participating in household functions (cooking, home making), basic self-care, leisure (reading, crafts), social engagement, and physical exercise. For persons with dementia, realigning the environment to meet cognitive and functional capabilities is particularly challenging but we have shown very possible (Trahan, Kuo, Carlson, & Gitlin, 2014). Additionally, we have shown that helping people with dementia engage in an activity of intrinsic meaning or value (zone of adaptation in Lawton's competence-environmental press model) reduces behavioral symptoms and functional dependence (New Ways for Better Days: Tailoring Activities to Persons with Dementia and Caregiveres; Gitlin et al., 2008; 2016).

Applying a similar perspective to depression and helping low-resourced African Americans reengage in activities of most interest to them, we have shown that we can enhance enhance their appraisals as to whether life is worth living, reduce depressive symptoms, and decrease functional disability (Gitlin et al., 2013). Thus, engagement in and of itself (versus new learning, or performing an activity correctly) appears to be a basic prescription (or "pill") for a better life (Parisi et al., 2015).

Care of the Caregiver

How the environment can support family caregiving remains a key theme in my research which has shown that there are ways to make life better for family caregivers, even in dementia care, the most distressful, elongated, and burdensome form of care provision. My focus in most of my caregiver interventions has been to examine characteristics of persons, their environments and caregivers and help families make modifications to realign all three domains. In doing so, we find that we can reduce caregiver burden, depressive symptoms, as well as a sense of mastery. We also show that modifying only the physical aspects of the home environment may ease the physical burdens of care but does not in itself reduce perceived burdens or enhance psychological wellbeing (Gitlin et al., 2010a).

The interventions I along with my teams have developed including Project Act, COPE, $Skills_2Care^R$ to name a few, have resulted in significant benefits for family members.

In summary, I have considered the socio-physical environment from its varied roles as the cause of behavioral or psychological outcomes of interest; as a moderator of a desired outcome(s), as a mediator of a desired outcome(s), as an outcome itself, or as the overall context in which behavioral, cognitive and affective processes occur or are shaped (Wahl & Gitlin, in press). More specifically, my interventions have targeted different quadrants and their respective domains of the Good Life model and seek to regulate person-environment alignments/interactions to achieve various adaptive outcomes including improving behavioral competencies, psychological wellbeing, perceived quality of life, and home safety and security (objective environmental conditions).

Taken as a whole, these interventions show that Environmental Gerontology has a front and center place in successful aging and specifically research, practice and policy concerning health care. An environmental framework and its associated constructs provide a critical balance to the overly somatic, pathophysiological understandings of aging and strive for cures that dominant our health research, care paradigms, and health delivery models and policies. Our research also suggests that Environmental Gerontology offers a positive message—there is always an opportunity to make life better even in the oldest of ages and for older adults with different impairment severities.

For this body of intervention work, I was most honored to have been nominated by Dr. Hans-Werner Wahl and then to receive in 2014, the M. Powell Lawton Award of the Gerontological Society of America. This was a highly personal award and recognition. As I had the serendipitous and great honor of working directly with Dr. Lawton, and the great fortune to be a colleague of Dr. Wahl, I viewed the award as testimony to the enduring values and traditions set forth by Dr. Lawton that I have tried to emulate and uphold. Here we see the intersection of autobiography and professional trajectory, chance and agency.

WHERE TO NEXT?

From my vantage point, I see two next steps in advancing Environmental Gerontology; measurement development and examining the environmental context for implementing evidence. Given the dearth of measures for evaluating facets of P × E dynamics, out of a necessity, I have had to participate in measurement development to examine home environments and psychosocial aspects relevant to home environmental modification oriented interventions (Gitlin, 2003).

Exemplars of measures we have developed include the Home Environmental Assessment Protocol (HEAP) to evaluate environmental hazards and supports for persons with dementia (Gitlin, Schinfeld, et al., 2002), the Task Management Simplification Index (TMSI; Gitlin, Winter, et al., 2002) to identify simplification strategies used by caregivers in managing dementia, the Perceived Change for the Better Index (PCI; Gitlin, Winter, Dennis, & Hauck, 2006) to evaluate caregiver perceptions as to whether everyday care challenges were improving, getting worse or staying the same, the Readiness to Change index (Gitlin & Rose, 2016) to evaluate level to which caregivers are ready to modify their own behaviors and home environments to address care challenges; the Caregiver Appraisal of Function and Upset (CAFU, Gitlin et al., 2005) to identify level of caregiver assistance provided with daily activities of living.

These measures however rely on self-report and single point in time measures, and thus have some inherent limitations. Although numerous important measures have been developed by others including the meaning of home (Oswald & Wahl, 2005), and P × E fit index for home accessibility (Iwarsson, Nygren, & Slaug, 2005), more in this area is very much needed; particularly ways to capture context in which behaviors occur and emotions are experienced and ways to capture P × E dynamics to better match clinically persons competencies and environmental conditions. Use of objective measurement approaches such as sensors, direct observations (video), and other measures (e.g., lighting and its impact on behaviors), and linking wellbeing with bio-physiological markers and health impacts would be important future research directions to more fully integrate an understanding of the role of the environment in successful aging.

Yet another direction is to expand upon the associated domains of the Good Life model. The model requires further explication and inclusion of a broader range of constructs including an update to and extension of activity of living skills which integrate environmental considerations and better capture gaps between "can do" and "does do."

As to implementation of evidence, as the policy, social and physical "context" is one of the most important drivers of scalability and uptake, I believe Environmental Gerontology has a lot to offer. We must find ways to more rapidly move proven psycho-social-environmental interventions into the world of every-day living and health care practices. Interventions are embedded in a layered ecology reflecting the proximal location of delivery (e.g., home), the surrounding area (e.g., neighborhood/community), a system of care delivery (e.g., home care), and reimbursement/policy (e.g., medicare, medicaid, long-term care). These layers reflect in part the context and policies of delivery and include the organizational capacity, culture and normative practices that may impact adoption and integration of interventions (Gitlin & Czaja, 2016). As such, an environmental perspective is critical to this enterprise.

CONCLUDING REFLECTIONS

I wrote this essay in part during a recent visit to Japan. In that country, the physical and social environment has a prominent role in the aesthetics and actions of daily life. I was immediately enthralled by the purposeful placement and arrangement of objects in living spaces, and the detailed attention to sensorial modalities including smell, look, and taste. Here the environment is not just backdrop or forgotten context, but foremost and integral to carrying out everyday activities, a prominent factor in wellbeing with objects and their handling and placement imbued with historical and cultural meanings, some apparent and others not. A trip outside the United States always reaffirms for me the critical role of Environmental Gerontology in aging, how environments are differentially recognized and have different roles rooted in historical, cultural and economic factors. These differences need explication as a way to understand and move forward the sociology and archeology of knowledge of the field and how it has advanced in any one geographic location. This volume may help to elaborate on the difference and sameness of the field's development and from which to offer next steps.

REFERENCES

Birren, J. E., & Schroots, J. J. F. (Eds.). (2000). *A history of geropsychology in autobiography*. Washington, DC: American Psychological Association.

Bolton, D. (2010). Conceptualisation of mental disorder and its personal meanings. *Journal of Mental Health*, *19*(4), 328–336.

Choi, S. W., Budhathoki, C., & Gitlin, L. N. (n.d.). Co-occurrence and predictors of three commonly occurring behavioral symptoms in dementia: Agitation, aggression, and rejection of care. *The American Journal of Geriatric Psychiatry*, 25.5(2017): 459–468.

Driscoll, J., & Teh, B. (2001). The potential of reflective practice to develop individual orthopeaedic nurse practitioners and their practice. *Journal of Orthopaedic Nursing*, 5, 95–103.

Gitlin, L. N. (1995). Why older people accept or reject assistive technology. *Generations*, *19*(1), 41–45.

Gitlin, L. N. (2003). Conducting research on home environments: Lessons learned and new directions. *The Gerontologist*, *43*(5), 628–637.

Gitlin, L. N., & Czaja, S. J. (2016). *Behavioral intervention research: Designing, evaluating and implementing*. New York, NY: Springer Publishing.

Gitlin, L. N., & Rose, K. (2016). Impact of caregiver readiness on outcomes of a nonpharmacological intervention to address behavioral symptoms in persons with dementia. *International Journal of Geriatric Psychiatry*, *31*(9), 1056–1063.

Gitlin, L. N., Harris, L. F., McCoy, M. C., Chernett, N. L., Pizzi, L. T., Jutkowitz, E., et al. (2013). A home-based intervention to reduce depressive symptoms and improve quality of life in older African Americans. *Annals of Internal Medicine*, *159*(4), 243–252. doi:10.7326/0003-4819-159-4-201308200-00005

Gitlin, L. N., Hauck, W. W., Dennis, M. P., & Schulz, R. (2007). Depressive symptoms in African American and White older adults with functional difficulty: The role of control strategies. *Journal of the American Geriatrics Society*, *55*(7), 1023–1030.

Gitlin, L. N., Hauck, W. W., Dennis, M. P., Winter, L., Hodgson, N., & Schinfeld, S. (2009). Long-term effect on mortality of a home intervention that reduces functional difficulties in older adults: Results from a randomized trial. *Journal of the American Geriatrics Society*, *57*(3), 476–481.

Gitlin, L. N., Hodgson, N., Jutkowitz, E., & Pizzi, L. (2010). The cost-effectiveness of a nonpharmacologic intervention for individuals with dementia and family caregivers: The Tailored Activity Program. *American Journal of Geriatric Psychiatry*, special issue on Depression and Dementia Care, *18*(6), 510–519.

Gitlin, L. N., Parisi, J. M., Huang, J., Winter, L., & Roth, D. L. (2017). Valuation of life as outcome and mediator of a depression intervention for older African Americans: The get busy get better trial. *International Journal of Geriatric Psychiatry*. [Epub ahead of print].

Gitlin, L., N., Piersol, C.V., Hodgson, N., Marx, K., Roth, D., Johnson, D., Samus, Q., Pizzi, L., Jutkowitz, E., & Lyketos, C. G. (2016). Reducing neuropsychiatric symptoms in persons with dementia and associated burden in family caregivers using tailored activities: Design and methods of a randomized clinical trial. *Contemporary Clinical Trials*, *49*, 92–102. doi:S1551-7144(16)30086-6 [pii]

Gitlin, L. N., Roth, D. L., Burgio, L. D., Loewenstein, D. A., Winter, L., Nichols, L., et al. (2005). Caregiver appraisals of functional dependence in individuals with dementia and associated caregiver upset: Psychometric properties of a new scale and response patterns by caregiver and care recipient characteristics. *Journal of Aging and Health*, *17*(2), 148–171.

Gitlin, L. N., Schinfeld, S., Winter, L., Corcoran, M., Boyce, A. A., & Hauck, W. (2002). Evaluating home environments of person with dementia: Interrater reliability and validity of the home environmental assessment protocol (HEAP). *Disability and Rehabilitation*, *24*, 59–71.

Gitlin, L. N., Winter, L., Burke, J., Chernett, N., Dennis, M. P., & Hauck, W. W. (2008). Tailored activities to manage neuropsychiatric behaviors in persons with dementia and reduce caregiver burden: A randomized pilot study. *American Journal of Geriatric Psychiatry*, *16*(3), 229–239.

Gitlin, L. N., Winter, L., Dennis, M. P., Corcoran, M., Schinfeld, S., & Hauck, W. W. (2002). Strategies used by families to simplify tasks for individuals with Alzheimer's disease and related disorders: Psychometric analysis of the task management strategy index (TMSI). *The Gerontologist*, *42*(1), 61–69.

Gitlin, L. N., Winter, L., Dennis, M. P., & Hauck, W. W. (2006). Assessing perceived change in well-being of family caregivers: Psychometric properties of the perceived change index (PCI) and responses patterns. *American Journal of Alzheimer's Disease and Other Dementias*, *21*(5), 304–311.

Gitlin, L. N., Winter, L., Dennis, M. P., Corcoran, M., Schinfeld, S., & Hauck, W. W. (2006). A randomized trial of a multi-component home intervention to reduce functional difficulties in older adults. *Journal of the American Geriatrics Society*, *54*(5), 809–816.

Gitlin, L. N., Winter, L., Dennis, M. P., Hodgson, N., & Hauck, W. W. (2010a). Targeting and managing behavioral symptoms in individuals with dementia: A randomized trial of a nonpharmacological intervention. *Journal of the American Geriatrics Society*, *58*(8), 1465–1474.

Gitlin, L. N., Winter, L., Dennis, M. P., Hodgson, N., & Hauck, W. W. (2010b). A biobehavioral home-based intervention and the well-being of patients with dementia and their caregivers: The COPE Randomized Trial. *Journal of the American Association*, *304*(9), 983–991.

Iwarsson, S. (2004). Assessing the fit between older people and their home environments–An occupational therapy research perspective. In H-W. Wahl, R. Scheidt & P. Windley (Eds.), *Annual Review of Gerontology and Geriatrics*, 23 (pp. 85–109). New York, NY: Springer Publishing.

Iwarsson, S., Horstmann, V., Carlsson, G., Oswald, F., & Wahl, H.-W. (2009). Person-environment fit predicts falls in older adults better than the consideration of environmental hazards only. *Clinical Rehabilitation*, *23*, 558–567.

Iwarsson, S., Nygren, C., & Slaug, B. (2005). Cross-national and multi-professional inter-rater reliability of the Housing Enabler. *Scandinavian Journal of Occupational Therapy*, *12*(1), 29–39.

Kales, H. C., Gitlin, L. N., Stanislawski, B., Marx, K., Turnwald, M., Watkins, D., Lyketsos, C. G. (2016). WeCareAdvisor™: The development of a caregiver-focused, web-based program to assess and manage behavioral and psychological symptoms of dementia. *Alzheimer Dementia and Associated Disorders*. [Epub ahead of print].

Laverdure, P. (2017). Using reflection to advance professional expertise: A novice-to-expert trajectory. *OT Practice*, *22*, 8–11.

Lawton, M. (1991). A multidimensional view of quality of life in frail elders. In J. Birren, J. Lubben, J. Rowe & D. Deutchman (Eds.), *The concept and measurement of quality of life in the frail elderly* (1st ed., pp. 4–27). Cambridge, MA: Academic Press.

Lawton, M. P. (1983). Environment and other determinants of well-being in older people. *The Gerontologist*, *23*(4), 349–357.

Lawton, M. P. (2000). Chance and choice make for a good life. In J. E., Birren, & J. J. F. Schroots (Eds.), *A history of geropsychology in autobiography* (pp. 185–196). Washington, DC: American Psychological Association.

Lawton, M. P., & Nahemow, N. (1973). Ecology and the aging process. In C. Eisdorfer, & M. P. Lawton (Eds.), *The psychology of adult development and aging* (pp. 619–674). Washington, DC: American Psychological Association.

Oswald, F., & Wahl, H-W. (2005). Dimensions of the meaning of home in later life. In G. D. Rowles, & H. Chaudhury (Eds.), *Home and identity in later life: International perspectives* (pp. 21–46). New York, NY: Springer Publishing.

Parisi, J. M., Roberts, L., Szanton, S. L., Hodgson, N. A., & Gitlin, L. N. (2015). Valued activities among individuals with and without cognitive impairments: Findings from the National Health and Aging Trends study (NHATS). *The Gerontologist, 57*(2), 309–318. doi:10.1093/geront/gnv144

Rubinstein, R. L. (1989). The home environments of older people: A description of the psychosocial processes linking person to place. *Journal of Gerontology: Social Sciences, 44*(2), S45–S53.

Schön, D. (1983). *The reflective practitioner* (1st ed.). New York, NY: Basic Books.

Swenor, B., Yonge, A., Goldhammer, V., Miller, R., Gitlin, L. N., & Ramulu, P. (2016). Evaluation of the home environment assessment for the visually impaired (HEAVI): An instrument designed to quantify fall-related hazards in the visually impaired. *BMC Geriatrics, 16*(1), 214.

Szanton, S. L., Leff, B., Wolff, J. L., Roberts, L., & Gitlin, L. N. (2016). Home-based care program reduces disability and promotes aging in place. *Health Affairs, 35*(9), 1558–1563.

Trahan, M. A., Kuo, J., Carlson, M. C., & Gitlin, L. N. (2014). A systematic review of strategies to foster activity engagement in persons with dementia. *Health Education & Behavior, 41*, 70S–83S.

Wahl, H-W., & Gitlin, L. N. (n.d.). Linking the socio-physical environment to successful aging: From basic research to intervention to implementation science considerations. In R. Fernandez-Ballesteros, J-M. Robine, & A. Benetos (Eds.), *The Cambridge Handbook of Successful Aging* [Manuscript submitted for publication]. London, UK: Cambridge Press.

Wahl, H-W., Fänge, A., Oswald, F., Gitlin, L. N., & Iwarsson, S. (2009). The home environment and disability-related outcomes in aging individuals: What is the empirical evidence? *The Gerontologist, 49*, 355–367.

Wahl, H-W., Oswald, F., Schilling, O., & Iwarsson, S. (2009). The home environment and quality of life related outcomes in advanced old age: Findings of the ENABLE-AGE Project. *European Journal of Ageing, 6*(2), 10.

CHAPTER 7

From Occupational Therapy to Environmental Gerontology

Susanne Iwarsson

ABSTRACT

Based on reflections on childhood experiences, my autobiography starts out from completing professional training as an occupational therapist. After academic studies in gerontology, I pursued PhD education in public health, with a specific interest in housing and health issues related to aging and disability. My early scientific work was concentrated to methodology development based on the notion of person-environment fit, with the Housing Enabler instrument as a recognized contribution. Crucial research career steps were establishing collaboration with public transport planning, and coordinating the ENABLE-AGE project engaging colleagues in five European countries. In addition to describing my research achievements over a period of 25 years, this chapter includes reflections on how unforeseen events boosted my development as an academic leader. Key facets include establishing the interdisciplinary research environment Centre for Ageing and Supportive Environments and the Swedish National Graduate School for Competitive Science on Ageing and Health. With home, health, and disability dynamics at the core, my research has expanded to focus on user participation in research, health promotion, and rehabilitation for specific diagnose groups, and environmental facets such as use of assistive technology. A challenge for coming years is to continuously reframe research priorities based on societal developments and challenges.

http://dx.doi.org/10.1891/0198-8794.38.109

BIOGRAPHICAL NOTES

Since 2003, Susanne Iwarsson is a professor at the Faculty of Medicine, Lund University, Sweden (LU); since 2005, she is the holder of Mary and Seved Ribbing's endowed chair in gerontology and care for older people. She has a PhD in medical science (1997) and is a registered occupational therapist (OT; 1979) with clinical experience in geriatrics and primary care. In 2014 she was appointed Doctor Honoris Causa at Riga Stradins University, Latvia.

Iwarsson is the Head of the research group Active and Healthy Ageing at the Department of Health Sciences, applying Environmental Gerontology perspectives to health sciences and neuroscience studying the aging individual's and population's opportunities for activity and participation in society. Iwarsson's publication record showcases the explicitly interdisciplinary and cross-national orientation of her work. She has been the main or co-supervisor of 19 completed PhD degrees and 6 licentiate degrees, in Sweden and abroad, and has a group of PhD students ongoing. Her academic leadership record includes a 6-year commitment as Pro-dean of the Faculty of Medicine and coordination of the Strategic Research Area of Neuroscience (MultiPark) at LU. Iwarsson is currently the Director of the Centre for Ageing and Supportive Environments (CASE), the Coordinator of the Swedish National Graduate School for Competitive Science on Ageing and Health (SWEAH), and the President of the Swedish Gerontological Society.

EARLY INFLUENCES

Although not consciously reflected upon when the decision was made, when looking back and reflecting upon my choice to become an OT, I am confident that it was influenced by the fact that I grew up close to a grandmother with severe disability due to Multiple Sclerosis. My grandmother Ingeborg was an extraordinary woman with a strong sense of autonomy, even if she was heavily dependent on others in practical everyday matters. Her disease developed early in life and despite numerous periods of high disease activity, she lived a long life until the age of 82. My grandmother—and later my parents, myself, and my younger brother—lived in a large farmhouse in southern Sweden with literally insurmountable environmental barriers such as high flights of stairs at all entrances (Figure 7.1). Still, grandmother's presence and active participation was never questioned in the family context—it was simply taken for granted that practical problems would be solved, and there was always somebody there to assist her in the tasks she was unable to do.

One situation—sometime in the 1960s—that I particularly remember was when my grandmother had decided to travel to Yugoslavia to enjoy the sun and

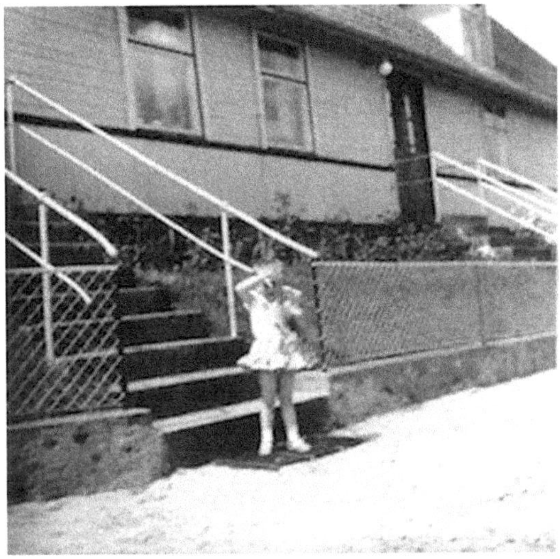

FIGURE 7.1 Susanne, 3 years old, standing in front of the high stairs of her childhood home.

warmth there. At that time, it was not common at all for people with severe disabilities to travel by air and accordingly, the assistance services were not well developed. My younger brother and I were both excited and frightened as father was allowed to drive our car out to the aircraft, park it immediately by the stairs and then carry grandmother on board. As to housing, one memory is when it was decided to adapt the balcony at my grandmother's apartment to make entrance possible from that direction since she was no longer able to use the stairs at the ordinary entrance. As was often the case, this kind of challenge turned into a family affair and the problems were readily solved by means of a ramp from the ground level up to the balcony. Overall, I remember repeatedly thinking that it was extremely impractical to be dependent on a clumsy wheelchair and on others in all kinds of problematic environments and everyday situations.

As already indicated, in hindsight I think that these early life experiences influenced my choice to become an OT, and have also been reflected in the line of research I have developed over the years. Adding the experiences from my years as a practicing OT this nurtured my curiosity regarding home, health, and disability dynamics. That is, many meetings with a wide range of clients in situations where their mobility, activity, participation, and overall quality of life were compromised by insufficient person-environment fit generated research questions that have formed my career as an environmental gerontologist.

NOTABLE PHASES AND DEVELOPMENTAL STEPS

When I graduated as an OT in 1979, my first clinical position was in geriatric long-term care. At that time, home care was barely developed in Sweden, and we had many hospitalized clients who nowadays would have been cared for mainly at home. Accordingly, it was very common and important for hospital-based OTs to contribute to make discharge and life at home possible for the clients. This was often demanding, not the least as the home environments of our clients were often loaded with environmental barriers. Adding to the complexity of returning back home after hospitalization, this was particularly true in the countryside where substandard housing was not uncommon.

After only a few years as a practitioner, I was challenged by a sense of lack of knowledge regarding aging. I felt a strong need to learn more and went to LU to study gerontology at the Department of Applied Psychology. At the same time, the health-care organization in Sweden developed toward more open forms of care. New positions were opened up, and I took the opportunity to leave the hospital context and start up a new OT service at a local primary health-care center. During a couple of years as a part-time university student I got acquainted with well-known theories of aging such as the activity theory (Havighurst & Albrecht, 1953), disengagement theory (Cumming & Henry, 1961) and gerotranscendence (Tornstam, 1997), and also learnt some basics of applied research. In particular, the activity theory resonated well with my OT background, but at that time I was not exposed to any of the aging theories explicitly oriented toward person-environment relations. Instead, I brought with me my OT theory background, emphasizing the importance of person-environment-task transactions for meaningful human occupation and health over the life span (Kielhofner, 2009; Wilcock & Hocking, 2015).

At that time in Sweden, the undergraduate education programs for health professionals were evaluated and debated, followed by significant change and development. From the late 1980s, opportunities for higher academic training for OTs emerged and I was curiously following this development. Utilizing my gerontology studies as a spring board, I was admitted to a complementary course in OT arranged by the Department of Community Health Sciences at the Faculty of Medicine at LU. The reason for this affiliation was that there were several senior scientists at this department, who were personally devoted to support a diversity of health professionals to qualify academically. With public health high on the political agenda in Sweden during this period, the courses provided were markedly oriented toward epidemiology, prevention, and health promotion. As I was at that time working as a district OT in primary health care, this orientation was new to me but very inspiring and served my clinical ambitions well. Moreover, I very much appreciated the interdisciplinary research environment including scholars in general practice, geriatrics, epidemiology, statistics, public health, nursing, physiotherapy, sociology, and psychology.

During this period of study, I defined a major research question that has inspired me since then: "What impact does the home environment have on activity and health for older people?" This question was based on my "clinical irritation" (Yerxa, 1979) emanating from the practice situations, where older clients whom I met as an OT, faced major challenges as they experienced the consequences of disease or injury. In community-based OT, housing adaptations and provision of assistive technology and related coaching and training are since long the major interventions used for problem solving (Ainsworth & de Jonge, 2011). My irritation was mostly based on the fact that even if people decided to move, even in newly built dwellings accessibility problems resulted in challenges to autonomy and independence in daily life (Iwarsson, 1997).

Making a long story short, strongly supported by mentors such as Dr. Bengt Scherstén and Dr. Åke Isacsson, after completing a course in community health of the medical program and publishing a first empirical study, I was admitted as a PhD student in community health science. Important influences by these early mentors were that they made great efforts to foster interdisciplinary thinking among the group of PhD students at the Department of Community Health Science at large, not only between professions and disciplines in medicine and health, but including behavioral and social sciences. Since at the department postdoctoral fellows as well as senior researchers representing this diversity were employed, working as an interdisciplinary team they were great role models for us students. Very uncommon for that time period Dr. Scherstén (MD, professor in general practice, Head of Department) nurtured a vision that not only physicians but all professionals working at primary health-care centers should have the possibility to develop academic skills and being able to contribute to the development of evidence-based practices. The department was well-known all across Sweden, not the least based on a high ambition for knowledge transfer activities targeting practitioners. Each year a well-attended conference was organized, including PhD students and all staff in the organization, preparation, and the program as such. We were exposed to media and encouraged to act independently to communicate research findings to different categories of knowledge users. Following this, based on an initiative of Dr. Isacsson, in the late 1990s together with OT PhD and PhD student colleagues, I contributed to the establishment of an annual conference to report our research findings. This conference series turned out as very successful and was in operation for more than 10 years. For sure, this kind of early training inspired me to develop competence and high ambitions for knowledge translation and user-oriented research

(Kylberg, Haak, & Iwarsson, 2017), today manifested in the profile of the research center on aging that I have the privilege to lead.

In 1997, I became the first OT graduating with a PhD at the Faculty of Medicine at LU. At that point, the academic development of the health professions in Sweden had evolved to the stage where all undergraduate programs were about to be integrated in the university system. In 1998, a new Division of OT was established at the Department of Clinical Neuroscience. Being the only OT with a PhD degree at the Faculty of Medicine, I was commissioned by the Faculty Dean to take the lead of the establishment of OT as an academic discipline at LU.

Personally, a very special situation arose shortly after my PhD graduation. My supervisor Åke Isacsson became seriously ill and died in 1999. I found myself in a demanding situation that was far too complex for a novice researcher. While there were other senior mentors around, none of them were acquainted with my research field, OT or aging research. Thus, I simply had to develop my own research track and at the same time lead the development of the new division and OT as an academic discipline. The pace in which all of this occurred turned out to be extraordinary. During this period, important support and encouragement was given by OT colleagues. Of particular significance was my day-to-day collaboration with Dr. Mona Eklund who had defended her PhD thesis in psychology, at the Faculty of Social Sciences at LU, only a few months earlier than me. We were both employed as senior lecturers at the new Division of OT at LU, and we have followed each other as colleagues through the years but with quite different research orientations. Taken together, this situation boosted my leadership training in an unforeseen manner—I learnt so much that has benefitted my development as an academic leader.

In 1999, I qualified as an associate professor, and in 2003, I was promoted to full professor in OT. Shortly thereafter, a very attractive senior position in gerontology financed by a private donation to the university was announced, and I could not resist the possibility to apply. Thus, in 2005, I was appointed as the holder of "Maria and Seved Ribbing's endowed chair in gerontology and care for the elderly." This position was favorably financed with a high level of autonomy; it was also entrusted with major responsibilities to develop an independent and strong research line that would satisfy the private donor.

During these years I successively developed cooperation with other researchers at LU, in particular with Dr. Agneta Ståhl at the Department of Technology and Society, Faculty of Engineering. This emanated from a contact made by her as my PhD thesis was made public. Since long, she had been engaged in research with older people in the field of public transport planning, and she was keen on developing collaboration starting out from our mutual research interests. In

2007, coordinating an interdisciplinary team of researchers at the faculties of medicine, engineering, and social sciences at LU we succeeded to receive 10 years of funding to establish CASE. This achievement was very important as it gave us the possibility to plan for long-term endeavors to develop our interdisciplinary research line.

KEY SCIENTIFIC CONTRIBUTIONS TO ENVIRONMENTAL GERONTOLOGY

Methodology for Housing Accessibility Assessments

As I was planning for my PhD thesis project, I had to overview and problematize the concept of accessibility and select a methodological approach appropriate for addressing my main research question (stated above). Starting out from my practical OT experiences based on housing adaptation services, this turned into a demanding process. As is often the case in research, my conclusion was that there was a need to define accessibility, find a theoretical base for it and also to develop an instrument with the capacity to validly capture the concept.

Searching the literature, I found Steinfeld et al.'s (1979) "Enabler" as a well-developed idea to describe accessibility as a function of person and environment. This caught my attention and interest, and I contacted Professor Edward Steinfeld to ask for his permission to use the Enabler concept as the starting point for the development of an instrument to capture accessibility. In parallel, I identified Lawton and Nahemow's Ecological Theory of Aging with the notion of person-environment fit and the docility hypothesis (Lawton & Nahemow, 1973) that seemed to work well as a theoretical base for my instrument development ambitions. At that time, my goal was to develop a scientifically sound instrument useful for the completion of my PhD thesis project. I embarked the journey of instrument development without any previous experience of such research, engaging OT colleagues and students in a first methodology study focusing on housing accessibility assessments (Iwarsson & Isacsson, 1996a). As I published my PhD thesis entitled "Functional capacity and physical environmental demand: Exploration of factors influencing everyday activity and health in the elderly population" (1997), it contained several empirical studies where the new instrument "Enabler" was used and successively validated (Iwarsson & Isacsson, 1996b, 1997). This instrument turned out to be attractive also for other researchers, and besides invitations for new research collaborations, I was encouraged by the fact that I received several rewards for my methodological contribution to the assessment and analysis of accessibility problems in the built environment. As we used the Enabler concept as a starting point also for instrument versions addressing environmental arenas beyond the housing environment (see e.g., Iwarsson, Jensen, & Ståhl, 2000), subsequently we coined the name Housing Enabler for the instrument that since then has gained considerable attention among environmental gerontologists, OTs, and other researchers and professionals. For an overview of the structure of the Housing Enabler, see Figure 7.2.

Within the European ENABLE-AGE project (see Iwarsson et al., 2007) the first large-scale effort to use the Housing Enabler in cross-national research was made (Iwarsson, Nygren, & Slaug, 2005). Subsequently, the instrument has been

First mark the functional limitations and dependence on mobility devices that you have observed. Then transfer the crosses to all the rating forms concerning environmental barriers.

Yes No
- ☐ ☒ A. Difficulty interpreting information
- ☐ ☒ B1. Visual impairment
- ☐ ☒ B2. Blindness
- ☒ ☐ C. Loss of hearing
- ☒ ☐ D. Poor balance
- ☐ ☒ E. Incoordination
- ☐ ☒ F. Limitations of stamina
- ☐ ☒ G. Difficulty in moving head
- ☐ ☒ H. Reduced upper extremity function
- ☒ ☐ I. Reduced fine motor skill
- ☐ ☒ J. Loss of upper extremity function
- ☐ ☒ K. Reduced spine and/or lower extremity function
- ☒ ☐ L. Dependence on walking aid(s) — A B C*: ☒ ☒ ☒
- ☐ ☒ M. Dependence on wheelchair — A B C*: ☐ ☐ ☐

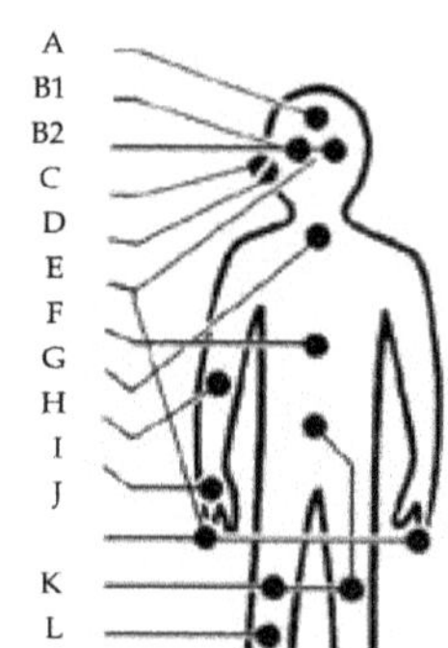

Section in the environmental component: A. Exterior surroundings. B. Entrance. C. Indoor environment

Mark the observed environmental barriers with a cross. Then circle the scoring points (1–4) found at the intersections between functional limitations etc. and environmental barriers. The total of these scores is a quantification of the magnitude of accessibility problems.

Personal component / functional profile	Yes / No	A	B1	B2	C	D	E	F	G	H	I	J	K	L	M	
	Yes				×	×					×			×		
	No	×	×	×			×	×	×	×		×	×		×	
A. Exterior surroundings	Bygg ikapp	A	B1	B2	C	D	E	F	G	H	I	J	K	L	M	RATI NG
General **A1.** Paths narrower than 1.5 m. *A width of 1.0 m is acceptable provided there are 1.5 m turning zones at least every 10 m.*	p. 304					3	3							3	3	☐ Yes ☒ No ☐ *Not rated*
A2. Irregular/uneven surface. (irregular surfacing, joins, slop ng sections cracks, holes; 5 mm or more).	p. 305		2	3		(1)	1		3				1	(3)	3	☒ Yes ☐ No ☐ *Not rated*
A3. Unstable surface (oose grave , sand, clay, etc). *Mark if it causes difficulties e.g. when using a wheelchair or rollator.*			2	3		3	3	2					1	3	4	☐ Yes ☒ No ☐ *Not rated*

FIGURE 7.2 Scoring principle of the Housing Enabler instrument.
Source: Reprinted with permission from Iwarsson and Slaug (2010).

translated to English as well as languages such as Finnish and Danish, including adaptation to the national guidelines for housing design in the countries involved (Helle et al., 2010). Recently, the instrument was adapted also to U.S. standards and tested for reliability in a small-scale study (Lien, Stegell, Slaug, & Iwarsson, 2015). At present—more than 20 years after the first steps of methodology development—I conclude that the development and successive refinement of the Housing Enabler instrument (Iwarsson, Haak, & Slaug, 2012) is regarded as one of my key scientific contributions to the field of Environmental Gerontology.

The most significant outcome from an Environmental Gerontology perspective on a personal level was that the Housing Enabler attracted the attention of several colleagues active in the field from outside Sweden. In late 2000, I was contacted by Professor Dr. Hans-Werner Wahl and Dr. Frank Oswald at Heidelberg University, Germany, asking me if I was interested in research collaboration on older people's home and health situation in a cross-national European context. Since I was overwhelmed with work as the Head of the Division of OT, the demands to develop and establish OT education and research at LU, and also without any knowledge and experience of international research collaboration, at first I was somewhat reluctant to their query. However, persistent as they were, they simply decided to come to Lund for a meeting—and this was the start of a fascinating collaborative endeavor that really introduced me and my research team to Environmental Gerontology. During a few hectic months in early 2001, including colleagues also from the UK, Hungary, and Latvia, with my coordination we developed the ENABLE-AGE project proposal for Framework 5 of the European Commission. I was not prepared for the successful outcome of that proposal, and was quite perplexed when I received a phone call from Brussels stating "Congratulations Dr. Iwarsson—you got every Euro you applied for." This was the start of a fantastic scholarly journey together with colleagues who will be my personal friends forever. Together, we experienced many challenges and developed a very creative and constructive working climate resulting in a project with outcomes and a scientific production of international recognition.

With the overall aim to examine housing and neighborhood environments and their importance for major components of healthy aging, the hallmark of the ENABLE-AGE project was the richness of variables covering objective and perceived aspects of housing, with a follow-up design including survey as well as in-depth studies. Overall, the results show that the home is an important support for activity, participation and health in very old age, and demonstrate that objective as well as perceived aspects of housing influence aspects of health. A major finding across studies is that environmental barriers per se do not have any significant influences on health, while accessibility problems (defined based on the notion of P-E fit) have. We also published first results on how housing-related control beliefs mediate the relationship between housing accessibility and activities of daily living (ADL) dependence. Regarding predictors for relocation, we show that depression, dependence on assistance in outdoor transportation, and housing-related control beliefs are significant. Moreover, data from a study on objective aspects of housing and mortality indicate that specific environmental barriers in entrances and close neighborhoods are significant. Adding to the complex picture of how very old people reason about housing and health changes, with a qualitative meta-synthesis we developed insights to the intertwined processes of turning-points, struggles, and negotiation characterizing living at home into very old age. Over the years, data from the ENABLE-AGE project were used in nine PhD theses, defended at the universities that were partners in the project. To date, approximately 50 original papers have been published based on the project (see e.g., Iwarsson et al., 2007; Oswald et al., 2007; see also Chapter 2, The Environment as Developmental Context: In All Ages but Certainly in Old Age). Recently, an overview with the ambition to synthesize the findings to facilitate knowledge translation was published (Iwarsson et al., 2016).

Extending My Research Trajectory to Out-of-Home Environments

One line of development originating from my early methodological work based on the Enabler Concept (Steinfeld et al., 1979) emanated from the evolving collaboration with Dr. Agneta Ståhl. Starting out with a joint publication where we problematized and outlined avenues for interdisciplinary research between OT and public transport planning (Iwarsson & Ståhl, 1999), during the years we have contributed to the knowledge development on older people's mobility, activity, and participation outside home (for an overview, see Iwarsson, Ståhl, & Löfqvist, 2013).

From Occupational Therapy to Environmental Gerontology

There are other examples of particular research projects that could be accounted for here, but I would rather like to summarize that moving beyond my basic professional orientation in OT to the multidisciplinary field of gerontology, in particular Environmental Gerontology, was a natural step for me. From a research and education perspective, I have always been more interested in contributing to problem solving and knowledge generation regarding the situation of people with disabilities and population aging than advocating for intradisciplinary scholarly developments. Moreover, from a conceptual and theoretical perspective, OT and Environmental Gerontology have much in common (Wahl & Iwarsson, 2007). While sometimes regarded as controversial in my attitude to intradisciplinary developments, over the years I have been told by colleagues from both fields that the interdisciplinary approach that I have been advocating and practicing has been instrumental for OT, as well as for Environmental Gerontology.

EVOLUTION IN RESEARCH FOCUS OVER TIME

Reflecting upon my research career in retrospect, the evolution in research focus over time is closely interlinked with the research focus I will have for the years to come. Most important in the light of my ambition to produce new knowledge that could make a difference in the everyday reality of people as they age, a cumulative approach to knowledge generation is also closely interlinked with practice topics of societal relevance for the future. With influences already in childhood, starting out from research questions evoked by cases of insufficient housing accessibility and resultant negative consequences for older people with functional limitations encountered as an OT in primary health care, 25 years later my primary research focus still is the home and health situation for older people. However, influenced by highly inspiring interdisciplinary and cross-national research cooperation, today my research focus is of course broader as well as deeper than the one I started out from. This multifaceted development includes: (1) successive evolution of research topics based on previous work; (2) increasing interdisciplinarity involving additional disciplines, as well as expansion of my methodological arsenal for research to include mixed-methods designs; (3) cross-national collaboration in Europe and beyond; (4) research involving individual, group, and population levels, focusing on "usual" aging in the community as well as vulnerable elders, such as those aging with chronic disease and/or disability; (5) user participation in research, including entrepreneurial and innovation approaches; and (6) engagement in graduate education and postdoctoral training at regional, national and international levels.

The complexity of home and health interactions is still a current research focus (see e.g., Nilsson, Ullén, Ekström, & Iwarsson, 2016), and the interplay of objective (e.g., housing standards, environmental barriers, accessibility) and perceived (e.g., usability, meaning of home, housing-related control beliefs) aspects of home (Nygren et al., 2007) is still intriguing. Related to such dynamics, another research focus that has evolved and produced new knowledge is older people's use and need of assistive technology, in particular, mobility devices (see e.g., Brandt, Iwarsson, & Ståhl, 2003; Pettersson, Brandt, Månsson Lexell, & Iwarsson, 2015; Sund, Iwarsson, Anttila, & Brandt, 2015). Moreover, this orientation and expertise area has also contributed to elaborations in research concentrated to environmental arenas such as outdoor pedestrian environments (for an overview, see Iwarsson et al., 2013), public facilities (Valdemarsson, Jernryd, & Iwarsson, 2005) and public transport contexts (Iwarsson et al., 2000;

Risser, Månsson, Lexell, Bell, Iwarsson, & Ståhl, 2015) as well as to research on physical activity among older people (see e.g., Rantakokko et al., 2010).

Over the years, together with many colleagues I have successively developed an explicitly interdisciplinary approach to research. This is not surprising as interdisciplinary research is increasingly being advocated for, not the least in Environmental Gerontology. In my opinion, however, the interdisciplinary research mission is far too often merely lip service and not actually manifested in reality. Together with senior and junior researchers from different disciplines I have made serious attempts to establish informal and formal structures for interdisciplinary research. This has resulted in some frustration and failures, but also in productive collaboration during many years. As to methodological approaches, this collaboration has led to a considerable extension of the methodological arsenal I am using, not the least inspired by the latest developments in mixed-methods research (see e.g., Creswell & Plano Clark, 2011).

Based on my personal experiences over the years, one key to success in interdisciplinary research is to identify and engage in long-term collaboration with senior scientists who truly share your commitment to such developments. Most important, interdisciplinary efforts must pass the languishing stage and turn into practical day-to-day efforts of visible and positive leaders. To be successful there is little room for prestige, but establishing the open, allowing and creative working climate that is necessary is easier said than done. As to the engagement of junior researchers, many are seriously interested in getting involved in interdisciplinary projects. Not the least in Environmental Gerontology with a multitude of perspectives and interacting factors relevant for virtually any problem or research question identified, interdisciplinary research environments seem to be popular. However, once PhD students and postdocs encounter the tensions and challenges that might arise when having to balance the requirements and standards of their "home discipline" with the uncertainty of where interdisciplinary developments might lead, frustration and stress are not uncommon. Developing new PhD student projects that require the input from different disciplines in the form of interdisciplinary supervision teams is one way we have found instrumental to overcome challenges. Moreover, in my opinion co-authored publications involving scholars from different disciplines, choosing target journals representing a wide range of disciplinary orientations, is another effective way toward interdisciplinary success. While it always can be debated whether researchers really succeed in their interdisciplinary ambitions, I am confident that we have demonstrated that interdisciplinary research collaboration in Environmental Gerontology is possible to achieve.

Another explicit personal ambition has been the development of cross-national research. Expanding our international collaboration over the years, in our research on home and health (Benzinger et al., 2014; Haak et al., 2015; Lien et al., 2015) as well as in our research involving assistive technology issues (Brandt et al., 2008; Löfqvist, Nygren, Brandt, Oswald, & Iwarsson, 2007; Sund, Iwarsson, Andersson, & Brandt, 2013), we have succeeded to include cross-national perspectives. Of particular importance for me personally is our studies describing and comparing the situation of older people in Sweden and Latvia (Horstmann, Haak, Tomsone, Iwarsson, & Gräsbeck, 2012; Kylberg, Löfqvist, et al., 2015), sparked by my early involvement in the establishment of an OT curriculum in Riga already in 1995. Having had the opportunity to interact with colleagues and study participants in a geographically nearby but socio-economically and politically distinctly different country has been invaluable to increase the awareness of the multitude of factors that influence the process of aging. Such collaboration has not only influenced my personal approach to international research collaboration and cross-national research but has also greatly influenced the cross-cultural awareness among the PhD students and young scholars in my research team.

As my early research career built upon my clinical experiences as a practicing OT, naturally my primary interest early on was the aging individual. More precisely, when I embarked on my PhD thesis project, the individual housing adaptation client was in focus. However, since I graduated with a PhD in community health science and had my main clinical experience from primary health care, already as a PhD student I was exposed to epidemiology, diagnosis groups, and population health perspectives. Consequently, over the years I have conducted research representing individual, group as well as population perspectives. As to study populations, I was influenced by clinical experiences as well as by the organizational affiliation of the Division of OT to the Department of Clinical Neuroscience at LU during 1998–2004. In addition, I was engaged in the coordination of the strategic research area of neuroscience (MultiPark) at LU from 2010–2014. These circumstances influenced my research group to mainly concentrate on diagnosis groups such as stroke and Parkinson's disease. While we are making progress in receiving some recognition to aging and environment issues in research fields heavily dominated by medical perspectives (see e.g., Nilsson, Haak, & Iwarsson, 2013; Norin, Slaug et al., 2016), overall it is demanding to get scholarly attention to Environmental Gerontology in such contexts. When it comes to the population level, we are struggling to bring issues of home and health into the public health domain. Introducing Environmental Gerontology perspectives in the broader epidemiological context is very challenging. However, we have some recent examples of contributions to the public health literature (Granbom, Iwarsson, Kylberg, Pettersson, & Slaug,

2016; Slaug, Schilling, Iwarsson, & Carlsson, 2015). Developing the cross-disciplinary skills necessary to be able to publish in a wide range of scientific journals is one example of where a personal background encompassing several disciplines is beneficial. However, the quest for profound integration of concepts, theories and methods at times is demanding and often challenging when it comes communicating with different parts of the scientific community. There is an obvious risk that such research could be criticized as superficial and not sufficiently anchored in the respective research orientation's paradigm, thus deserving constant attention and monitoring of quality of your own work.

With the establishment of CASE at LU in 2007, together with colleagues I embarked on a journey toward explicit user participation in research. Reflecting upon this orientation from a personal perspective, since the start of my academic career it has stood clear that it is important for me that research and practice application are intertwined. In the original proposal for long-term funding of the center, operational goals for user participation were posed. During the last 10 years, we have successively developed a model including a formalized Board of Users, several completed or ongoing projects with active user participation in different stages of the research process (see Kylberg, Haak, et al., 2015), and structured knowledge translation activities. In the present situation I am very much enjoying a rapidly increasing interest from older people's organizations and policy makers, with a large amount of invitations to engage with them as expert, project partner, workshop leader, or lecturer. From a personal point of view this is encouraging and also providing great opportunities for skills development regarding interaction with knowledge users. Importantly, the junior colleagues of my research team and CASE are constantly being exposed to the challenges and benefits of having many opportunities to train and learn about user participation in research.

We have developed several projects where we also approached entrepreneurship and innovation, thus extending our approach to user participation to include public agencies and industry. One example is my private company established in 1997, engaging in methodology training based on the Housing Enabler, for practitioners and researchers in Sweden and other countries (Iwarsson et al., 2012). Another example is the development of an app for user-driven housing provision, developed together with researchers and users in four EU countries (Haak et al., 2015) engaged in the EC-financed Innovage Project. At present, based on our empirical work and literature studies (Kylberg, Haak, et al., 2015) together with colleagues at three additional universities in southern Sweden, we are developing a novel research program devoted to understanding user participation in research.

Running in parallel with these different but intertwined lines of development, is an increasing interest for and engagement in graduate education at regional, national and international levels. PhD students well integrated in the research activities of my research group and CASE constitute an important and valuable category of coworkers. Starting out as a cosupervisor of several PhD students directly after my own PhD graduation, over the years I have learnt so much from those that I have had the privilege to work with. Subsequently, nurtured particularly by the development of a graduate school integrated with CASE, I have also been engaged in systematic efforts to establish teaching and learning environments for junior researchers. As a scientific enterprise, these developments include international publication efforts (see Iwarsson, 2013). In turn, this has led to engagement as a co-supervisor or examiner also for PhD students at other universities in Sweden and abroad, in particular asking for my competence in Environmental Gerontology. The latest developments include the establishment of the SWEAH, including engagement in the International Summer School on Ageing (Barbarella et al., 2016) and postdoctoral courses open to young scholars worldwide.

POTENTIAL IMPLICATIONS OF SCHOLARLY AND APPLIED RESEARCH CONTRIBUTION TO ENVIRONMENTAL GERONTOLOGY AND THE AGING SOCIETY AT LARGE

Over the years, I have had continuous encouragement from the science community as well as from practitioners and users of the kind of knowledge produced by my research team and CASE. This has resulted in national and international recognition including commissions and awards speaking to the relevance of this research. In particular, the Housing Enabler methodology has gained recognition, not only as a research tool, but also as an influence for practitioners to apply more structured approaches to the assessment of person-environment fit at individual level. We have also succeeded in influencing public policies on housing in Sweden, where the government on several instances has commissioned us to produce research-based reports for national housing policies. Occasionally, we have had such queries also from other EU countries. The explicit user orientation of our research has resulted in much attention from user organizations and public agencies, and we have indications of an increasing interest also from relevant industry.

To what extent these interests from different groups of knowledge users will actually contribute to positive developments for the aging population and society at large is beyond what we as researchers are able to judge and foresee. While I am satisfied with the signs of interest and appreciation I am noting, at the same time like most research colleagues, I am frustrated by the fact that it is very challenging and time consuming for research to influence the societal development and the situation for the aging individual and population. Personally, I am struggling with the balance between scientific rigor and the time it takes to produce and present solid and valid results on the one hand, and the demands from societal actors to collaborate and contribute with research-based knowledge at a pace that does not always allow for research quality on the other.

As to research contributions to Environmental Gerontology, I interpret the increasing number of invitations for scholarly contributions to national and international conferences and other activities as a signification of the relevance of my research for the field. I am receiving positive and reassuring feedback that my practice background as an OT as well as my health science orientation contribute to the diversity and interdisciplinarity of Environmental Gerontology. Also, even if it is challenging to get some attention to Environmental Gerontology perspectives in the realms of clinical and public health research, I have aspirations to be able to provide increased attention to environmental dynamics related to aging among those with disease and/or disability also in the medical context.

EMERGENT CHALLENGES AND RESEARCH TASKS FOR ENVIRONMENTAL GERONTOLOGY FOR THE UPCOMING YEARS

As a member of the core team of the EC-funded coordination action project FUTURAGE (Walker, 2011), I had the privilege to work together with researchers and knowledge users of aging research in the most extensive consultation ever undertaken in Europe in this field. The project was based on the following basic assumptions: multidisciplinarity, user engagement, a life-course perspective, a person-environment perspective, the importance of diversity and intergenerational relationships, knowledge exchange, and technological innovation. The outcome of FUTURAGE was a roadmap outlining the major priority themes for future aging research. Speaking to the relevance of further endeavors in Environmental Gerontology, several of the basic assumptions resonate with central premises in the field, and one of the seven priority themes identified was "aging well at home and in community environments." While some time has passed since the final FUTURAGE report was published, in my opinion, the research priorities set out under this theme are still relevant and well worth considering. One important insight, based on input from users engaged in FUTURAGE as well as on the results of one of our recent studies (Haak et al., 2015), is that although the home environment is very important as we age, today's senior citizens emphasize the importance of neighborhoods. That is, there is a need for research on the everyday environments of aging including not only the dwelling as such, but also the out-of-home environments as important arenas for activity and participation. This resonates well with the research orientation at CASE, and is promising not the least at the prospect of future research funding. A cross-cutting dimension identified in the FUTURAGE as important for home and community environments was the rapid technology development, and one recommendation was to initiate more research on physical-spatial-technical environments. Such research is underway (see e.g., Chiatti et al., 2015), but much remains to be accomplished in this complex area of inquiry. Turning to issues of migration, being much more prominent now than when the FUTURAGE Roadmap was launched, there is a need for research on new cohorts of older people crossing national and cultural borders and the many implications of such situations. Overall, while population aging to a major extent is positive and many people will enjoy active and healthy aging, there are vulnerable subgroups that deserve more research investments (Walker, 2011), not the least from an Environmental Gerontology perspective. Examples are people with dementia and other cognitive disorders, frail older people and their carers, refugees, and people with psychiatric diagnoses.

Turning to the basics of science, while there are good examples of theoretical ambitions in current Environmental Gerontology, there are needs as well as strong possibilities to move into further theoretical development. Notably, the ENABLE-AGE Project has produced a multitude of publications on home and health dynamics in very old age (Iwarsson et al., 2016), constituting a solid empirical base that should be utilized for theory building. So far, we have not made much use of this potential, and it is a personal goal of mine to also contribute theoretically in this area. Medicine and health sciences—that is, where I come from professionally and research-wise—are often empirically rich but theory poor while the social and behavioral sciences can be viewed as theory rich but not always rich in terms of empirical studies. However, strong scientific progress requires that empirical and theoretical developments go hand in hand (Jaccard & Jacoby, 2010). The strong empirical developments seen in Environmental Gerontology should be utilized for theoretical development and refinement, and there are also examples of existing theories that require empirical testing.

Having been engaged in methodology development of relevance for Environmental Gerontology during many years, I still see needs for continuous endeavors to arrive at an optimized methodology arsenal for this very broad and complex field of inquiry. Current limitations are limited sample sizes in quantitative studies, unbalanced datasets with a paucity of high quality data on several environmental dimensions, and insufficient treatment of cultural and socio-economic specificities and differences. As there is a paucity of data collection instruments that are available in reliable and valid versions in different languages, the possibilities for cross-national research are limited. A largely unexplored methodological domain is the possibility to utilize census data and large public registers for research on housing and health along the process of aging, thus taking trends in demography, economy and welfare service developments into account in complex modeling. As to qualitative methodologies, in my opinion more should be done to develop meta-analytic strategies that would result in the much needed accumulation of knowledge in Environmental Gerontology. Finally, there is underutilized power in the combination of methods, and in a complex research field such as Environmental Gerontology the strongly evolving mixed-methods paradigm (see Creswell & Plano Clark, 2011) deserves more attention. However, no matter if researchers use all their time and effort for methodology studies, there are always more to be done. Thus, it is necessary to strike a balance between the methodological efforts and empirical research in its own right, to produce new knowledge on important matters.

As to changes for or benefits to society, the impact of Environmental Gerontology to a large extent remains to be demonstrated. The field has seen a strong progression, but the process of translation of new knowledge to practice and society at large is slow. The needs and preferences of the diverse aging population are new and rapidly changing, but far from being met by society. One avenue often advocated for addressing this situation is user participation in research. However, the positive and potentially negative effects of participatory research approaches are largely unknown and the evidence in terms of outcomes is weak (Shippee et al., 2013). Research needs relevant for Environmental Gerontology include determining which user groups and individuals should be involved and how. Furthermore, there is a need for development of valid methods for evaluation of research with user participation (Kylberg et al., 2017). Moreover, there are ethical challenges and dilemmas not addressed (Backhouse et al., 2016), and the resources needed for such research deserve consideration. Summing up on open question and emergent challenges for Environmental Gerontology, while upholding a critical and independent mindset, we must continuously reconsider and reframe our priorities based on current and future societal developments and challenges.

REFERENCES

Ainsworth, E., & de Jonge, D. (2011). *An occupational therapist's guide to home modification practice*. Thorofare, NJ: Slack Incorporated.

Backhouse, T., Kenkmann, A., Lane, K., Penhale, B., Poland, F., & Killett, A. (2016). Older care-home residents as collaborators in research: A systematic review. *Age and Ageing*, *45*(3), 337–345.

Barbarella, F., Chiatti, C., Di Rosa, M., Lamura, G., Martin-Matthews, A., Papa, R., & Svensson, T. (2016). Launching an interdisciplinary "International Summer School on Ageing" (ISSA): Aims, methodology, and outcomes. *Educational Gerontology*, *42*(4), 253–264.

Benzinger, P., Iwarsson, S., Kroog, A., Beische, D., Lindemann, U., Klenk, J., & Becker, C. (2014). The association between the home environment and physical activity in community-dwelling older adults. *Aging Clinical and Experimental Research*, *26*(4), 377–385.

Brandt, Å., Iwarsson, S., & Ståhl, A. (2003). Satisfaction with rollators among community-living users: a follow-up study. *Disability and Rehabilitation*, *25*(7), 343–353.

Brandt, Å., Löfqvist, C., Jónsdottir, I., Sund, T., Salminen, A-L., Werngren-Elgström, M., & Iwarsson, S. (2008). Towards an instrument targeting mobility-related participation: Nordic cross-national reliability. *Journal of Rehabilitation Medicine*, *40*(9), 766–772.

Chiatti, C., Rimland, J. M., Bonfranceschi, F., Maseray, F., Bustacchini, S., Cassetta, L., & Lattanzio, F. (2015). The UP-TECH project, an intervention to support caregivers of Alzheimer's disease patients in Italy: Preliminary findings on recruitment and caregiving burden in the baseline population. *Aging and Mental Health*, *19*(6), 517–525.

Creswell, J. W., & Plano Clarke, V. L. (2011). *Designing and conducting mixed methods research* (2nd ed.). Thousand Oaks, CA: Sage Publications.

Cumming, E., & Henry, W. E. (1961). *Growing old: The process of disengagement*. New York, NY: Basic Books.

Granbom, M., Iwarsson, S., Kylberg, M., Pettersson, C., & Slaug, B. (2016). A public health perspective to environmental barriers and accessibility problems for senior citizens living in ordinary housing. *BMC Public Health*, *16*(1), 1–11.

Haak, M., Slaug, B., Oswald, F., Schmidt, S. M., Rimland, J. M., Tomsone, S., et al. (2015). Cross-national user priorities for housing provision and accessibility–Findings from the European innovAge project. *International Journal of Environmental Research and Public Health*, *12*(3), 2670–2686.

Havighurst, R. J., & Albrecht, R. E. (1953). *Older people*. New York, NY: Longmans, Green.

Helle, T., Nygren, C., Slaug, B., Brandt, Å., Pikkarainen, A., Hansen, A-G., et al. (2010). The Nordic Housing Enabler: Inter-rater reliability in cross-Nordic occupational therapy practice. *Scandinavian Journal of Occupational Therapy*, *17*(4), 258–266.

Horstmann, V., Haak, M., Tomsone, S., Iwarsson, S., & Gräsbeck, A. (2012). Life satisfaction in older women in Latvia and Sweden–Relations to standard of living, aspects of health and coping behaviour. *Journal of Cross-Cultural Gerontology*, *27*(4), 391–407.

Iwarsson, S. (1997). *Functional capacity and physical environmental demand. Exploration of factors influencing everyday activity and health in the elderly population.* (Doctoral thesis, Department of Community Health Sciences). Lund University, Sweden.

Iwarsson, S. (2013). A critical analysis of a master course in gerontology. *Education*, *3*(6), 325–332.

Iwarsson, S., Haak, M., & Slaug, B. (2012). Current developments of the Housing Enabler methodology. *British Journal of Occupational Therapy*, *75*(11), 517–521.

Iwarsson, S., & Isacsson, Å. (1996a). Development of a novel instrument for occupational therapy assessment of the physical environment in the home–A methodologic study on "The Enabler." *Occupational Therapy Journal of Research*, *16*(4), 227–244.

Iwarsson, S., & Isacsson, Å. (1996b). Housing standards, environmental barriers in the home and subjective general apprehension of housing situation among the rural elderly. *Scandinavian Journal of Occupational Therapy*, *3*(2), 52–61.

Iwarsson, S., & Isacsson, Å. (1997). Quality of life in the elderly population: an example exploring interrelationships among subjective well-being, ADL dependence, and housing accessibility. *Archives of Gerontology and Geriatrics*, *26*(1), 71–83.

Iwarsson, S., Jensen, G., & Ståhl, A. (2000). Travel Chain Enabler: Development of a pilot instrument for assessment of urban public bus transport accessibility. *Technology and Disability*, *12*(1), 3–12.

Iwarsson, S., Löfqvist, C., Oswald, F., Wahl, H-W., Slaug, B., Schmidt, S., et al. (2016). Synthesizing ENABLE-AGE research findings to suggest evidence-based home and health interventions. *Journal of Housing for the Elderly*, *30*(3), 330–343.

Iwarsson, S., Nygren, C., & Slaug, B. (2005). Cross-national and multi-professional inter-rater reliability of the Housing Enabler. *Scandinavian Journal of Occupational Therapy*, *12*(1), 29–39.

Iwarsson, S., & Slaug, B. (2010). *Housing Enabler–A method for rating/screening and analyzing accessibility problems in housing. Manual for the complete instrument and screening tool* (2nd ed.). Sweden: Veten & Skapen HB.

Iwarsson, S., & Ståhl, A. (1999). Traffic engineering and occupational therapy: A collaborative approach for future directions. *Scandinavian Journal of Occupational Therapy*, *6*(1), 21–28.

Iwarsson, S., Ståhl, A., & Löfqvist, C. (2013). Mobility in outdoor environments in old age. In G. Rowles & M. Bernard (Eds.), *Environmental gerontology: Making meaningful places in old age* (pp. 175–198). New York, NY: Springer Publishing.

Iwarsson, S., Wahl, H-W., Nygren, C., Oswald, F., Sixsmith, A., Sixsmith, J., et al. (2007). Importance of the home environment for healthy aging: Conceptual and methodological background of the European ENABLE-AGE Project. *Gerontologist*, *47*(1), 78–84.

Jaccard, J., & Jacoby, J. (2010). *Theory construction and model-building skills*. New York, NY: Guilford Press.

Kielhofner, G. (2009). *Conceptual foundations of occupational therapy practice*. Philadelphia, PA: F. A. Davis Company.

Kylberg, M., Haak, M., & Iwarsson, S. (2017). Research with and about user participation: potentials and challenges. *Aging Clinical and Experimental Research*. doi:10.1007/s40520-017-0750-7

Kylberg, M., Löfqvist, C., Tomsone, S., Phillips, J., Liepina, Z., & Iwarsson, S. (2015). A European perspective on the service delivery systems for assistive technology–differences and similarities between Latvia and Sweden. *Journal of Cross-Cultural Gerontology*, *30*(1), 51–67.

Lawton, M. P., & Nahemow, L. (1973). Ecology and the aging process. In C. Eisdorfer & M. P. Lawton (Eds.), *The psychology of adult development and aging* (pp. 619–674). Washington, DC: American Psychological Association.

Lien, L. L., Stegell, C. D., Slaug, B., & Iwarsson, S. (2015). Assessment and analysis of housing accessibility: Adapting the environmental component of the housing enabler to United States applications. *Journal of Housing and the Built Environment*, *31*(3), 565–580.

Löfqvist, C., Nygren, C., Brandt, Å., Oswald, F., & Iwarsson, S. (2007). Use of mobility devices and changes over 12 months among very old people in five European countries. *Aging Clinical and Experimental Research*, *19*(6), 497–505.

Nilsson, M., Haak, M., & Iwarsson, S. (2013). Housing and health: Very old people with self-reported Parkinson's disease versus controls. *Parkinson's Disease*, *2013*. doi:10.1155/2013/710839

Nilsson, M. H., Ullén, S., Ekström, H., & Iwarsson, S. (2016). The association between indicators of health and housing in people with Parkinson's disease. *BMC Geriatrics*, *16*(146), 1–8.

Norin, L., Slaug, B., Haak, M., Jörgsensen, S., Lexell, J., & Iwarsson, S. (2016). Housing accessibility and its associations with participation among older adults living with long-standing spinal cord injury. *Journal of Spinal Cord Medicine*, *29*(3), 147–156.

Nygren, C., Oswald, F., Iwarsson, S., Fänge, A., Sixsmith, J., Schilling, O., et al. (2007). Relationships between objective and perceived housing in very old age. *Gerontologist*, *47*(1), 85–95.

Oswald, F., Wahl, H-W., Schilling, O., Nygren, C., Fänge, A., Sixsmith, A., et al. (2007). Relationships between housing and healthy aging in very old age. *Gerontologist*, *47*(1), 96–107.

Pettersson, C., Brandt, Å., Månsson Lexell, E., & Iwarsson, S. (2015). Autonomy and housing accessibility among powered mobility device users. *American Journal of Occupational Therapy*, *69*(5), 1–9.

Rantakokko, M., Iwarsson, S., Hirvensalo, M., Leinonen, R., Heikkinen, E., & Rantanen, T. (2010). Unmet physical activity need in old age. *Journal of the American Geriatrics Society (JAGS)*, *58*(4), 707–712.

Risser, R., Månsson Lexell, E., Bell, D., Iwarsson, S., & Ståhl, A. (2015). Use of local public transport among people with cognitive impairments–A literature review. *Transportation Research Part F: Traffic Psychology and Behaviour*, *29*, 83–97.

Shippee, N. D., Domecq Garces, J. P., Prutsky Lopez, G. J., Wang, Z., Elraiyah, T. A., Nabhan, M., et al. (2013). Patient and service user engagement in research: a systematic review and synthesized framework. *Health Expectations*, *18*(5), 1151–1166.

Slaug, B., Schilling, O., Iwarsson, S., & Carlsson, G. (2015). Typology of person-environment fit constellations: A platform addressing accessibility problems in the built environment for people with functional limitations. *BMC Public Health*, *15*(1), 1–13.

Steinfeld, E., Schroeder, S., Duncan, J., Faste, R., Chollet, B., Bishop, M., et al. (1979). *Access to the built environments: A review of the literature.* Washington, DC: Government Printing Office.

Sund, T., Iwarsson, S., Andersson, M. C., & Brandt, Å. (2013). Documentation of and satisfaction with the service delivery process of electric powered scooters among adult users in different national contexts. *Disability and rehabilitation: Assistive Technology*, *8*(2), 151–160.

Sund, T., Iwarsson, S., Anttila, H., & Brandt, Å. (2015). Effectiveness of powered mobility devices in enabling community mobility-related participation: A prospective study among people with mobility restrictions. *PM & R*, *7*(8), 859–870.

Tornstam, L. (1997). Gerotranscendence: The contemplative dimension of aging. *Journal of Aging Studies*, *11*(2), 143–154.

Valdemarsson, M., Jernryd, E., & Iwarsson, S. (2005). Preferences and frequencies of visits to public facilities in old age–A pilot study in a Swedish town center. *Archives of Gerontology and Geriatrics*, *40*(1), 15–28.

Wahl, H-W., & Iwarsson, S. (2007). Person-environment relations in old age. In F. Fernandez-Ballesteros (Ed.), *Geropsychology. European Perspectives for an Aging World* (pp. 49–66). Göttingen, Germany: Hogrefe & Huber Publishers.

Walker, A. (Ed.). (2011). *FUTURAGE–A road map for European ageing research.* Sheffield, UK: University of Sheffield.

Wilcock, A., & Hocking, C. (2015). *An occupational perspective of health* (3rd ed.). Thorofare, NJ: Slack Incorporated.

Yerxa, E. (1979). The philosophical base of occupational therapy. In *Occupational Therapy: 2001 AD* (pp. 26–30). Rockville, MD: American Occupational Therapy Association.

CHAPTER 8

Home Thoughts

Sheila Peace

ABSTRACT

As a Past President of the British Society of Gerontology, I found my own academic home as a social geographer within the multidisciplinary field of Environmental Gerontology. This chapter reflects the personal growth of a researcher while developing a body of scientific work exploring the interface between people as they age and the valued concept of home. Research areas are overlapping focusing on quality of life, person–environment interaction, and the meaning of context to self-identity within—care homes, supportive and mainstream housing, the micro kitchen environment, and the wider community. Through developing mixed methods research participatory approaches are recognized when making research evidence available beyond academia. In addition, the importance of temporality to understanding continuity and change is central and environmental biographies have pioneered a layered approach to aging in place and the understanding of home through global to local experiences. The value of research application and influence on policy and practice is an on-going mission and the chapter concludes by reviewing the contribution made to this area. Finally, as an autobiographical piece aspects of my own life as a woman with a unique history of family, education, employment, health, and wellbeing offer a parallel perspective on aging, opportunity, and place.

BIBLIOGRAPHICAL NOTES

". . . home in its broadest sense is a physical, social, psychological (Easthope, 2004; Sommerville, 1997), as well as political, environment where an individual's

http://dx.doi.org/10.1891/0198-8794.38.131

life history with all its relationships contextualized in time and space becomes a part of unpacking meaning and exploring continuity and change" (Peace, 2015, p. 447). This quote from a recent publication concerning the meaning of home in later life provides a starting point for this chapter which is autobiographical, to a degree chronological and certainly reflective utilizing research not only concerning the lives of older people living in care homes, supportive and domestic housing, and their interactions in the wider community but through individual experience across the past 40 years. The ways in which personal identity is embodied within environments change through historical time and are activated through spatial relations. This process supports my own journey.

Becoming An Environmental Gerontologist

I am a baby-boomer born in the UK in 1952. At present I would call myself an environmental gerontologist living in north London as part of a family of four with a son and a daughter in their mid-late 20s and edging to a degree of retirement. I was born into a British family with an English father, a Welsh mother and an elder sister who lived in south-west suburban London. There are a number of threads that come together here. I am told that I first went to Wales at 2 months old which continued every year to this different homeland where Nana and Granpa, and then Nana lived surrounded by great aunts and uncles and their family. The cultural difference and working class environment of the council house in the small mining village in the valley in South Wales provided a freedom that was totally unlike the London suburbs. In Wales, my sister and I could walk unaccompanied to the wooded foothills of what seemed mountains to me, whereas in London, the street was the play area, children became friends but family lives were more distant, more private and detached.

School life began very locally at a Church of England Primary school with under 180 children. I passed the 11-plus exam at the end of primary education and asked to attend the same school as my older sister; a bilateral girls school (part Grammar, part Secondary). We were the first generation to go to university and as I had been chosen to be "head girl" of school, it was hoped for and expected. However, perhaps I found early leaderships skills demanding and one poor examination result led me to retake the exam and then spend 9 months working, an unplanned "gap year." Determination got me to university in the end and I returned to Wales in 1971, to study geography at what was then the University College of Swansea. I am a social geographer by first discipline with urban studies a special interest especially urban ecology, social construction of space, and residential mobility. I valued the eclectic mix of geography, sociology, and psychology, especially environmental, through authors such as Buttimer (1969), Jacobs (1961), Lynch (1960), Pastalan and Carson (1970), Sommer

(1969), moving methodologically from quantitative social area analysis to qualitative understanding of individual behavior.

During my undergraduate years, I became a community service volunteer and worked with Age Concern Swansea (now Age UK) setting up a Good Neighbour scheme encouraging local residents to support older people in their streets. This was a public beginning to my interest in the lives of older people. I was also asked if I would visit Mrs E living on Townhill, a large council housing estate overlooking Swansea Bay. Later I would reflect on Mrs E in discussions of the meaning of home when understanding attachment to place. This was her immediate environment in the mid-1970s:

> For the past three years Mrs E has slept in the living-room; her single bed placed next to the front window surrounded by a sofa, two armchairs, the television, a small table and a large sideboard covered in photos of her daughter and grandchildren and stacked high with books, magazines and letters. (Peace, 1988, p. 218)

Later, this picture conjured comparisons with myself. It describes a woman living in one room, her bed brought downstairs and in a domestic sense "out of place." I remember we talked of this for when I was a teenager, home was a semidetached house called a "chalet bungalow" in style as it had two bedrooms upstairs and one downstairs. I was offered the downstairs room and tried to make it mine but never got used to sleeping downstairs when everyone else was upstairs. It didn't work and so I returned to sharing with my sister. This was a direct experience of environmental psychology compared across the life course.

Though not actively sought, my experiences of ageing and place continued. As a student, I spent summer holidays working, first, as a domestic and then a care assistant, at Percy Gardens Old People's Home in the London Borough of Sutton. Care staff were always needed and students with limited training fitted in. This institutional setting with 60 residents was run by the Local Authority and managed by a nursing Matron. About half of the residents had a room of their own while in some rooms there were up to four beds. There was a "sick bay," a hospital style environment, for people with poor health. During the day, most residents spent time sitting in communal lounges and I learned the expected rules about the worlds of staff and residents. It was here that I continued talking with older people who were not family members, learnt a little about their lives, and recognized that for many, this environment was not their "real" home, but part of the provision for long-term care then provided by the state. The comparison between Mrs E and the residents of Percy Gardens was more than symbolic.

Following my undergraduate degree, I was awarded a University of Wales scholarship to undertake a PhD from 1974–1977. My PhD supervisor, urban studies expert David.T. Herbert (Herbert & Johnston, 1976) responded positively when I suggested bringing under-researched areas ageing and social geography together to explore issues of place in later life. Not being an ageing specialist, Professor Herbert advised drawing upon local scholars Chris Harris (Rosser & Harris, 1965) and Bill Bytheway (Bytheway, 1977). My thesis became a community-based study of the spatial mobility and neighborhood interaction of older people living in mainstream housing and care homes in five contrasting neighborhoods in Swansea (Peace, 1977) aiming to understand tensions between integration/segregation by age and place attachment influenced by Rosow (1967) and Lawton (1970). Methods included semistructured interviews and activity mapping with 273 older people (226 living in mainstream housing, 47 care home residents) plus comparison of cognitive mapping to define place and reported activity. This was an early British attempt to define "images of the city" by older people and develop mixed methods a practice that became central to my future research.

Perhaps not surprisingly, fieldwork convinced me that practical application of research findings was key and that I should train to become a community development worker. Fortunately, I was convinced that I should finish my PhD first and then make that decision. My PhD examiner was Tony Warnes, a geographer who later became an eminent social gerontologist in the UK (Warnes, 1982, 2009). Then at Kings College London, he invited me to hear Graham Rowles talk about his research for *Prisoners of Space? Exploring the Geographical Experience of Older People* (Rowles, 1978). I was drawn to Graham's in-depth qualitative approach to the study of environment and ageing and soon, Rowles' work became something I always read. Tony also encouraged me to join the British Society of Gerontology (BSG) which began in 1971. On joining in 1978, I felt that I had found an academic home outside geography with 300 to 400 like-minded people.

SHARED INTERESTS, INTERDISCIPLINARY RESEARCH, AND INNOVATIVE METHODS

"Gerontology is by definition multidisciplinary, probably one reason why it is so satisfying to certain people" (Lawton, 2000, p. 195). This quote rings true in my case; BSG members come from a range of social science disciplines and professional practice. As someone without an academic training in gerontology, I have always been eclectic aiming to pick things up as I go along from wherever is most appropriate, from gerontology texts to those from other allied disciplines. My thesis shows that I had already discovered the work of American scholars Golant, Regnier, Schooler, Lawton drawing on the environmental docility hypothesis and the ecology of ageing theory.

As a post-doc researcher, I moved into the world of contract research naively confident that "something would turn up." Something did turn up as I moved between academic and voluntary organizations. In 1980, then research officer at MIND (National Association for Mental Health), I was privileged to be awarded the first international 1-year internship with the International Federation on Ageing (IFA) at their office then based at AARP in Washington D.C. For someone who had made only brief trips to parts of western Europe this was a true adventure from working alongside Bill Kerrigan, Charlotte Nusberg and Mary Jo Gibson, to meeting with Robert Butler at National Institute on Aging and hearing his ideas of life review. As well as desk research concerning the needs and status of older women for a UN briefing (Peace, 1981), I chose to focus on alternative ways of living in later life—home-sharing, shared housing, and co-housing which were extremely limited in the UK. Due to IFA/AARP networks, I was able to share interests in inclusive architectural and interior design, living with others (familial and non familial), access to alternative housing, and methodological developments from those with different perspectives. I met with Tom Byerts then at HUD, Sandy Howell at MIT both embracing the architectural angle, I was invited to teach with Jeanne Bader in Minneapolis, to learn from activist Maggie Kuhn in Baltimore, who was living in intergenerational shared housing, and then to spend time with psychologist Powell Lawton at the Philadelphia Geriatric Centre. Talking with Powell, one of my academic heroes, we discussed alternative housing arrangements and introducing qualitative methods to understand behavior and the different levels through which the interface between environment and later life are realized and which his book *Environment and Aging* (Lawton, 1980) captured. Reflecting on his kindness to an unknown British scholar; we went on to run a symposium on "Micro-environmental Issues in Housing for the Elderly" at the XIIIth International Congress of Gerontology/IAGG in New York in 1985 and he later contributed to our book *Private Lives in Public Places* (Willcocks et al., 1987). Although I could have sought to stay in the United States, I went back to the UK in 1981 and Powell Lawton and I continued to correspond.

I came home due to a research tender concerning the design of care homes from the Works Division (policy group and architectural department) of the Department of Health and Social Security (DHSS; now Department of Health, DH) that had come to the Survey Research Unit (SRU) at the North London Polytechnic. I had worked at the SRU briefly in the late 1970s on a feasibility study of quality of life of older people living in care homes and was contacted in the United States regarding the new proposal initially liaising with colleagues at a distance during a time when email was not available. At that point, care homes for older people were run primarily by local authorities and were either large adapted buildings or designed in relation to ministerial building guidance (DHSS & Welsh Office, 1973). This research was to inform new building regulations and was to involve 100 local authority-run old people's homes across England where 1,000 residents and 400 members of staff would be asked about the ways in which they wished to live and the quality of their living and working environments. For someone with my interests, this was a project not to be missed.

We were awarded the contract and I returned to work with multidisciplinary colleagues—Dianne Willcocks, sociologist; Leonie Kellaher, social worker and anthropologist; Jim Ring, statistician; and myself former social geographer and now social gerontologist. Our diversity in terms of methodological expertise was to prove a strength. While the DHSS were keen to base policy change on quantifiable data, they agreed that qualitative research from detailed studies in four of the 100 care homes, exploring the internal and external lives of residents through nonparticipant observation, in-depth interviews and locational surveys would provide important materials. The triangulation of these detailed assessments of four homes alongside quantifiable material from 100 homes proved a powerful tool when discussing the research (Kellaher, Peace, & Willcocks, 1990). The team therefore combined survey research and ethnographic research learning from each other.

While we were part of the Survey Research Unit, we decided that our expertise in environment and ageing needed to be recognized. In 1983, we set up the Centre for Environmental and Social Studies in Ageing (CESSA) based solely on contract research. CESSA was to run for over 20 years at what later became London Metropolitan University. At that time, the term environmental gerontologist was not common either nationally or internationally. The core team grew through new projects but maintained a mixed-method approach throughout its lifetime and beyond as members went to work elsewhere but continued to research collaboratively.

This is also the point to say that gender, health, and wellbeing are central to my own personal narrative. Married in 1983, to Steve Buzzard, bio-chemist turned primary school teacher and leader, I was to have our first child in 1986. Three years later, I suffered from pancreatitis being hospitalized and resulting in a weakened immune system. In 1990, I moved to a secure full-time teaching post at The Open University (OU), the UK's national distance learning university founded in the 1970s where the contexts of later life were central to my teaching modules. In 1991, our second child was born and unfortunately, following maternal diabetes I developed Type 1 diabetes learning to live with insulin dependency and a long-term condition. Domestic life and home working became a part of my every day, with the one adapted to suit the other. This synergy sometimes led a professional career to dominate a private space even though it enabled the continuity of research and maintained my morale. It became even more important as in December 1998, a head-on car crash led to a brain injury and short-term memory loss. Following further hospitalization I was to spend 2 years coming back into part-time and then full-time employment at The OU. This was a time where without the support of my family and colleagues I may not have continued in academia.

During the 1990s, two of my PhD students at The OU, both mature students with experience of professional practice, made important contributions to my research. First, I was joined in 1993 by Caroline Holland, also a geographer by first degree with experience in housing management, who through oral history methods brought to our understanding of home the value of undertaking housing histories (Holland, 2000). This work encouraged the development of a life-course approach to attachment to place. Second, in 1996, John Percival was awarded a studentship cofunded by housing association, The Anchor Trust, to study the quality of life of older people living in sheltered housing. A trained social worker, John developed particular skills in understanding the role of domestic space in daily routines (Percival, 2002) and later worked with me on a study of kitchen living (see p. 140). Following her studentship, Caroline continued to work on her thesis while undertaking part-time research concerning small residential care homes then operating in the UK for four or less residents. We continued to test the meaning of home in different settings showing how institutional practices could continue within mainstream domestic settings creating an environment with greater similarity to a guest house than facilitating the agency of many personal home experiences (Peace & Holland, 2001).

AN OPPORTUNITY FOR INNOVATIVE METHODS AND RESEARCH DEVELOPMENT

During this time the UK's Economic and Social Research Council began to support research on ageing through the "Growing Older" program (1999–2004)—and Leonie, Caroline, and I were successful in gaining funding for collaborative work across two Higher Education Institutions focusing on "Environment and Identity" (1999–2003). This research brought together several strands of thinking: how do people define environment in later life? What is the association between self-identity and environment? And how might this differ for people living in a range of mainstream housing, supportive housing, and care homes in rural/urban localities? All issues arising through earlier studies. My return to academic life through this research led to reflection on how life history affects understanding of contemporary context; methods needed to embrace the concept of time; how the questions of academics, participants, and policy makers concerning housing needs vary, and the importance of developing participatory research approaches.

This was a qualitative study utilizing ethnographic methods with 54 respondents and 9 focus groups from 3 authorities in southern England. Through groupwork we heard the views of older people regarding how environment affected their lifestyle, life quality, and wellbeing. We used thematic analysis of these discussions to elicit common responses and develop a tool that we called the "facets of life wheel" (Peace, Holland, & Kellaher, 2006, p. 26)—a board with a moveable wheel divided into eight themes with suggested prompts (Figure 8.1) that respondents could use to determine where they might start an in-depth interview. All the themes were given equal weight. The academic team did not direct the conversation but ended the session asking a number of basic characteristic questions to enable some comparability. These were listed in boxes on either side of the wheel and related to structured questions. Interestingly, most participants covered a majority of the topics identified and were pleased to talk at length; the board focusing attention. Since this research, we have used an

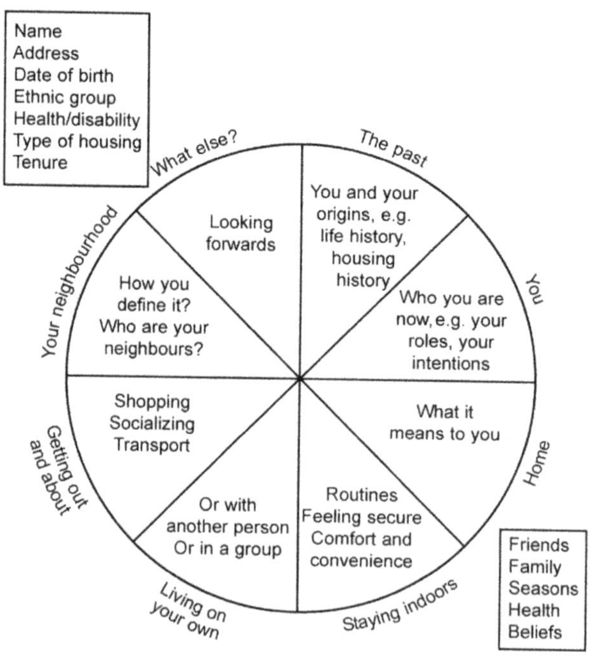

FIGURE 8.1 Facets of life wheel.
Source: Peace et al. (2006).

adapted version in qualitative research concerning the lives of people with "high support needs" (Katz, Holland, Peace, & Roberts, 2011) and an oral version for research with visually impaired older people (Peace, Katz, Holland, & Jones, 2016). In both cases, the original issues raised were less open-ended with more detail given to "health" and "support" and participants could add topics to the conversation.

The first chapter of the book from this research (Peace et al., 2006) is called "Placing the Self" and reviews literature that inspired us when discussing how an individual creates meaning for themselves in their situation, context, and setting. Given our backgrounds it is not surprising that we drew upon Lawton, Rowles, Rubinstein, and Golant from gerontology in the United States as well as Goffman, Bourdieu, Lefebvre, Baltes and Baltes, Massey, and Laws. While home is the focus for this chapter, our findings demonstrate a layered environmental approach to ageing in place from global to local where we tried to understand "how people create, or constantly try to create, a life of quality that meets their expectations" (Peace et al., 2006, p. 154). We created environmental biographies that captured temporal change and embraced complex definitions of home from the underpinnings of homeland through migration to the personal experience of embodiment, acceptance and comfort that you may find in one room. This research allowed us to see how unique perceptions of "environment" and "self-identity" may stand alone and then gain greater value through coming together.[1] The diversity of contexts studied led us to define the concept of "option recognition" (Peace et al., 2006, p. 129) where it was possible to see how person–environment (P-E) interaction experienced through daily routines, coping skills and competence within the complexity of different social, physical/material and psychological environments may present a "tipping point" for change leading some to make an informed move, some to a crisis situation, and others to "stay-put" (Peace, Holland, & Kellaher, 2011).

Two further extremes of environmental experience were studied during the noughties reflecting my deliberate wish to consider aspects of environment and ageing within different spatial contexts–community space and a room in everyday housing. At what I now see as a meso spatial level, I returned to my community survey routes through the Joseph Rowntree Foundation's public places program. Here our focus was intergenerational social interaction in the town of Aylesbury, Buckinghamshire (2004–2006) using nonparticipant observation to record patterns that were not only diurnal, but also seasonal. The only way to facilitate this research was through seeking community coresearchers who were

[1]Five respondents were filmed in their contemporary environment capturing aspects of personal biography through oral history (see Peace et al., 2006).

trained to observe certain sites throughout the town; one recording a narrative of interactions and the other mapping individuals (see Clark, Holland, Katz, & Peace, 2009; Holland, Clark, Katz, & Peace, 2007; Peace, 2013). Forty-six volunteers, aged 16 to 73 years, contributed to this research and through their data collection we were able to discuss temporal patterns within and between different age groups and how spaces were dominated, contested, and avoided reporting findings to local policy makers.

The environmental biography was also researched at the micro level of P-E interaction. In the second major initiative on ageing research run by the UK Research Councils in the New Dynamics of Ageing Programme (2008–2015), a funding call concerning "Nutrition and Ageing" led to a "sandpit" (retreat) where multidisciplinary scholars from nutritionists to engineers came together. To be part of this event my proposal focused on my personal experience of coping with Type 1 diabetes and concerns over kitchen design in the domestic environment as people get older. Eventually, the *Transitions in Kitchen Living* study brought together former student John Percival and I at The OU, and members of the Loughborough University Design School—ergonomists and designers. The kitchen became the most intense study of one micro environment that I have been part of. My experience of multidisciplinary research was to extend from interdisciplinary working in the social sciences to the field of inclusive/universal design.

The teams brought different skills, sharing, and learning each other's methods and supported by an Advisory Group including an Occupational Therapist, kitchen designer and lighting expert. We developed Holland's earlier housing history methods to focus on the experience of the kitchen across the life course for the 48 participants who worked with us in a detailed qualitative study. This purposive sample of 31 women and 17 men, living across the range of UK housing types from flats to terrace to detached, ranged in age from their 60s to 90s with dates of birth from 1919 to 1946. Their personal histories embraced the development of kitchen equipment in the UK and gender, ethnicity and social class informed life-course experiences. These interviews were followed by an ergonomic assessment of contemporary design, activity profiling and an interview concerning everyday kitchen living. The research was innovative and is continuing to be reported (Maguire et al., 2014; Peace, 2016) identifying not only a working example of the environmental docility hypothesis as changes in reach, dexterity, accessibility, vision highlight issues for design and adaptation/modification, but also how the kitchen embodies home living, often gender specific and represents a predictor of "option recognition" for those for whom the kitchen has been deserted becoming the provenance of home carers.

RESEARCH WITH APPLICATION

This chronological review shows how I have always felt that research should have some practical application. If I had become a community development worker the opportunity to work for change may, or may not, have been more immediate. As researchers, such change is not always within your power. For example, I go back to the national care homes study and the political environment in which it took place. In 1979, the UK elected a conservative government under Margaret Thatcher, staying in office for 11 years. During the 1980s, supplementary benefits for "board and lodgings" enabled people to spend funding on care home places run by the voluntary and private sectors. Since that time the independent sector has dominated care home provision in the UK. In the early 1980s, the government also deregulated the building development of care homes; building guidance was no longer published and we were invited to disseminate the research findings ourselves.

Perhaps unsurprisingly, given my comments concerning shared bedrooms in the 1970s, having a private room was the major change requested by residents. In talking to people about the move from their own home to a care home often via a hospital stay, having somewhere to create a sense of "home" was important this being the last place many would live. Recognizing the need for a design solution the research team proposed a "residential flatlet" which could be a single room with *en suite* bathroom and enough space to sit comfortably. Of course, while the use of this room would be very dependent on the management of the home and staffing, the team wanted to provide an environment that could at least provide a basis for empowerment.

The growth of independent care home services led to regulation through the *Registered Homes Act 1984* and the development of good practice guides and national minimum standards including research-based environmental changes. During the 1980s, the London-based think tank, Centre for Policy on Ageing, developed the code of practice "Home Life" (1984, revised 1996) with the Advisory group including Leonie Kellaher. In 1996, it was acknowledged that care homes were often not purpose-built and that major conversions would be expensive leading to deferred changes. However, residents should be offered a single room or the choice of sharing if requested. It is interesting to note that a paper on long-term care in 2013 shows that 93.8% of care homes (residential and nursing) have singles rooms and 73.5% with *en suite* WCs (Laing, 2014). For researchers who can trace the history of such change, 30 years have passed and this is seen as "upgrade of existing facilities rather than replacement of old stock with new facilities" (Laing, 2014, p. 12). This is just one example of the way in which research influences the built environment at a national scale.

CONTRIBUTIONS TO THE FIELD OF ENVIRONMENTAL GERONTOLOGY

While the interface between environment and ageing continues to be acknowledged, environmental gerontologists are reconsidering the need for theoretical and methodological development (Scheidt & Schwarz, 2013) at a time when other disciplines sit within and aside gerontology more recently finding ageing a relevant issue. While geographic gerontology emerges (Skinner, Andrews, & Cutchin, n.d.), I remain a gerontologist with an environmental perspective who recognizes the continuing challenge of ageism, and partners other disciplines to contribute to successful ageing. During the "noughties" members of the BSG with European colleagues developed the third edition of the text book *Ageing & Society* (Bond, Peace, Dittmann-Kohli, & Westerhof, 2007), and I worked with Hans-Werner Wahl, Heidrun Mollenkopf and Frank Oswald on the "Environment and Ageing" chapter. This was an important association through which I became part of the EuroAge Roadmap team for research on Environment and Ageing in EU Framework 8 with meetings in Heidelberg and Lund (March, June 2009).

Future challenges for theoretical development initially outlined in our work from 2007:

- Better integration of environmental docility and proactivity
- Better integration of the micro and macro level of analysis
- Better integration of temporality
- Better integration of physical and social environment
- Better integration of ongoing cohort dynamics
  (Peace et al., 2007, p. 211)

provides a framework to discuss a contribution to Environmental Gerontology. As a team-worker the contributions considered here are collective and also reflect the work of Leonie Kellaher and Caroline Holland. Within the E & I research the construction of "environmental biographies" that have a holistic life course perspective even though presently based primarily on cross-sectional research across cohorts are pioneering. We have developed innovative methods that capture temporality through oral history; engaged with layers of environmental experience and recognized the importance of routines within the every day which have similarities with Golant's (2003) discussion of "time" and "behavior." Other projects have focused either at the micro environment of the kitchen or the meso environment of the Aylesbury Community defining macro as addressing issues of globalization. Our mixed and participatory methodologies recognize "ongoing cohort dynamics" either through comparison of people spanning a 40-year period or through taking an intergenerational position to situate wider integration. We have seen the value of participatory research that involves the lay public as co-researchers while maintaining research rigor through training and support.

EMERGENT CHALLENGES–MEANING OF HOME FOR THE FUTURE

To conclude, this autobiographical account has foregrounded areas where our research could be taken further. In particular, I would like to see continuing research concerning the concept of "option recognition" especially through longitudinal research to understand how the meaning of home may be adapted, reassessed or reformulated within different types of place and space across later life. This work should inform social policy which in the UK has long supported the view held by many older people that they wish to live independently in their current home for "as long as possible." For some older people, many living alone or caring for a partner, this environment may no longer be "a comfort zone" needing either modification to the physical environment or greater possibility for social engagement to avoid isolation and loneliness and maintain wellbeing. Here we note how our thinking parallels Golant's views on residential normalacy and theoretical model of individual-environment congruence (Golant, 2012, 2015). This is where the feasibility of options beyond the nuclear family from intergenerational living to co-housing needs to be explored addressing issues relating to the housing market, equity and tenure alongside gendered, ethnic, and cultural preferences. I see Environmental Gerontology as central to future research that continues to highlight the context in which we live our lives as we grow older. My home, a ground floor flat in an Edwardian house in north London, is already showing its positive and negative attributes. A recent bicycle accident found my husband with broken bones and some corridors too narrow for the "gutter rack" zimmer he had to negotiate; but neither of us want to leave the city our location is more important. As an older academic, I will continue to add to this discussion from my writing hut at the bottom of the garden (Peace, n.d.).

REFERENCES

Bond, J., Peace, S., Dittmann-Kohli, F., & Westerhof, G. (2007). *Ageing in society* (3rd ed.). UK: Sage Publications.

Buttimer, A. (1969). Social space in interdisciplinary perspective. *The Geographical Review*, *59*(3), 417–426.

Bytheway, B. (1977). Problems of representation in 'The three generation family study'. *Journal of Marriage and Family*, *39*(2), 243–250.

Clark, A., Holland, C., Katz, J., & Peace, S. (2009). Learning to see: Lessons from a participatory observation research project in public space. *International Journal of Research Methodology*, *12*(4), 345–360.

Department of Health and Social Security & Welsh Office. (1973). Local authority building note no.2. *Residential accommodation for elderly people* (pp. 1–21). London, UK: Author.

Easthope, H. (2004). A place called home. *Housing Theory and Society*, *21*(3), 128–138.

Golant, S. M. (2003). Conceptualizing time and behaviour in environmental gerontology: A pair of old issues deserving new thought. *The Gerontologist*, *43*(5), 638–648. doi:10.1093/geront/43.5.638

Golant, S. M. (2012). Out of their residential comfort and mastery zones: Toward a more relevant environmental gerontology. In Scheidt, R. J., & Schwarz, B. (Eds.), *Environmental gerontology: What now?* (pp. 26–43). London, UK: Routledge.

Golant, S. M. (2015). *Aging in the right place*. Baltimore, MD: Health Professions Press.

Herbert, D. T., & Johnston, R. (Eds.). (1976). *Social areas in cities*. London, UK: John Wiley.

Holland, C. A. (2000). *Housing histories, older women's experiences of home*. (Doctoral dissertation). Milton Keynes: The Open University.

Holland, C., Clark, A., Katz, J., & Peace, S. (2007). *Social interactions in urban public places*. UK: Policy Press/Joseph Rowntree Foundation.

Jacobs, J. (1961). *The death and life of great American cities*. New York, NY: Random House.

Katz, J., Holland, C., Peace, S., & Roberts, E. (2011). *A better life: What older people with high support needs value*. Retrieved from https://www.jrf.org.uk/report/better-life-what-older-people-high-support-needs-value

Kellaher, L., Peace, S., & Willcocks, D. (1990). Triangulating data. In S. M. Peace (Ed.), *Researching social gerontology: Concepts, methods and issues* (pp. 115–128). London, UK: Sage Publications.

Laing, W. (2014). *Strategic commissioning of long term care for older people: Can we get more for less?* London, UK: LaingBuisson. Retrieved from http://www.laingbuisson.co.uk/Portals/1/Media_Packs/Fact_Sheets/LaingBuisson_White_Paper_LongTermCare.pdf

Lawton, M. P. (1970). Assessment, integration and environments for older people. *The Gerontologist*, *10*(1), 38–46. doi:10.1093/geront/10.1_Part_1.38

Lawton, M. P. (1980). *Environment and aging (The Brooks/Cole Series in Social Gerontology)*. Monterey, CA: Brooks/Cole Publishing Company.

Lawton, M. P. (2000). Chance and choice make a good life. In J. Birren & J. J. F. Schroots (Eds.), *A History of Geropsychology in Autobiography* (pp. 185–196). Washington, DC: American Psychological Association.

Lynch, K. (1960). *The image of the city*. Harvard, MA: MIT Urban Studies Series.

Maguire, M., Peace, S., Nicolle, C., Marshall, R., Simms, R., Percival, J., & Lawton, C. (2014). Kitchen living in later life: Exploring ergonomic problems, coping strategies and solutions. *International Journal of Design*, *8*(1), 73–91.

Pastalan, L. A., & Carson, D. H. (1970). *Spatial behaviour of older people*. Ann Arbor, MI: University of Michigan Press.

Peace, S. (1977). *The elderly in an urban environment: A study of spatial mobility in Swansea.* (Doctoral dissertation). University College of Swansea: South Wales.

Peace, S. (1981). *An international perspective on the status of older women.* Research Monograph, International Federation on Ageing, Washington D.C.

Peace, S. (1988). Living environments for the elderly. 2: promoting the 'right' institutional environment. In N. Wells & C. Freer (Eds.), *The ageing population: Burden or challenge?* (pp. 217–234). Basingstoke, UK: Macmillan.

Peace, S. (2013). Social interaction in public places and spaces: A conceptual overview. In G. Rowles & M. Bernard (Eds.), *Environmental gerontology: Making meaningful places in old age* (pp. 25–50). New York, NY: Springer Publishing.

Peace, S. (2015). Meanings of home and age. In J. Twigg, & W. Martin (Eds.), *Routledge handbook of cultural gerontology* (pp. 447–454). London, UK: Routledge.

Peace, S. (2016). Age-inclusive design–A challenge for urban living? In C. Bates, R. Imrie, & K. Kullman (Eds.), *Care & design: Bodies, buildings and cities* (pp. 18–32). London, UK: John Wiley & Sons.

Peace, S. (n.d.). *Environment and ageing: Place, space and materiality* [Manuscript in preparation]. Bristol, UK: Policy Press.

Peace, S., & Holland, C. (2001). Homely residential care: A contradiction in terms. *Journal of Social Policy*, *30*(3), 393–410.

Peace, S., Holland, C., & Kellaher, L. (2006). *Environment and identity in later life.* Maidenhead, UK: Open University Press.

Peace, S., Holland, C., & Kellaher, L. (2011). Option recognition in later life: Variations in ageing in place. *Ageing & Society*, *31*(5), 734–757.

Peace, S., Katz, J., Holland, C., & Jones, R. L. (2016). *Understanding the lives of older people with vision impairment.* Retrieved from http://www.pocklington-trust.org.uk/project/understanding-lives-older-people-vision-impairment

Peace, S., Wahl, H. W., Oswald, F., & Mollenkoph, H. (2007). Environment and ageing: Space, time and place. In J. Bond, S. Peace, F. Dittmar-Kohli, & G. Westerhof (Eds.), *Ageing in society* (3rd ed., pp. 209–234). London, UK: Sage Publications.

Percival, J. (2002). Domestic spaces: Uses and meanings in the daily lives of older people. *Ageing & Society*, 22(6), 729–749.

Rosow, I. (1967). *Social integration of the aged.* New York, NY: Free Press.

Rosser, C., & Harris, C. (1965). *The family and social change: A study of family and kinship in a South Wales town.* London, UK: Routeldge & Kegan Paul.

Rowles, G. (1978). *Prisoners of space? exploring the geographical experience of older people.* Boulder, CO: Westview Press.

Scheidt, R., & Schwarz, B (Eds.). (2013). *Environmental gerontology: What's now?* UK: Routledge, Taylor Francis.

Skinner, M., Andrews, G., & Cutchin, M (Eds.). (n.d.). *Geographical gerontology: Concepts and approaches* [Manuscript in preparation]. UK: Routledge.

Sommer, R. (1969). *Personal space: The behavioural basis of design.* Upper Saddle River, NJ: Prentice-Hall Inc.

Sommerville, P. (1997). The social construction of home. *Journal of Architecture and Planning Research*, *14*(3), 226–245. Retrieved from http://www.jstor.org/stable/43030210

Warnes, A. M (Ed.). (1982). *Geographical perspectives on the elderly*. Chichester, UK: John Wiley & Sons.

Warnes, A. M. (2009). International retirement migration. In Uhlenberg, P. (Ed.), *International handbook of population aging* (pp. 341–356). New York, NY: Springer Publishing.

Willcocks, D., Peace, S., & Kellaher, L. (1987). *Private lives in public places: A research-based critique of residential life in local authority old people's homes with a foreward by M. Powell Lawton*. London, UK: Tavistock Publications.

CHAPTER 9

Housing for Older Adults

A Personal Journey in Environmental Gerontology

Jon Pynoos

ABSTRACT

Personal experiences, observations, and empathy have often been my touchstones to identify problems and solutions in Environmental Gerontology. I have been influenced by the lives of people who I have known, places I have visited, and colleagues (including my wife Elyse Salend) with whom I have worked over the years. As a second generation researcher in the field, I have been fortunate to have known the pioneers who were generous with their time and supportive of my efforts. Several approaches underlie my work. First, as a result of growing up in the 1960s, I have been committed to social justice. Second, my research is translational in that it has attempted to impact policy, programs, and practices. Third, the inherent complexity of societal issues on which I have focused (e.g., housing, aging in place, long-term care, fall prevention, age-friendly communities) has led to my collaborating with colleagues from many disciplines. Fourth, context matters as history, values, people, and politics play a large role in shaping the built environment. Fifth, research in other countries has broadened my perspective and enriched my life. At the core of my concerns has been the disconnect between housing and long-term care that makes it difficult to support older frail persons who want to age in place. The lack of essential housing features and services disproportionally affect those with low incomes who have

http://dx.doi.org/10.1891/0198-8794.38.147

had limited housing choices. Aided by grants, I have analyzed a wide range of housing options, explored many facets of supportive housing, and honed in on home modifications. An integral part of my career has been teaching, mentoring others, applying lessons I have learned to my own environment, and advocating for better policies.

BIOGRAPHICAL NOTES

I had not intended to become an environmental gerontologist, but have always been interested in housing. My father was a civil engineer who, during WWII, designed military aircraft. While working on Howard Hughes' Spruce Goose, he invented the nail gun. Afterward, he became a contractor, specializing in custom homes in Southern California, many of them by designers who would later be on the roster of master architects. I went out with him on many jobs, and as a teenager, worked as a laborer helping to build them. The most famous architect with whom my father collaborated was the American Frank Lloyd Wright who at the time was 84 years old.

In celebration of Wright's "Sixty Years of Living Architecture," my father constructed an exhibit space in which dozens of architectural models and drawings became a reality. The exhibit space was next to Wright's Hollyhock House in Barnsdall Park in Los Angeles. I remember it well because of the very low ceilings (Mr. Wright was not a tall man) and wooden dining room chairs in which you had to sit very straight—a parent's dream. Mr. Wright was very upset if in *any* of *his* houses a single piece of furniture had been moved or anything altered. Reflecting back, his rigid attitude was antithetical to adapting the environment as a way of coping with physical and cognitive changes. He also told me to throw away my glasses, a crazy thing to tell a 9-year old *kid* with vision problems.

Given that background and my interest in design, I might have become an architect (actually my parents thought I would become a doctor), but drawing was then a prerequisite for admission into an architecture program, and I was not very proficient at it. Instead, as an undergraduate, I first chose economics and then the program in Urban and Regional Planning at Harvard's Graduate School of Design. This was during the mid-1960s when there was a pushback from top-down schemes of urban renewal and highways that dislocated low-income persons, including the elderly whose social networks were damaged, and in some cases, destroyed. As Herbert Gans, one of my professors pointed out, even though proponents of urban renewal painted a picture of blight and dilapidated housing, "The slum was home, providing the support of neighbors and relatives" (Wilson, 1966, p. 584). Marc Fried (1966) concluded that those displaced by urban renewal grieved for their lost homes (pp. 357–379).

In opposition to the top-down approach, I was involved in a "bottom-up" movement of advocacy planning in which the clients of urban planners were community groups and neighborhood organizations. I became Assistant Director of the Harvard Urban Field Service (UFS) run by Chester Hartman, a faculty member with expertise in housing and a strong commitment to social justice. A controversial program in the School of Design, UFS gave credit to students who worked in teams with faculty members on cutting edge projects that were at the time considered antiestablishment. These included opposing several urban renewal projects that threatened to destroy low-income neighborhoods and developing a physical modernization plan with resident control for an 1,100-unit public housing project in Boston. I subsequently edited, along with classmate Robert Schafer and Chester Hartman, *Housing Urban America* (Pynoos, Schafer, & Hartman, 1973, 1980), a widely read book that focused on housing problems of and policies for low-income persons. It touched on housing for the elderly only tangentially, noting that as subsidized family housing lost momentum, changes in housing subsidies led to a growth of housing designed specifically for the elderly, considered to be the worthy poor. Unfortunately that effort too was short lived.

BECOMING AN ENVIRONMENTAL GERONTOLOGIST

My journey in Environmental Gerontology began in 1966 with a tap on the door of my Cambridge apartment into which I had just moved. My neighbor introduced herself as Dorothy Burr Benton. A spry, 73-year-old dressed in silk brocade, she asked me to join her for tea. We lived in the Jarvis, a stately brick apartment building on Everett Street that was intergenerational. Mrs. B—as we called her—was a refined, articulate, intensely independent woman, a divorcee who'd raised a daughter alone, and worked for and later volunteered checking on elderly shut-ins for the Red Cross. Her apartment decor was understated with beautiful Victorian furniture, much of which she had inherited. The environment was a source of meaning, belonging, history, security, comfort, and socialization for Mrs. B and her visitors, somewhat like a time capsule to a different time and place. Mrs. B's afternoon teas brought together a cross-section of Cambridge society—old and young, affluent and low income, gay and straight, different races and ethnicities.

As our friendship deepened, I started to ponder what it was like to be an older person trying to live independently. As she entered her 80s, I began to see the Jarvis through her eyes: how the three flights she had to climb for lack of an elevator took their toll; how the fire marshal's order to remove a dumb waiter made grocery shopping infinitely harder. At 94, Mrs. B fell in her apartment having tripped over a foot-rest in the evening on the way to the bathroom. She had in place a phone system to check on her: The Red Cross called in the morning and her niece in the evening. In this one instance, the system failed. Mrs. B waited 12 hours for help to arrive, her telephone inches out of reach. Deemed too frail to return to the Jarvis, she was consigned to a stark white-walled nursing home in which she shared a room with a woman who had dementia. She wrote me from the facility: "Hard as it is to believe, I am no longer mistress of all that I survey. If you can imagine anything more ridiculous than my being dictated to, you have a sense of how things have changed."

Serendipitously, one of my first jobs during the summer was as a graduate research assistant for Sandra Howell, a Professor at MIT on a project that led to her brilliant book, *Designing for Aging: Patterns of Use* (Howell, 1980). It is based on a series of case studies in which she analyzed how older persons interact with their home environments, accompanied by photographs illustrating how they used the spaces. This approach has been useful in reflecting on my own experiences and conveying information about the environment and aging. Although I did not realize it at the time, as part of my assignment, I was reading and summarizing articles from pioneers in the field such as Powell Lawton, who later had an enormous impact on my work and influenced my career.

Soon thereafter, as part of the research for my PhD dissertation while I was a fellow at the Joint Center for Urban Studies of MIT and Harvard, I spent 6 months at large public housing projects in Boston and New York City, analyzing the operations of overburdened agencies charged with responsibility for housing low-income people and promoting integration in cities riddled with deep racial and ethnic problems. Later published as *Breaking the Rules: Housing Bureaucracy and Reform in Public Housing* (Pynoos, 1986), it analyzed how rules intended to reduce racial discrimination were implemented at a very large housing project of the Boston Housing Authority with a high proportion of minority residents and which, because of its size, often had vacancies. The rules were set up such that if applicants refused assignment they would be dropped to the bottom of the waiting list.

Based on data analysis, interviews, observations, and policy analysis that included historical context (methods that I have used in much of my research), I found that instead of following the rules, managers often exercised discretion by making exceptions based on individual applicant circumstances. Among those favored were white elderly applicants who wanted to live in smaller buildings in other parts of the city. My research supported Michael Lipsky's contention that it is the action of street-level bureaucrats rather than high-level officials who make policy. I have revisited these issues several times in my career related to mixing older persons and younger persons in federally assisted housing (Parrott &

Pynoos, 1996), the service needs of older persons on waiting lists for federally assisted housing, and the fairness of the system for housing elderly tenants.

After finishing my PhD, instead of accepting a faculty appointment I was offered at the University of Southern California's (USC) School of Urban and Regional Planning, with Mrs. B's encouragement, I became Executive Director of the newly formed nonprofit Minuteman Home Care/Area Agency on Aging in the suburbs of Boston. Minutemen's mission was to keep frail seniors in their own homes as long as possible. With funding from the U.S. Administration on Aging, it provided services to older persons in a 16-town region stretching from Arlington to Harvard. I recall that a member of Minuteman's Executive Board interviewing me for the job, looked at my resume, and said: "It looks like you are thinker and not a doer. We need a doer." I responded that I always felt it was important to think before I did something. They hired me.

However, he was correct. I didn't know what to do. But I was resourceful and called Elyse Salend, the Director of nearby Mystic Valley Home Care that had been running for almost 2 years to get advice about such matters as how to select sites for nutrition programs, what qualifications to look for in a case-management supervisor, and what services to provide. When we were married several years later, the joke was that I was marrying into money because her agency had a bigger budget than mine. Thirty-eight years later, we are both still working in the field of aging as are our two daughters, Jessica and Rebecca, who is also exploring aging and urban planning. Our son Josh took a different course: juvenile justice.

The Minuteman experience was an invaluable lesson about the challenges of organizing and planning services so that older persons could stay at home, what in the United States became referred to as "aging in place." It involved organizing support from sectors such as health, social services, transportation, and housing. Each had its own eligibility requirements, reporting system, and level of reimbursement or funding. Over time, Minuteman produced a regional plan for the area and delivered a range of services including home-delivered meals, transportation, information and referral, legal services, and programs (e.g., exercise, social, cultural). The linchpins were case managers who visited older people in their homes to conduct assessments and coordinate the care that they needed.

Although it was obvious that many older clients were living in homes with barriers, lacked supportive features, and were at risk of accidents, there was little we could provide beyond installing grab bars. Regardless, they did not want to leave. Part of the problem was few choices; only one large subsidized housing complex for low-income seniors was operating in the entire region, where we opened a meal site for residents and the community. These meals and our services enabled residents to stay much longer than otherwise would have been possible. In many ways, our Minuteman program laid the foundation for "supportive housing," a topic that I researched later in my career. We even went so far as to run a pilot project that brought nursing home residents to the meal site where they would eat and participate in social activities with other seniors. Unfortunately, this effort turned out to be very costly and we couldn't afford to continue the van transportation.

After 3 years as Director of Minuteman, I accepted the position of Special Assistant for Planning, Research and Demonstration Projects under Jim Callahan, Secretary of the Massachusetts Department of Elder Affairs. Jim was a role model of how to operate as a change agent for social change both within government and as an academic. He became my mentor and a long-term friend who encouraged me in my career. My experience as director of an agency and at the state level provided me with an invaluable grounding in housing, aging, services, and planning.

RETURNING TO ACADEMIA: RESEARCH AT USC

When Jim Callahan left Elder Affairs for Brandeis University, I began looking for a new endeavor. At that juncture, Victor Regnier, who 5 years earlier served on USC's School of Urban and Regional Planning's search committee, contacted me about an exciting new position to teach courses on public policy and oversee community programs at USC's Leonard Davis School of Gerontology. After a series of interviews with faculty, representatives of agencies, older members of the Andrus Volunteers, and Dean James Birren, I was offered and accepted the position of assistant professor in charge of community programs. It fit well with my experience at Minuteman in terms of trying to make a difference in the lives of older persons. Jim Birren made me the same offer as other faculty: a fishing license for obtaining grants to carry out research projects!

My major concern has been that the long-term care system is too often disconnected from housing and thus fails to support frail elderly in the community. At the same time, conventional housing lacks essential features and services that support safety, health, independence, caregiving, and social interaction.

As indicated above, personal experiences, observation and empathy are often my touchstones to identify problems and solutions. Several approaches underlie my research. First, I am firmly rooted in translational research and always interested in practical impact. Second, complex housing problems are often best addressed by involving persons from several disciplines. Third, context matters as history, values and political realities play a large role in policy.

Translational Research

Taking a cue from Powell Lawton, I have worked at the intersection of research, practice, and policy (Lawton, 1980). In keeping with my background in urban planning, I have consistently turned research findings, into formats to reach and influence a broad audience including policy makers, government officials, housing developers/sponsors, program administrators, practitioners, older persons, and their families.

Interdisciplinary Research

I have been fortunate over the years to have worked with many talented, innovative, and creative colleagues from a variety of fields: architecture (e.g., Victor Regnier, Jon Sanford, Maggie Calkins), interior design (Evelyn Cohen), planning (e.g., Tridib Banerjee, Dick Duncan), social welfare (e.g., Jim Callahan, Rob Hudson, Fernando Torres-Gil), social work (e.g., Susan Enguidanos), public policy/administration (e.g., Phoebe Liebig, Bob Myrtle), sociology (Don Redfoot), occupational therapy (e.g., Anna Nguyen, Liz Ainsworth, Dory Sabata), kinesiology (Debbie Rose) pharmacy (Brad Williams), medicine (e.g., Larry Rubenstein), geography (Steven Golant), and, of course, gerontology itself (e.g., Caroline Cicero, Bernard Steinman, Christy Nishita, Emily Nabors, Julie Overton, Rachel Caraviello). Much of my research has been under the umbrella of Centers for which, with the help of Maria Henke, I obtained multiyear funding: the National Resource Center on Housing and Long Term Care, the National Resource Center on Supportive Housing and Home Modifications, and the Fall Prevention Center of Excellence.

Social Justice and Context

I have moved between micro- and macro-level analyses, trying to understand connections between the two. I also place great importance on context and history. For example, with the support of a Guggenheim Fellowship, I have chronicled how trends, events, demographics, and politics have influenced government's role in subsidized housing for the elderly and the types of housing that have emerged (Pynoos, Kendig & Nishita, 2007; Pynoos & Nishita, 2006). As noted earlier, despite a perception that older persons in the United States have been considered the "deserving poor," successful housing programs for low- and moderate-income elderly have been underfunded and often eliminated. At the same time, senior housing for middle and upper income housing has proliferated.

HOUSING

When I first entered the field of aging, housing was perceived as a domain separate from health and long-term care. In the United States, there was housing for the elderly such as the federally funded Section 202 program but it was in short supply and intended for low-income persons who could live independently. It was assumed that as older persons became more frail, unless they had strong family support and the money to purchase services, they would move along a continuum from conventional housing to other settings such as board and care and nursing homes. However, as the costs of long-term care rose and research confirmed the desire of older persons to live in more conventional housing, pressure increased to make other settings including homes, apartments, and senior housing more physically supportive and connected with services (Pynoos, Feldman, & Ahrens, 2004; Vasunilashorn, Steinman, Liebig, & Pynoos, 2012).

Although I had considerable expertise in housing policy and planning, I knew less about design for the elderly. Fortunately, I filled that gap through teaching courses with Victor Regnier and working with him on our book *Housing the Aged: Design Perspectives and Policy Considerations* (Regnier & Pynoos, 1987) that won the Phi Kappa Phi Award. Through that project and at meetings of GSA, I met Powell Lawton, Gerry Weisman, Michael Hunt, and Leonard Heumann. As a person with severe visual problems stemming from keratoconus and cornea transplants, I was especially drawn to Lee Pastalan's work that simulated effects of vision loss.

Housing Options: Choices for Older Persons

I have conducted extensive research on a broad range of housing options because of the importance of older persons having choices, a key element of elder friendly communities (Alley, Liebig, Pynoos, Banerjee, & Choi, 2007). These studies analyzed who is served, how they have been developed, their impact on friendship formation, community building, participation in activities, wellbeing, and use cost effectiveness. These options have included home sharing, house matching, board and care homes, assisted living, accessory dwelling units, supportive housing, continuing care retirement communities (CCRCs), housing for persons with Alzheimer's disease and AIDS, and naturally occurring retirement communities (NORCs).

The NORC research has a special meaning because it was carried out in a 4,200 apartment community where I grew up in the 1950s called Park La Brea in Los Angeles. Initially occupied by families with children, it was not planned for older persons who in the 1990s accounted for over 20% of its population. We found that it was not meeting their needs for safety, physical access, emergency preparedness, social activities, and services for frail older persons who had become isolated and depressed. In response to our study, new programs were created involving roles for volunteers, leadership training, a talk line, transportation, and home modifications (Enguidanos, Pynoos, Siciliano, & Diepenbrock, 2010).

An International Perspective

I have been fortunate in that the Davis School has been a gateway for my international research on housing and aging in countries such as England, Australia, Japan, and Cuba. For example, in 1988, I met Dr. Tony Broe, a geriatrician from Sydney who, after visiting the School, invited me to Australia for 6 months as the RSL Visiting Professor at the School of Medicine to conduct research on the housing and service needs of veterans. My family lived in a small house on the grounds of a mental health hospital of which the only remaining residents were elderly living in a locked and fenced institutional building. Fittingly, after we left, our place was turned into a group home for them. I was especially impressed on home visits with geriatricians at their awareness of the home environment, how closely they worked with occupational therapists to make changes and efforts to bring services to hostels, a type of housing for the elderly. In Australia I met many colleagues such as Anna Howe, Liz Ainsworth, and Hal Kendig, with whom I worked on research over the years.

Soon after returning, I was off to Japan as a Fulbright scholar, to study housing for the elderly. My sponsor, a professor of Architecture, had arranged for us to live in a small Japanese house in a neighborhood of Tokyo. When he realized the young age of our children, he installed a lower handrail on the narrow spiral staircase (designed to save space) so they could more safely climb to the second floor. Of course, we slept on futons. The Fulbright provided me with an opportunity to study first-hand a country at the beginning of a population transition as it faced a rapid increase in the proportion of older persons. It was evident in the building of CCRCs (we stayed in one for a week), a universal designed house for a researcher at the Tokyo Metropolitan Center for Gerontology who had polio as a child, the development of technology, and home modifications of existing housing.

Such experiences were the impetus for an international meeting of experts that Phoebe Liebig and I organized at the Leonard Davis School followed by the publication of *Housing Frail Elders: International Policies, Perspectives and Prospects* (Pynoos & Liebig, 1995). According to all accounts, it was a path-breaking book of original chapters written by researchers from Europe, Israel, and the "New World" that underscores the importance of addressing the shelter and supportive services for the elderly. It also emphasizes that the movement has been occurring at different rates and forms in specific countries.

Following a similar format, I worked with the Visiting Nurses Association of New York to organize a conference of experts from United States to drill down on how to better coordinate services and housing in the United States. A book edited by myself, Penny Feldman, and JoAnn Aherns, *Linking Housing and Services for Older Adults: Obstacles, Options and Opportunities* (Pynoos et al., 2004) was based on the papers and presentations. One major recommendation was reversing the misguided policy during the early 1980s that, in the name of cost-cutting, required 20% of new units in subsidized housing for the elderly be built as studios instead of one bedroom and a reduction of common spaces. The studios lack sufficient space for caregiving and smaller common spaces have been inadequate for dining, services and activities.

Aging in Place in the Home and Community

I have viewed aging in place as a phenomenon, a preference, and an increasingly important subject of public policy. The preference to age in place is related to psychological attachment, security, familiarity, and the meaning of home itself (Chaudhury, 1999), and the community. It increases from 78% of adults between 50 and 64 years of age and 95% for age 75 and older, the group for whom aging in place is most problematic. At Minuteman, I had the opportunity to explore how home and community-based services help older persons to age in place and the difficulties of organizing assistance that crossed the boundaries of health, services, and transportation. But it turns out that the environment is equally as important and challenging.

Lawton and Nahemow (1973) pointed out the negative effects that result from an imbalance between the demands of the environment and the functioning level of the individual. Nowhere is this more apparent than in the homes where older persons live and spend most of their time. My friend and colleague, Patrick Hare, aptly referred to them as "Peter Pan" housing, designed for persons who will never grow old. Research corroborated the problem: less than 10% of housing units had supportive features such as ramps, grab bars, and handrails and only slightly over 1% had sink, faucet, cabinet modifications, and wall socket/light switch adaptations (Struyk & Katsura, 1988). Such housing also often had inadequate lighting. Overall, much of the housing we have built is poorly suited for older persons with balance, mobility, hearing, memory, and vision limitations to carry out activities and instrumental activities of daily living (ADL's and IADL's). I remember seeing one older lady precariously trying to get down the outside seven stairs of her apartment building to go shopping by placing her walker sideways just ahead of her as she went.

A major limitation in the United States has been that federal laws and regulations such as the Fair Housing Amendments Act of 1998, intended to provide basic accessibility in housing, does not apply retroactively, covers only housing of four units or more, and overlooks many features that would help older persons as they age (Pynoos, Nishita, Cicero, & Caraviello, 2008). Consequently, it leaves out the majority of homes and apartments in which older persons live. Over the years, I have been a proponent of creating programs that would support aging in place in order to give older persons a choice of staying in their home, apartments, and communities. Toward that end, I have spent considerable effort to move it higher on the public policy agenda as well as to raise the awareness of older persons, and their families about how to make it more possible. Our online Executive Certificate in Home Modifications program has trained over 1,000 professional and practitioners from a variety of fields such as occupational therapy, gerontology, social work, and remodeling.

Home Modifications

Home modification (HM) refers to adapting the environment to increase use, safety, security, health, social interaction, and independence. Surveys of older persons have suggested that such factors as affordability, inability to make the changes oneself, and not having a trusted person to make changes, present barriers to older persons modifying their homes (AARP, 2000). Many older persons do not think that they need them or don't perceive that they will make a difference. But there are also psychological and aesthetic considerations. In one of our studies, an occupational therapist that assessed an older woman's home reported that she was willing to put a grab bar in the back bathroom that was rarely used but not in the front bathroom for guests and where she took baths. She did not want to reveal the extent of her disability nor a shiny grab that clashed with her décor. It therefore came as no surprise that after I conducted an assessment of President Ronald Reagan's home because of his advancing Alzheimer's disease, that Mrs. Reagan had me send my recommendations to her interior designer.

In order to explain the process of HM, we developed categories to reflect different types of environmental changes. These include changes that are additive, subtractive, transformational, and behavioral (Figure 9.1; Pynoos, Steinman, Nguyen, & Bresette, 2012).

Additive modifications refer to new supportive features or structural changes. Because they often require professional installation by contractors or remodelers, the cost may be relatively expensive compared to other types of changes. *Subtractive* modifications involve the removal of items or hazards and tend to be less expensive as well as easier for individuals to implement on their own. *Transformative* modifications include restructuring the existing environment to facilitate the use of space and features. *Behavioral* modifications include avoidance or adoption of specific behaviors. Faced with climbing up steep stairs to his bedroom on the second floor, which he described as the equivalent of climbing Mt. Everest, one older gentleman told us he slept on the couch on the first floor. Similarly, those who can't shop or don't cook may rely on home-delivered meals. In accordance with Lawton and Nahemow's (1973) ecological model of person–environment fit, behavioral modifications recognize the

Home Modification Categories					
Type	Role	Purpose	Execution	Cost	Example
Additive	Accommodate physical changes	Improve access/safety	Contractors; remodelers	$ - $$$$	Grab bars in bathrooms; installing wheelchair ramp
Subtractive	Remove hazards	Increase safety	Older person	$	Remove throw rugs; clearing clutter
Transformative	Facilitate space use	Improve access/safety	Contractors; remodelers	$ - $$$$	Widening doorways; clearing passages
Behavioral	Avoidance/adoption of specific behaviors	Reduce stress; increase safety	Older person	$ - $$	Sponge bath instead of bathing in bathtub; sleeping on lower level

FIGURE 9.1 Categories of home modification.
Source: Pynoos et al. (2012).

potential of behavior change as a means to reestablish equilibrium between the capabilities of individuals, and their environments.

England, Australia, and Japan have made home modification a priority. For example, Japan has a National Long Term Care Insurance program that provides funds for modifications such as installing handrails or grab bars, addressing different levels of floors, modifying doors and replacing old Japanese style toilets with Western style fixtures (Makigami & Pynoos, 2002). Similar to other countries, however, debates continue about prosthetic versus preventative approaches.

The United States has been far behind, especially in assisting low-income older persons. Our studies have found that Medicare and Medicaid pay for some medically necessary assistive devices, but only limited home modifications. Despite a variety of Medicaid waivers, Community Development Block Grants and Older Americans Act Title III funds, they are often unreliable. They also vary from one geographic area to another due to state and local policies. It is difficult to patch together funds from a variety of programs that have different eligibility requirements, caps on the amount spent per person, and limited types of HMs that are covered. Several more comprehensive programs such as PACE (Program of All-Inclusive Care for the Elderly) and Money Follows the Person with responsibility for the health and community-based care of frail older persons include HMs. Over a decade ago, I suggested that what might make a difference is evidence indicating the cost effectiveness of HM for health and long-term care services. A major breakthrough along these lines is CAPABLE (Community Aging in Place, Advancing Better Living for Elders), a program developed at Johns Hopkins that involves a team of an occupational therapist, a nurse and a handyman has demonstrated that visits and a modest package of home modifications averaging $1,300 can improve functioning and save health-care expenditures (Szanton, Leff, Wolf, Roberts, & Gitlin, 2016). These type of programs need to be brought to scale. Funds are also needed to insure retrofitting and proper maintenance of multiunit residential buildings.

While immediate needs often dictate HM, we have explored other approaches that can lead consumers to think ahead. For example, a project that we conducted with the Hartford Insurance Company, which employs several gerontologists, found that providing their claimants, who had suffered major damage to either their kitchen or bathroom with information about universal design, resulted in significant changes than they otherwise would not have considered (Beck et al., 2016). On the basis of this research the Hartford has instituted a program of incentives for universal design.

Fall Prevention

I had been long interested in falls but never expected it to be a major phase in my career. I knew from my own experience and the earlier case of Mrs. B, that falls could result in serious injuries that jeopardize older persons' ability to age in place. Our work on HM included identification of environmental problems that could contribute to falls and recommendations for corrective action. Serendipity of the Archstone Foundation having funded much of our efforts in aging in place and HM, Mary Ellen Kullman invited us to be part of an interdisciplinary team to address falls in a more comprehensive manner. In essence, she was the matchmaker of what became the Fall Prevention Center of Excellence (FPCE). Our strength was the involvement of five institutions: USC (Jon Pynoos) UCLA/VA (Larry Rubenstein, Josie Kramer), Cal State Fullerton (Debbie Rose), and the California Department of Public Health (Barb Alberson). FPCE's major activities included raising awareness, developing interventions, building CA state coalitions, and training professionals and students. FPCE designed a fall prevention model (InStep) that varied the intensity (high, medium, and low) of three components (medical risk assessment, exercise, and home modifications). Results indicated that overall, the high and medium intensity were most effective in reducing the incidence of falls. Home assessments conducted by occupational therapists and social workers, were comparable, while those only done by older persons/family members were much lower (Kramer et al., 2014).

While the traditional research has been exciting and worthwhile, I have especially enjoyed creating and testing programs in which Emily Nabors, Julie

Overton, Anna Nguyen, Maria Henke and I tried to think outside of the box. For example, *FP Connect* involved fire department emergency responders, an untapped resource, in conducting fall-related home assessments when going out to the homes of older persons. We commissioned *The Falling Monologues*, five semi-humorous vignettes written and performed by older actors and actresses, to raise the consciousness about fall prevention, the environment, and behavior. They have been performed by groups around the country and are on YouTube. *Beyond Space and Beyond Time* were exhibits in donated retail space in shopping malls that showcased attractive home modifications, a universal designed kitchen, new technology and bathroom innovations. A universal-designed dollhouse_shrunk the exhibits to appeal to young and old alike, stimulating conversations among different generations.

Housing, aging in place, home modifications, and fall prevention are linked. The underlying foundation for research in these areas is my background in urban and regional planning. Almost all conventional housing and neighborhoods were not built with older persons in mind. Their lack of basic accessibility and supportive features make it difficult for older persons to function and put them at risk of falling. This is even true in suburban areas built after WWII for single families in suburban areas. However, in the United States and many other countries, there is a strong desire to age in place. Hence, the need for more widespread availability of home modifications and, for those who need to move, a variety of supportive housing options in age friendly communities.

PUTTING RESEARCH INTO PRACTICE

I have had the opportunity to test what I have learned about the environment in my own personal life. For example, I modified a small structure in the back of our house into a “granny” (or in this case a “grandpa”) flat to accommodate my father-in-law Harry who came from the East to live with us. He had a feeding tube because of throat cancer and was at high risk of falling because his gait was very irregular. Ed Steinfeld and Victor Regnier, well-known environmental gerontologists, graciously drew up a floor plan and specs based on the principles of universal design. It included features such as nonglare lighting, a walk in shower with a temperature control valve to avoid scalds, a light switch and panic button near the bed, nonskid tile in the bathroom, a lever handle faucet, flat carpet glued to the floor, and grab bars near the raised toilet. I discovered the difficulty of finding appropriate products and materials; the lack of guidelines about how to proceed and the challenge of creating an environment that took into account Harry’s particular needs. Harry’s back house was attractive and residential. He lived with us for five years, carrying out his ADLs and IADLs independently. It always warmed my heart to find Harry and our young son Josh back there doing what they both liked best: watching baseball games together on a large TV we had installed. Every month a nurse came to clean out Harry's feeding tube and remarked that people with his health problems were usually in nursing homes. Harry told her that he was able to enjoy his three grandchildren because of the care we provided and the attention paid to the design of where he was living. The two went hand in hand. Fortunately, he never fell. I now wonder, as I grow older, if I will be living in the back house because of the reality that in the early 1980s, we purchased an older home with many accessibility problems.

In my role as a Board Member of Menorah Housing Foundation, a nonprofit provider of Section 202 housing for elderly, I have supported changes that would make life easier and safer for residents, staff and caregivers. Based on my experience with Harry and state of the art design in housing for the elderly, new buildings have only walk-in showers. In all buildings, enhanced nonglare lighting was installed and thresholds removed. These changes have universally drawn praise.

CONTRIBUTIONS

My work has helped break down the barriers between housing and long-term care, establish the home as a long-term care site of the future, spur research about aging in place and housing options for older persons, lay the groundwork for studies demonstrating the efficacy and cost savings of HM, and develop new models of fall prevention. Along the way I have not only written books and articles, but also produced materials and training programs for professionals, practitioners, caregivers, older persons, and family members. I am especially proud of my advocacy for policy changes through my publications, testimony before Congressional Committees, service on National Science Foundation's Task Force on Human Factors, and the California Commission on Aging. As a delegate at three White House Conferences on Aging I was able to get propositions passed in favor of supportive housing, aging in place, home modifications and fall prevention. But my most important legacy is through the students for whom I have been a mentor and with whom I have continued to collaborate on research and test new models.

FUTURE RESEARCH

We have made great strides in conducting research about housing, aging in place, HM, and fall prevention. We need more case studies of people living in their homes over time in terms of what changes they make and their view about the meaning of home. In addition, it would be helpful to have longitudinal data on housing features in both housing and health datasets instead of just one-time special studies. In a time of potentially less government support it will be especially important to preserve the housing that exists, develop new technologies and products that make it easier to age in place, protect older persons in areas where gentrification is occurring, and scale up evidence-based programs so they are more available.

I have recorded over 40 hours of interviews with Mrs. B, and now is the time to finish transcribing them and to write an oral history of her life. Similarly, I have taped interviews of pioneers in the field of housing for the elderly that I want to update as the basis for a book on the social history of housing for the elderly. I have several research projects underway related to home modifications, fall prevention, and universal design. In addition, I am part of research initiative to assess how permanent supportive housing can address geriatric syndromes for older persons who are homeless.

CLOSING OBSERVATIONS

I had not consciously intended to be in the field of aging, let alone Environmental Gerontology. But fortunately, I took American poet Robert Frost's proverbial "road less travelled" (in a poem that I heard him read during my first year in college) "and that has made all the difference." Looking back we have made considerable progress in both understanding and creating better housing for the elderly. But the rapid aging of the world's population and the increasing likelihood of living into advanced old age, challenges us to develop new models and policies that better link housing with services and health care. A critical element is to create policies that result in more accessible, supportive, and affordable housing in the first place and to modify existing homes so that older people can age in place. This underscores the importance of the right to housing.

REFERENCES

AARP. (2000). *Fixing to stay: A national survey of housing and home modification issues*. Washington, DC: Author.

Alley, D., Liebig, P., Pynoos, J., Banerjee, T., & Choi, I. (2007). Creating elder-friendly communities: Preparations for an aging society. *Journal of Geriatric Social*, *49*(3), 1–18.

Beck, P., Enguidanos, S., Rahman, A., Nabors, E., Tracton-Bishop, B., Olshevski, J., & Pynoos, J. (2016). Making universal design modifications following a homeowners insurance claim. *Journal of Housing for the Elderly*, *30*(3), 237–252.

Chaudhury. H. (1999). Self and reminiscence of place: A conceptual study. *Journal of Aging and Identity*, 4(4), 231–253.

Enguidanos, S., Pynoos, J. Siciliano, M., & Diepenbrock, L. (2010). Integrating community services within a NORC: The Park La Brea Experience. *Cityscape: A Journal of Policy Development and Research*, 12(2), 29–45.

Fried, M. (1966). Grieving for a lost home: Psychological costs of relocation. In J. Q. Wilson (Ed.), *Urban renewal: The record and the controversy* (pp. 359–379). Cambridge, MA: MIT Press.

Howell, S. (1980). *Designing for aging: Patterns of use*. Cambridge, MA: MIT Press.

Kramer, B. J., Creekmur, B., Mitchell, M. N., Rose, D., Pynoos, J., & Rubenstein, L. Z. (2014). Community fall prevention programs: Comparing three InStep models by levels of intensity. *Journal of Aging and Physical Activity*, 22(3), 372–379.

Lawton, M. P. (1980). *Environment and aging*. Boston, CA: Brooks/Cole.

Lawton, M. P., & Nahemow, L. (1973). Ecology and the aging process. In C. Eisdorfer & M. P. Lawton (Eds.), *The psychology of adult development and aging* (pp. 619–674). Washington, DC: American Psychological Association.

Makigami, K., & Pynoos, J. (2002). The evolution of home modification programs in Japan. *Ageing International*, 27(3), 95–112.

Parrott, T., & Pynoos, J. (1996). Uncommon ground: The politics of mixing older persons and younger persons with disabilities in federally assisted housing. *The Gerontologist*, 36(4), 518–529.

Pynoos, J. (1986). *Breaking the rules: Bureaucracy and reform in public housing*. New York, NY: Plenum Press.

Pynoos, J., Feldman, P., & Ahrens, J. (Eds.). (2004). *Linking housing and services for older adults: Obstacles, options, and opportunities*. New York, NY: The Haworth Press.

Pynoos, J., Kendig, H., & Nishita, C. (2007). *Housing*. In J. R. Birren, V. Marshall, T. Cole et al. (Eds.), *Encyclopedia of gerontology* (pp. 709–719). Oxford: Elsevier.

Pynoos, J., & Liebig, P. (Eds.). (1995). *Housing frail elders: International policies, perspectives, and prospects*. Baltimore, MD: Johns Hopkins University Press.

Pynoos, J., & Nisihita, C. (2006). Elders and the right to housing. In R. Bratt, M. Stone & C. Hartman (Eds.), *A right to housing: Foundation for a new social agenda* (pp. 279–295). Philadelphia, PA: Temple University Press.

Pynoos, J., Nishita, C., Cicero, C., & Caraviello, R. (2008). Aging in place, housing and the law. *The Elder Law Journal*, 16(1), 77–106.

Pynoos, J., Schafer, R., & Hartman, C. (Eds.). (1973). *Housing urban America*. New York, NY: Aldine.

Pynoos, J., Schafer, R., & Hartman, C. (Eds.). (1980). *Housing urban America* (2nd ed.). New York, NY: Aldine.

Pynoos, J., Steinman, B., Nguyen, A., & Bresette, M. (2012). Assessing and adapting the home environment to reduce falls and meet the changing capacity of older adults. *Journal of Housing and the Elderly*, 26(1), 137–155.

Regnier, V., & Pynoos, J. (Eds.). (1987). *Housing and the aged: Design perspectives and policy considerations*. New York, NY: Elsevier.

Struyk, R. J., & Katsura, H. (1988). Aging at home: How the elderly adjust their housing without moving. *Journal of Housing for the Elderly*, *4*, 1–192.

Szanton, S., Leff, B., Wolf, J., Roberts, L., & Gitlin, L. (2016). Home-based care program reduces disability and promotes aging in place. *Health Affairs*, *35*(9), 1158–1563.

Vasunilashorn, S., Steinman, B. A., Liebig, P. S., & Pynoos, J. (2012). Aging in place: Evolution of a research topic whose time has come. *Journal of Aging Research*, *2012*, 1–6.

Wilson, J. Q. (1966). *Urban renewal: The record and the controversy*. Cambridge, MA: MIT Press.

CHAPTER 10

The Role of Community and the Environment in the Lives of Older People

Understanding Local and Global Social Change

Chris Phillipson

ABSTRACT

This chapter provides an overview of the various strands of my research on community and environmental perspectives on aging and later life. Following an outline of biographical influences and early work in critical gerontology, the chapter provides examples from research (with a variety of colleagues) covering themes relating to family and community life in old age, the impact of social exclusion, and the development of transnational communities. The chapter then reviews subsequent work on the impact of globalization on urban life, and research on the theme of "age-friendly cities." The chapter concludes with a summary of future research agendas for Environmental Gerontology.

BIOGRAPHICAL NOTES

Engaging with ideas associated with "community" and "the environment" has been an important part of my career as a sociologist working in the field of aging. Research on this topic played a significant role in my initial training and induction as a sociologist. There was then a period devoted to other research interests

http://dx.doi.org/10.1891/0198-8794.38.165

before a return to community-related concerns in the middle and later phases of my career. In this chapter, I will provide some biographical background to explain the origins of my interests; indicate some of the main themes developed in my research; review a number of findings which have emerged from different studies; and summarize my own priorities for future research. The chapter begins by reflecting on the extent to which my interest in community and environmental issues link with aspects of my personal history and development as a sociologist.

BACKGROUND AND TRAINING

In terms of origins, I was born in 1949 in London, UK, spending my first 13 years living in the suburb of Harrow-on-the-Hill. Both my parents had been born in London. My father was an aircraft engineer whose family came from the East End (around Poplar and Bow), an area where he retained extensive family ties. When I was 13 the family moved, for a variety of reasons, to Cornwall, a mainly rural area in the southwest of England, where my mother had strong family connections. Socialization into an urban and then a rural community certainly provided a sense of the contrasting experiences and opportunities which neighborhoods could provide. Of more immediate importance, however, at least from a biographical perspective, was the disruption to my education which ultimately led me to leave school soon after the age of 15, going to work on farms for a couple of years before attending agricultural college. In fact, it soon became clear during my time at the college that my interests were moving in an opposite direction to working on the land. In what kind of direction was unclear to me at the time, but I was at least fortunate to be given good advice that I should resume my studies and attempt to widen my career options.

I made a relatively brief return to full-time education (studying at a local technical college) to pick up sufficient qualifications to get into higher education, but even at this point I was unsure (a) whether this was a sensible thing to do (no one else in the family had done it before—a common experience among working-class/lower middle-class families at the time); or (b) what I should study. As a result, I decided to delay any decision and spent a year as a community service volunteer (CSV; see Chapter 8, Home Thoughts) working in a large (c. 800 beds) psychiatric hospital, located in Somerset, a rural county in the southwest of the UK. CSV was a national organization which sent young people to projects around the UK (and overseas), typically to communities where different kinds of help and support were required. The purpose of my own project was to forge links between the hospital—which was set in the countryside—and the nearest town (some 10 miles distant).

In many ways, it was an overwhelming task for someone completely unprepared for the complexity of the relationships and issues faced by the hospital. But the experience did leave many lasting impressions which were almost certainly influential in the career path which I finally chose to adopt. Two aspects were of particular importance: first, a large proportion of patients in the hospital were older people, most of whom had spent years—decades in many cases—confined to the "back wards" of the hospital and were victims of the kind of "institutionalization" memorably described by Irving Goffman (1961) (whose work I had briefly studied at technical college). The conditions experienced by older patients were dreadful in terms of the lack of any facilities or personal care: completely dehumanizing in many ways, obvious even to a neophyte such as myself.

But another dimension to my experience at the hospital was also to assume long-term significance. My stay coincided with the rise of what came to be known as the "antipsychiatry movement," led in the UK by R. D. Laing ([1960] along with David Cooper and others) whose book *The Divided Self* had an enormous influence on many of my generation and especially those of us who had first-hand experience of psychiatric institutions. I was unaware of the book when I began working in the hospital but was introduced to it by a day patient who came into a club I was running (one designed to get patients and public to get together for coffee) brandishing a copy of the book and suggesting that there might be better things I could do with my time. The theme of *The Divided Self* was that "madness" was better understood as a "lived experience" (e.g., reflecting disturbed family dynamics) rather than an underlying biological/genetic disorder. "Madness" in essence should be taken out of the realm of individual pathology and into a broader understanding of how society itself (notably the family) treats/scapegoats particular individuals. I found the arguments in the book difficult to understand at the time but I was attracted to the case being made. Moreover, it chimed well with my growing sense that a better understanding of "society" and the social changes (and conflicts) which were happening at the time would be worth pursuing: hence my move into studying for an undergraduate degree in sociology.

SOCIOLOGICAL TRAINING

I had just scraped sufficient qualifications to get into higher education and was successful in an application to Birmingham Polytechnic to undertake a 4-year degree in the subject. I was already committed to applied research and this particular program had a year-long placement in community organizations, combining an undergraduate degree in sociology with qualification as a community worker. The early 1970s was an exciting time to be a student: immersion in studies for sure but numerous opportunities to be engaged in various forms of community and political action (the war in Vietnam was at its height and demonstrations in London were for me as with many others almost a weekly event). The development of community-related interventions became highly significant in the late 1960s/early 1970s, with a particular focus on inner-city areas affected by high levels of economic and social deprivation (see, e.g., Craig, Derricourt, & Loney, 1982; Leonard, 1975).

During my time as an undergraduate, I had become increasingly interested in issues affecting older people. This reflected, as previously noted, my work in the psychiatric hospital but as an undergraduate I spent time as a voluntary worker in a geriatric hospital (as it was then called) located in an inner-city part of Birmingham. Conditions in the hospital were extremely poor, with crowded wards and a sense of despair and alienation among the elderly patients. A study of their experiences and social attitudes toward older people more generally formed the subject of my undergraduate dissertation. Writing the dissertation fired my enthusiasm for research and I was fortunate to be awarded a 3-year studentship to study for a PhD, at the Department of Sociology and Social Policy at Durham University. The University proved to be an inspired choice in many respects. The department was led by Philip Abrams, a fine social scientist who had written extensively on the history of sociology (Abrams, 1968) but was also—during my time in Durham—leading important work on the sociology of neighboring (Bulmer, 1986) and research on the commune movement in Britain (Abrams, McCulloch, Abrams, & Gore, 1976). The department also developed a close interest in the mining communities which had dominated the industrial landscape of Durham, as well as shipbuilding—an industry which had been of particular importance in the North-East of England.

My doctoral research, which examined the transition from work to retirement among men from different occupational groups, reflected growing interest in community aspects of ageing. The study comprised 100 tape-recorded interviews: 25 miners; 25 men living in an inner-city community in Newcastle; 25 car workers; and 25 architects. The purpose of the research was to examine how different class and occupational contexts influence retirement, but with the intersection with community—both geographical and occupational—also important. The work drew upon my reading of earlier community studies (see further in the following text), which had stressed the importance of immersing oneself in the life of the community. In the case of the miners, for example, I lived in the adjacent mining village to the one I studied, spent time in the pubs and clubs, and also went underground in a working mine at one point (Phillipson, 1980, 1987).

DEVELOPING CRITICAL GERONTOLOGY

Following completion of my doctorate, interest in community and related issues were put to one side while I completed a number of projects focused on evaluating the benefits of preretirement education, investigating health promotion for older people, and developing what became known as "critical gerontology" in association with scholars such as Carroll Estes in the United States and Alan Walker in the UK.

This strand of my work—which has been prominent throughout my career as a researcher—developed from publication of my book *Capitalism and the Construction of Old Age* (Phillipson, 1982). The book—which reflected my interest (which has remained) in Marxist political economy—contributed to ideas which had started to emerge in the 1970s and early 1980s around the "social construction of ageing." After publication of the book I came across the work of Carroll Estes (her study *The Ageing Enterprise* [1979] was a great influence on my own work) and also papers by Alan Walker (1980, 1981). Along with others, we started corresponding and writing about what came to be termed the "political economy perspective on ageing" (later critical gerontology). Estes (1991, p. 19) defined this approach as follows:

> A political economy perspective on aging and old age emphasizes the broad implications of economic life for the aged and for society's treatment of the elderly. It is a systematic view predicted on the assumption that old age can only be understood in the context of problems and issues of the wider social order. Significantly, the aged are not treated as a homogenous group or category. Rather a key element is the analysis of the implications of class, gender, and race for all aspects of the definition and management of the elderly.

A subsequent strand of work in critical gerontology (developed with Carroll Estes but also with Jan Baars and Dale Dannefer) concerned the impact of globalization on older people, illustrated through greater inequalities within and between societies, and the impact of economic austerity arising from financial instabilities associated with globalization. These issues were reviewed in Baars, Dannefer, Phillipson, and Walker (2006) and in various symposia at conferences, notably those of the Gerontology Society of America. To help expand work in critical gerontology, I founded, with a number of colleagues, in the early 1980s, the Centre for Social Gerontology, at Keele University, devoted to pursuing critical perspectives, with a particular focus on questions relating to social theory, community surveys, and action research.

DEVELOPING COMMUNITY AND ENVIRONMENTAL RESEARCH

My first major opportunity for research relating to community and neighborhood arose from securing substantial funding (in the late 1990s), from the UK Economic and Social Research Council, for a project investigating postwar changes in the family and community life of older people. The inspiration for the research came from the British tradition of community studies, represented by work carried out by Young and Willmott (1957), Townsend (1957), Willmott and Young (1960) and Frankenberg (1966) (see, further, Phillipson & Thompson, 2008). This body of research had come under attack during the 1970s and 1980s, with concerns expressed about lack of rigor and generalizability (Crow & Allan, 1994).

By the 1990s, however, interest in community issues had come back on the agenda, in part driven by awareness of the influence of environmental factors in contributing to poverty and related problems affecting many urban areas (Taylor, 2004). My own experience of community action in the 1970s, studies such as those by Young and Willmott (1957), and the development of area-based interventions to tackle poverty (Loney, 1985), all confirmed my view that the idea of community was still valuable as a framework for "thinking about" and analyzing social issues (Morgan, 2008). Crow (2002, para.1.3) highlights the ability of community research to: ". . . reveal the local expression of macro-social forces and their impact on ordinary people's everyday activities as they are lived out in the locality." This may be of particular significance for communities undergoing changes associated with economic recession, high levels of in- or out-migration, or urban regeneration—issues which became especially significant for researchers in the 1980s and 1990s.

The above concerns were especially relevant for the study which was eventually published as *The Family and Community Life of Older People* (Phillipson, Bernard, Phillips, & Ogg, 2001). The idea behind the research was to revisit three areas which had been the subject of major community studies carried out in the late 1940s and during the 1950s: Bethnal Green, in the London Borough of Tower Hamlets (the subject of research by, among others, Townsend, 1957; Young & Willmott, 1957); suburban Woodford (also London; Willmott & Young, 1960); and the metropolitan borough of Wolverhampton (Sheldon, 1948). The starting point for the research was the question: *how different was it to be an older person in the late 20th century in comparison with the late 1940s and 1950s?* To help answer this question the research drew upon Frankenberg's (1966) observation that the early community studies had demonstrated that older people were surrounded by what he termed an "*environment of kin*." This phrase was used to develop a number of specific research questions which could be tested though different types of data collection and field work. The resulting study interviewed 627 older people across the three areas, with a follow-up qualitative phase of interviews with people 75 and over as well as those identified as important within their networks.

Social Change and Urban Neighborhoods

The results from the research have been reported elsewhere (Phillipson et al., 2001), the main question examined in this chapter is the extent to which this type of research aids understanding of the changes affecting urban neighborhoods. One answer would be to refer back to the point made by Crow (2002) above, namely, that thinking about how the lives of older people are shaped and connected to immediate local contexts (as well as national and transnational ones) remains an important task for sociology in general and Environmental Gerontology in particular. Bell and Newby's (1971, p. 18) comment about community research in the 1950s and 1960s that: ". . . there is no study that has demonstrated that nobody has any local relationships," remains accurate. Indeed, given demographic changes since that period, with the increased proportion of older people in the community, it is almost certainly the case that neighbourhoods have become more important with older people having *more* rather than fewer local relationships. There is therefore a strong case for seeing how these complement or substitute for other kinds of ties. Arguably, this can only be done by examining people's lives in local contexts, exploring the full range of individuals, groups, and organizations through which everyday life is built and maintained (Crow & Allan, 1994).

In addition, and linked to the above, drawing comparisons with communities at different time periods can allow some important points about social change to be developed. For example, our own study of Wolverhampton suggested the maintenance of a form of "local extended family." In this instance, our findings suggested that ties to kin and neighborhood had undergone less fragmentation than might have been expected since the baseline study. On the other hand, there was also a suggestion that for people losing a tie of central significance in their lives (for example with the death of a spouse or partner) there often appeared fewer "strong" relationships to fall back upon. Indeed, this itself reflected an important finding that in comparison with the 1950s, the "couple relationship" had moved center stage, with older people (men in particular) more often viewing their partner as a confidant (Jamieson, 1998), this in sharp contrast with the tension between husband and wives conveyed in studies of English working-class communities in the 1950s carried out by Townsend (1957) and Dennis, Henriques, and Slaughter (1956).

Finally, and following on from the above, a further argument for community studies and restudies might be linked with Morgan's (2008) advice that communities are still "good to think with" because of the way they help us frame and analyze sociological questions. Here, the argument for some form of restudying might be that immersion in how communities were studied in the past, and the conclusions they came to, provide us with a template for anchoring findings from the present. Thus the particular findings about family life in Bethnal Green, Wolverhampton and Woodford in the 1950s assisted us in thinking about the continuities and changes revealed in studies of these areas at later points in time. Indeed, the powerful image which these studies had conveyed of "family groups" operating in support of older people directly helped focus on what might have changed over the intervening time period. The conclusions of our research suggested a mixture of positive and negative changes since the baseline studies. With different points of emphasis, the lives of older people in Wolverhampton and Woodford demonstrated involvement with diverse social networks, some family-focused, others comprising a mixture of family, friends, and leisure associates. These continued to provide the mainstay of supportive needs, emotional as well as practical. At the same time, our finding about a new "type" of old age was also important: that is the shift from an old age experienced largely within family groups to one (following the work of Wellman, 1990) framed within "personal communities." This insight was also important in shifting our perspective from one which viewed older people as dependants within their family circle to active participants within a larger network, one to which they both provided as well as received support (Phillipson et al., 2001).

SOCIAL EXCLUSION AND COMMUNITY LIFE

One important finding from the family and community life study concerned the pressures on older people within minority ethnic groups. This was especially the case in Bethnal Green, where at the time of the study around 50% of the population comprised ethnic minorities, of which the Bangladeshi population formed the majority. Our own study included a small number of older people originally from Bangladesh who we found to be living in conditions of considerable hardship (Phillipson, Al-Haq, Ullah, & Ogg, 2000). These households also included female spouses, usually much younger than their husbands, together with a large number of dependent children. The issues raised by the interviews led me to develop another study, funded by the Nuffield Foundation, focused on first generation Bangladeshi women living in Tower Hamlets: *Women in Transition: A Study of the Experiences of Bangladeshi Women Living in Tower Hamlets* (Phillipson, Ahmed, & Latimer, 2003). The research interviewed 100 women aged 35 to 55 who had come to Britain in the 1970s and 1980s; carried out group interviews with women in their late teens and early twenties; as well as interviews with relevant community organizations. The study was concerned with examining issues about intergenerational and transnational support, with a particular focus on a group of women caring for older husbands (60 plus in most cases) as well as young children.

Both the family and community life research and the study of female migrants from Bangladesh reinforced interests relating to the effects of neighborhood deprivation on older people. This led to funding from the Economic and Social Research Council for a project: *Older People in Deprived Neighborhoods: Social Exclusion and Quality of Life in Old Age* (2000–2003), led by Thomas Scharf, with myself, Allison Smith, and Paul Kingston (Scharf, Phillipson, Smith, & Kingston, 2002; Scharf & Smith, 2004; Smith, 2009). An important aspect of the project was exploration of the link between *social exclusion*—defined as detachment from key institutions in society—and residence in particular types of neighborhood. The importance of the geographical dimension had been emphasized by Madanipour, Cars, and Allen (1998, p. 22) who suggested that the various components of social exclusion can combine to "create acute forms of exclusion that find a spatial manifestation in particular neighborhoods."

Following the above, a survey was made of 600 older people living in 9 deprived neighborhoods in three English cities: Liverpool, Manchester, and the London Borough of Newham. An important finding was confirmation of a link between neighborhood exclusion and exclusion from different types of social relations. At the same time, notwithstanding exclusionary pressures, many of the older people interviewed also developed strategies of control that enabled them to rise above concerns about safety and related issues. This was especially evident in the strategies developed by participants in order to reduce their feelings of insecurity, including reducing the risk of victimization by avoiding dangerous settings and situations, managing risks through precautionary behaviors, and engaging in collective action aimed at community safety.

MIGRATION AND TRANSNATIONAL TIES

An important finding from both the *Women in Transition* and *Social Exclusion* research concerned the significance of "*transnational ties*" and the links maintained with relatives among the different minority ethnic groups represented in both of the studies. Awareness of the increasing importance and impact of transnational migration on community life was a significant insight gained from the research, one which was reinforced by my increasing interest in issues relating to the impact of globalization on local communities (see further below). A clearer understanding of the relationship between social exclusion, migration, and globalization was to come through collaboration on a series of papers with my colleague Tine Buffel. I was privileged to comment upon various papers she was writing for her doctoral dissertation—subsequently published as *Experiences of Place and Neighbourhood in Later Life: Developing Age-Friendly Communities* (Buffel, 2012). This book proved influential for my own work in highlighting the link between various traditions within Environmental Gerontology and work on neighborhood issues in critical gerontology.

An initial avenue for exploring the neighborhood and globalization connection came through the experience of migrant communities. In Buffel and Phillipson (2011) we drew upon datasets from Belgium and England to examine the daily lives of migrants living in inner-city neighborhoods. The concern of the research was to examine: first, how older migrants created a sense of "home" in their current neighborhood? Second, what were the constraints which might prevent them from creating a sense of home? Third, how did migrants maintain transnational ties, and what significance did these have for experiences of place? The research explored these questions through qualitative interviews with older migrants from Morocco and Turkey (living in Brussels), and older migrants from Somalia and Pakistan (living respectively in Liverpool and Manchester).

The transnational lifestyles and discontinuous life-course patterns of many of the respondents interviewed introduced various complexities in relation to the experience of space and place. Moreover, the study areas illustrated environmental pressures linked to urban change and deprivation, these having the potential to undermine people's "feelings of home" within their neighborhood (Chaudhury & Rowles, 2005). Despite these constraints, an important finding from the study was the extent to which participants strived to transform their physical environment into a meaningful place with a sense of attachment to "home." This local attachment was especially evident in people's narratives about memories and experiences that had accumulated about their neighborhood, with two recurring themes emerging across the study areas: first, the proximity of members of their own cultural community which offered opportunities for developing social networks and realizing common social bonds; and, second, access to (ethnic) amenities. The paper suggested that the narratives of older migrants do not represent the voices of people who have had life-long settled lives (Becker, 2003). The structure of the migrants' life course may be seen as "discontinuous" (Torres, 2006), with key biographical events—such as marriage, having children, establishing a home—often occurring in a less predictable order as compared with non-migrants. Given this context, establishing secure and meaningful places may assume particular importance, with the achievement of what Rowles (1983) termed "*social insideness*" providing both continuity and support. The role of neighborhood and community in the construction of home among first-generation migrants was further explored in Buffel and Phillipson (2016b), with an additional paper examining the issue of how migrants negotiate "space" within urban communities affected by spatial segregation and local inequalities (Buffel & Phillipson, 2015).

GLOBALIZATION AND BELONGING

Research on local and transnational communities helped to shape my own thinking about questions concerning belonging and identity in the context of global social change. A paper exploring sociological perspectives on the experience of place and community in old age (Phillipson, 2007) argued that although the impact of globalization on aging was starting to be explored at a political and economic level (e.g., Baars et al., 2006), issues relating to place and the environment had received considerably less attention. The argument advanced was that the influence of globalization at a local level should be incorporated within social gerontology and environmental perspectives in particular. The paper suggested that work around the theme of globalization provided a way of rethinking issues about ageing and the environment, especially in relation to questions of community, environment and identity.

The importance of these developments was viewed in terms of posing new questions about people's sense of belonging to, and integration with, particular communities and environments (see, further, Savage, Bagnell, & Longhurst, 2005). In particular, the paper advanced a theoretical argument that it was important to distinguish between, on the one hand, those able to choose and identify with particular locations, which are viewed as consistent with and affirmative of their own biographies and life histories; and, on the other hand, those who experience rejection or exclusion from their locality and who see neighborhood change as incompatible with their own view of themselves and their peers. To put this another way: while some groups of older people can actively reshape communities which are meaningful to them in old age, others are relatively disempowered from the option of managing community and neighborhood change. The key change over the past 50 years may lie precisely in the social division that has opened up between these two groups: those that have expanding lifestyles options, and those whose experiences of their neighborhood are dominated by marginalization and alienation.

DEVELOPING AGE-FRIENDLY CITIES

Much of the above research was eventually brought together in a variety of studies, developed in collaboration with my colleague Tine Buffel, exploring the issue of what the World Health Organization (2007) defined as "age-friendly cities and communities" (Buffel, 2012; Buffel et al., 2014; Buffel & Phillipson, 2016a). A focus of this research was an attempt to integrate work in the field of Environmental Gerontology and urban sociology, with developing policies to support age-friendly cities. This work was greatly assisted by funding from the UK Economic and Social Research Council to establish a network of researchers working on age-friendly cities. The aim of the International Network on Population Ageing and Urbanisation (INPAU) was to, first, bring together researchers from a variety of countries in Asia, Europe, and the United States, to develop research on the relationship between ageing and urbanization; second, to provide a critical perspective on developing age-friendly communities and to assess new ways of approaching the issue of ageing and urbanization; third, to identify age-friendly strategies and initiatives designed to improve the lives of older people; and fourth, to identify ways in which older people themselves can be involved in the coproduction of age-friendly policies and practices (see, further, Buffel, 2015).

One important output from INPAU has been an edited volume (Buffel, Handler, & Phillipson, 2018) which combines theoretical perspectives from Environmental Gerontology, case studies examining the application of age-friendly work, and the presentation of a range of policy proposals. Reflecting the influence of critical gerontology, the volume also has a "Manifesto for Change" which sets out a new framework for developing age-friendly cities, one which acknowledges the impact of widening inequalities and economic austerity affecting cities and communities across the world.

FUTURE RESEARCH AGENDAS FOR ENVIRONMENTAL GERONTOLOGY

In terms of future priorities for my own research, I would highlight three areas that are likely to form major areas of interest. First, I remain committed to testing the idea that the concept of "community" is still "good to think with"; indeed, knowing how communities work or fail to work will be essential if current policies which promote the value of "*ageing in place*" are to be realized. Crow (2002) has made the point that, accepting the various difficulties associated with community sociology, such research has "a solid track record as a testing ground for general theories of social change [and in revealing] the active engagement of individuals and groups in the re-making of their social worlds." Moreover, in focusing on the impact of social change, community studies offer a way forward in terms of examining how macro-sociological and economic forces such as globalization work on the ground, influencing the daily life of older people as well as the neighborhoods in which they live.

Second, ideas about developing age-friendly cities and communities have come into favor among local authorities, nongovernmental organizations, and voluntary organizations, across both the global north and south. However interest and activity has expanded but with limited research testing the benefits or otherwise of this type of work. Given this, tackling the impact evaluation gap will be crucial for the next phase of developing age-friendly work. Applying mixed methods will be particularly important to identify who benefits from age-friendly initiatives and why; as well as measurement of the impact on traditionally excluded groups. Encouraging comparative studies examining the various approaches to building age-friendly communities in different social, political, and economic contexts should also be an important element of future research.

Finally, I am especially committed to developing links between urban sociology and related disciplines on the one side and that of Environmental Gerontology on the other. The intention here is to build upon arguments explored in Phillipson (2010) and in Buffel and Phillipson (2016a) which examine pressures on urban environments (e.g., gentrification, decline of social housing), and their impact on particular groups of older people. These papers suggested that although work on environmental aspects of aging has an impressive literature to its name, research has remained detached from work analyzing the powerful global and economic forces transforming the physical and social context of cities. Remedying this will require integration of Environmental Gerontology with a range of disciplines, urban sociology for one, but also urban economics, urban design and architecture, and human geography.

CONCLUSION

Finally, what kind of future is there for community and environmental studies of the kind discussed in this chapter, research which has been a preoccupation for much of my own career? On the surface at least, a strong case can be made for social investigations, working from within particular localities and neighborhoods. Ties—virtual or otherwise—may well spill out well beyond geographical borders. But loyalties and identities may still be framed within defined territories—increasingly so given pressures experienced at a national and global level. Moreover, for some groups—notably older people and certain minority ethnic groups—the spaces represented by neighborhoods continue to be essential for security and quality of life.

But challenges for community studies and by implication Environmental Gerontology may also be identified. Pressures facing certain communities given rising inequalities and economic austerity will require new types of fieldwork and research methodologies. Working in areas experiencing tension and violence, driven in part by the fragmentation of local institutions, will require new ways of thinking about and understanding community change. Researchers may need to take more risks to gain access to certain types of groups: Venkatesh's (2008) work in an abandoned housing project in Chicago, researching drug dealers and gangs, provides one illustration. Developing distinctive fieldwork strategies aimed at different minority ethnic groups will be essential. Collaborative research—especially with newly arrived migrant groups—would seem especially desirable. Some of the best ethnographies of city life have, arguably, emerged from solitary walkers, for example, Lyle (2008) in San Francisco, and Sinclair (1997) in London. And the ecology of urban areas—with the "social separation of the affluent and impoverished" (Klinenberg, 2002, p. 231) presents a challenge for undertaking community studies. But the argument for such work remains compelling: People's lives remain touched to at least some degree by their immediate environment; for some it represents *the* main focus of their life. Using the idea of "community" to understand social connections and social divisions is likely to continue as an important feature of work in Environmental Gerontology for many years to come.

ACKNOWLEDGMENTS

I am grateful to the many researchers who have participated in the studies discussed in this paper, in particular: Nilufar Ahmed, Miriam Bernard, Jim Ogg, Judith Phillips, Allison Smith, and Thomas Scharf. Jan Baars, Dale Dannefer, and Carroll Estes have been inspiring colleagues (and great friends) in the project to develop a critical gerontology. I owe a particular debt to Tine Buffel whose outstanding work in Environmental Gerontology has enormously influenced my own thinking. In particular, her work on community empowerment and coproduction with older people represents a significant advance in thinking about the possibilities and potential of a critical Environmental Gerontology.

REFERENCES

Abrams, P. (1968). *The origins of british sociology 1834–1914: An essay with selected papers.* Chicago, IL: University of Chicago Press.

Abrams, P., McCulloch, A., Abrams, S., & Gore, P. (1976). *Communes, sociology and society.* Cambridge, UK: Cambridge University Press.

Baars, J., Dannefer, D., Phillipson, C., & Walker, A. (Eds.). (2006). *Aging, globalization and inequality*. New York, NY: Baywood Publishing.

Becker, G. (2003). Meanings of place and displacement in three groups of older immigrants. *Journal of Aging Studies, 17*(2), 129–149.

Bell, C., & Newby, H. (1971). *Community studies*. London, UK: George Allen and Unwin.

Buffel, T. (2012). *Experiences of place and neighbourhood in later life: Developing age-friendly communities*. Brussels: VUB Press.

Buffel, T. (Ed.). (2015). *Researching age-friendly communities: Stories from older people as co-investigators*. Manchester, UK: The University of Manchester Library.

Buffel, T., Handler, S., & Phillipson, C. (2018). *Age friendly cities and communities: A global perspective* [Manuscript submitted for publication]. Bristol, UK: Policy Press.

Buffel, T., McGarry, P., Phillipson, C., De Donder, D., Dury, S., De Witte, N., et al. (2014). Developing age-friendly cities: Case studies from Brussels and Manchester and implications for policy and practice. *Journal of Aging and Social Policy, 26*(1–2), 52–71.

Buffel, T., & Phillipson, C. (2011). Experiences of place among older migrants living in inner-city neighbourhoods in Belgium and England. *Diversité Urbaine, 11*(1), 13–37.

Buffel, T., & Phillipson, C. (2015). Negotiating urban space: Older people and the contestation of generational and ethnic boundaries. In R. Wanderbeck & N. Worth (Eds.), *Intergenerational space* (pp. 314–328). London, UK: Routledge.

Buffel, T., & Phillipson, C. (2016a). Can global cities be age-friendly cities? Urban development and ageing populations. *Cities, 55*, 94–100.

Buffel, T., & Phillipson, C. (2016b). Constructions of 'home' among first generation migrants living in Belgium and England. In K. Walsh & L. Näre (Eds.), *Transnational migration and home in older age* (pp. 63–74). London, UK: Routledge.

Bulmer, M. (Ed.). (1986). *Neighbours: the work of Philip Abrams*. Cambridge, UK: Cambridge University Press.

Chaudhury, H., & Rowles, G. D. (2005). Between the shores of recollection and imagination: Self, aging, and home. In G. D. Rowles & H. Chaudhury (Eds.), *Home and identity in late life: International perspectives* (pp. 3–20). New York, NY: Springer Publishing.

Craig, G., Derricourt, N., & Loney, M. (1982). *Community work and the state: Towards a radical practice*. London, UK: Routledge Books.

Crow, G. (2002). Community studies: Fifty years of theorization. *Sociological Research Online, 7*(3). Retrieved from http://www.socresonline.org.uk/7/3/crow.html

Crow, G., & Allan, G. (1994). *Community life: An introduction to local social relations*. Hemel Hempstead, UK: Harvester Wheatsheaf.

Dennis, N., Henriques, F., & Slaughter, C. (1956). *Coal is our life: An analysis of a Yorkshire mining community*. London, UK: Tavistock.

Estes, C. (1979). *The aging enterprise*. San Francisco, CA: Josey Bass.

Estes, C. (1991). The new political economy of aging: Introduction and critique. In M. Minkler & C. Estes (Eds.), *Critical perspectives on aging: The political and moral economy of growing old* (pp. 19–36). New York, NY: Baywood Publishing Co.

Frankenberg, R. (1966). *Communities in Britain.* Harmondsworth: Penguin Books.

Goffman, I. (1961). *Asylums: Essays on the social situation of mental patients and other inmates.* New York, NY: Random House.

Jamieson, L. (1998). *Intimacy: Personal relationships in modern societies.* Cambridge, UK: Polity Press.

Klinenberg, E. (2002). *Heat wave: A social autopsy of disaster in Chicago.* Chicago, IL: University of Chicago Press.

Laing, R. D. (1960). *The divided self: An existential study in sanity and madness.* Harmondsworth: Penguin Books.

Leonard, P. (1975). *The sociology of community action.* Keele, UK: University of Keele, Sociological Review Monograph.

Loney, M. (1985). *Community against government: British community development project, 1968–78: A study of government incompetence.* London, UK: Heinemann Education.

Lyle, E. (2008). *On the lower frequencies: A secret history of the city.* Brooklyn, NY: Soft Skull Press.

Madanipour, A., Cars, G., & Allen, J. (1998). *Social exclusion in european cities: Process, experiences and responses.* London, UK: Jessica Kingsley.

Morgan, D. H. J. (2008). Are community studies still 'good to think with'. In R. Edwards (Ed.), *Research families and communities: Social and generational change* (pp. 25–40). London, UK: Routledge.

Phillipson, C. (1980). Boredom in Benwell. *New Age*, Winter 29–32.

Phillipson, C. (1982). *Capitalism and the construction of old age.* London, UK: Macmillan.

Phillipson, C. (1987). The transition to retirement. In G. Cohen (Ed.), *Social change and the life course* (pp. 156–184). London, UK: Tavistock Books.

Phillipson, C. (2007). The 'elected' and the 'excluded': Sociological perspectives on the experience of place and community in old age. *Ageing and Society*, *27*, 321–342.

Phillipson, C. (2010). Growing old in the "century of the city." In D. Dannefer & C. Phillipson (Eds.), *The sage handbook of social gerontology* (pp. 597–606). London, UK: Sage.

Phillipson, C., Ahmed, N., & Latimer, J. (2003). *Women in transition: A study of the experiences of Bangladeshi women living in Tower Hamlets.* Bristol, UK: Policy Press

Phillipson, C., Al-Haq, E., Ullah, S., & Ogg, J. (2000). Bangladeshi families in Bethnal Green: Older people, ethnicity and social exclusion. In T. Warnes, L. Warren, & M. Nolan (Eds.), *Care services for later life* (pp. 273–290). London, UK: Jessica Kingsley.

Phillipson, C., Bernard, M., Phillips, J., & Ogg., J. (2001). *The family and community life of older people.* London, UK: Routledge.

Phillipson, C., & Thompson, P. (Eds.). (2008). Whither community studies? A special issue on researching community studies past and present. *International Journal of Social Science Methodolology*, *11*(2), 87–91.

Rowles, G. (1983). Place and personal identity in old age: Observations from Appalachia. *Journal of Environmental Psychology*, *3*(4), 299–313.

Savage, M., Bagnall, G., & Longhurst, B. (2005). *Globalization and belonging*. London, UK: Sage.
Scharf, T., Phillipson, C., Smith, A., & Kingston, P. (2002). *Growing older in socially deprived areas*. London, UK: Help the Aged.
Scharf, T., & Smith, A. (2004). Older people in urban neighbourhoods: Addressing the risk of social exclusion. In C. Phillipson, G. Allan, & D. Morgan (Eds.), *Social networks and social exclusion: Sociological and policy perspectives* (pp. 162–179). Surrey, UK: Ashgate.
Sheldon, J. H. (1948). *The social medicine of old age*. London, UK: Oxford University Press.
Sinclair, I. (1997). *Lights out for the territory*. London, UK: Granta Books.
Smith, A. (2009). *Ageing in urban neighbourhoods*. Bristol, UK: Policy Press.
Taylor, M. (2004). Community issues and social networks. In C. Phillipson, G. Allan, & D. Morgan (Eds.), *Social networks and social exclusion: Sociological and policy perspectives* (pp. 205–218). Farnham, UK: Ashgate.
Torres, S. (2006). Culture, migration, inequality, and 'periphery' in a globalized world: Challenges for ethno- and anthropogerontology. In J. Baars, D. Dannefer, C. Phillipson & A. Walker (Eds.), *Aging, globalization and inequality. The new critical gerontology*. New York, NY: Baywood.
Townsend, P. (1957). *The family life of old people*. London, UK: Routledge.
Venkatesh, S. (2008). *Gang leader for a day*. New York, NY: The Penguin Press.
Walker, A. (1980). The social creation of poverty and dependency in old age. *Journal of Social Policy*, *9*(1), 49–75.
Walker, A. (1981). Towards a political economy of old age. *Ageing and Society*, *1*(1), 73–94.
Wellman, B. (1990). The place of kinfolk in personal community settings. In B. Wellman (Ed.), *Families in community settings: Interdisciplinary settings*. New York, NY: Haworth Press.
World Health Organization. (2007). *Global age-friendly cities: A guide*. Geneva: Author.
Willmott, P., & Young, M. (1960). *Family and class in a London suburb*. London, UK: Routledge & Kegan Paul.
Young, M., & Willmott, P. (1957). *Family and kinship in East London*. London, UK: Routledge and Kegan Paul.
Young, M., & Willmott, P. (1957). *Family and class in a London suburb*. London, UK: Routledge and Kegan Paul.

CHAPTER 11

A "Good Fit"

Professionally Aging in Small Kansas Towns

Rick J. Scheidt

ABSTRACT

In this chapter, Rick Scheidt shares episodes and eras marking his professional lifetime in the ecology of aging. In particular, he reflects on his experiences with two ground-breaking field studies of small-town rural elders. The first, a study of nearly 1,000 rural elders across 18 small Kansas towns, was the first major survey to assess community-level environmental influences on the mental health of older rural residents. Perhaps most significant, contrary to bucolic rural stereotypes, distinct perceptual views of local environments were linked to diverse patterns psychological well-being among these individuals. The second—the "ghost town study"—used a transactional model to capture multilevel environmental gains and losses experienced by elders aging-in-place in declining and dying towns. This includes a 30-year case study of the dynamics of place-deconstruction and place-making within a single endangered rural village. The author shares his appreciation of several positive contributors to Environmental Gerontology, including M. Powell Lawton, Victor Regnier, Paul Windley, Carolyn Norris-Baker, Roger Barker, Rudolf Moos, and Benyamin Schwarz.

BIOGRAPHICAL NOTES

My introduction to environmental *psychology* came in 1968 when, as a master's student in clinical and social psychology, I discovered a copy of Roger Barker's

http://dx.doi.org/10.1891/0198-8794.38.183

(1968) *Ecological Psychology* on the desk of my major professor, Harrison Madden, at California State University, Fresno. His words were to the effect: "That's a book you must read." Though I had encountered Kurt Lewin's theory in coursework on personality, it was my first *serious* exposure to the environment component of Lewin's classic formula, B = f (Person, Environment). Barker's "behavior setting" construct remains, in my view, the most significant theoretical and operational advance in environmental psychology for understanding behavior-in-milieu. In particular, I remember the basic message in the book's prologue:

> Psychology knows much about the physical properties of the environmental probes its uses for (studying) distal objects of perception, for example, and of energy-changes at receptor surfaces. But (. . .) it has excised these environmental elements from the complexities of the real-life settings in which they occur, from ball games, from symposia meetings, from turnpikes, from arithmetic classes. The result is, inevitably, that the science of psychology has had no adequate knowledge of the psychologist-free environment of behavior. The view is not uncommon among psychologists that the environment of behavior is a relatively unstructured, passive, probabilistic arena of objects and events upon which man behaves in accordance with the programming he carries about within himself. (Barker, 1968, p. 4)

My view of the study of behavior was permanently changed by Barker's approach. Like many students of my day, I had been trained largely in the mold that Barker chided, where the environment, to paraphrase Barker, was relevant largely as a near-the-skin experimental stimulus. My personal notions of why people behave the way they do widened. I found a "good fit" within the contextual paradigm (I could not imagine that 10 years later, Barker would serve a consultant role on two projects targeting rural aging.). After completion of master's studies, I entered the new social psychology program at the University of Nebraska-Lincoln. In addition to social psychology, I trained heavily in developmental studies as well as sociology. My commitment to the study of behavior "in situ" added a year to my doctoral studies. At one point, I considered conducting dissertation research on the language of stigmatization and creation of dependency scripts for elders in long-term care. Due to a series of influential incidents, I focused instead on an 18-month field study of the social construction of deviance and stigmatization among occultists and other religionists (Scheidt, 1974). I fell in love with field research. There was no doubt, following this experience, that field research "fit" my preferences, skill set, and personality well. My first academic appointment was in the psychology department at a private liberal arts college located in New York, located along the hilly banks of the upper Hudson River. From the outset, my desire to conduct field research was constricted by the campus-based teaching duties. Though I was interested in teaching and enjoyed the students, I grew increasingly concerned that I might never be able to conduct serious research situated in an undergraduate college largely devoted to teaching. Yes, I should have thought of that going in. Also, though I admitted it to very few, I missed the wide open spaces offered by more western states. I was a flat-lander.

During my brief stay in New York, a series of publications began to flow from the Life Span Developmental Psychology program at West Virginia University. I had an immediate interest in the attention given to the adult end of the life span. I read hungrily through the available volumes of the multicolored Academic Press series on life-span developmental psychology. In the spring of 1975, I placed a call to K. Warner Schaie, then Director of the Research Institute at the Ethel Percy Andrus Gerontology Center at the University of Southern California: Did he have an available postdoctoral or fellowship position in his lab? The timing was serendipitous. I told Schaie of my interest in "situationism" and contextual influences on behavior. He related that earlier in the day, his *Seattle Longitudinal Study of Intelligence* team had discussed the pursuit of ecological ("real world") validity of measures of intelligence. Whether due to coincidence or to a new environmental Zeitgeist, we were on the same page. Within a few months we (including my spouse and our 3-year-old twin daughters) were living in Santa Monica, California, and I was training as a postdoctoral fellow under Warner's mentorship at the Andrus Gerontology Center in Los Angeles.

THE ANDRUS GERONTOLOGY CENTER

As anticipated, the Andrus Gerontology Center was filled with bright, creative, extremely well-trained professionals in virtually every active arena of aging-related research. Most appealing, everyone was speaking "aging." My research with Warner Schaie explored ways to represent objective and subjective elements of everyday environments in assessments of intelligence and competence (Scheidt & Schaie, 1978). Warner was brilliant, creative, and accommodative. One of the important primers in my training was Eisdorfer and Lawton's (1973) recently edited volume, *The Psychology of Adult Development and Aging*. Most significant, it included Lawton and Nahemow's (1973) chapter, "Ecology and the Aging Process," which presented the now-classic Competence-Press model. I was struck by the efficiency of the model for displaying alternative adaptive outcomes resulting from interactions of "terms of the organism" with "terms of the environment." Excited by this work, I had an immediate desire to know more about Lawton and his work, a wish rewarded soon after my departure from Andrus.

A fortunate arrangement of office locations at the Andrus Center provided me an opportunity to deepen my exposure to Environmental Gerontology. Warner's lab was located next to that of Victor Regnier, Lab Chief for Environmental Studies (see Chapter 14). Regnier was a lean, extremely bright, and constantly-in-motion architect. His life seemed driven by grant deadlines. Victor's neurons were permanently locked in the "rapid fire" mode. He put ideas together more quickly than anyone I had encountered. Prior to this time, my training focused almost solely on the social environment. Victor introduced me to the behavioral design paradigm (e.g., Regnier, 2003). I was struck by the sheer sensibility of designing environments around behavioral needs and more specifically, of introducing environmental accommodations to aid the changing needs of older adults. Moreover, the paradigm dealt directly with the individual-environment interactions discussed in the Competence-Press model. The built environment became more than mere "background" for me as a psychologist; it now rushed to the foreground as a significant determinant of behavioral dysfunction and behavior change. I had entered the Andrus Center as a social psychologist; I left Andrus with a sapling's knowledge of Environmental Gerontology and life-span human development though I felt reasonably well grounded in the psychology of aging.

TO KANSAS

Though offered a fellowship to remain at Andrus, I opted for family-related reasons to accept a job at Kansas State University in 1976 as a life-span developmental psychologist. I was responsible for developing a curriculum treating the last two-thirds of the life span, the years extending from young adulthood through the later years. Or, in terms expressed by some of my child development colleagues, I was charged with handling the period of "left over life"—referring to the then-prevailing view that very little of developmental interest occurred after the formative years of youth (see Scheidt [2016] regarding my early experiences with the structural and paradigmatic ageism prompting this belief). There was an expectation, of course, that I would establish a funded research program in the same arena.

Following a suggestion offered by Victor, I made contact with Dr. Paul Windley, an Associate Professor of Architecture at K-State. Paul was already part of the "Housing and Environment for Aging Project" (1971–1975) spearheaded by The Gerontological Society of America; I was also familiar with his work, "Theory Development in Environment and Aging" (Windley, Byerts, & Ernst, 1975). Upon meeting Paul, I knew at once that we had the potential to be compatible teammates. Our personalities and areas of training were complimentary.

Paul was an introvert, rather reserved and shy. I am an extravert, more socially assertive. Paul had a phlegmatic demeanor; I am more of a worrier. Paul was a quiet and solitary thinker; I believe that ideas are enriched and advanced through discussion. Paul was an architect, trained in behavioral design in Lee Pastalan's program at the University of Michigan (if pressed, Paul referred to himself as a behavioral ecologist). I was a psychologist, pursuing my learning curve at the upper end of the developmental continuum. Paul was a man of faith; in contrast, I believe we are "lost in the stars." We agreed that each of us had much to bring to a common research pursuit in environmental aging. We agreed that the success of interdisciplinary collaboration requires *knowing who you are* and what you are bringing to the table, feeling comfortable in your own skin, and being self-aware of your limitations. We were able to talk openly with one another about our relationship when we hit inevitable sticking points in our work. Thus began one of the most personally and professionally satisfying experiences of my career.

STARTING WHERE YOU ARE

Residing in Kansas, we began by following the maxim of field research to "start where you are." The starting point for our collaboration was the simple fact that Kansas is a highly rural environment. In the mid-1970s, there was very little research focusing on rural elders, much less research examining how rural context influences psychological wellbeing. In 1978, our first and most major collaboration resulted in a National Institute of Mental Health (NIMH)-funded 2-year face-to-face interview study of almost 1,000 elderly residents across 18 small Kansas towns. At the most general level, the purpose was two-fold: What is the status of psychological wellbeing of these elders? How much of the diversity in psychological wellbeing is predicted by the personal, physical, and psychosocial environments in these communities? This study as well as a more micro-environmental NIMH-funded follow-up produced answers to both of these questions and many more. It also provided us with a bounty of research lessons and professional experiences that come from being completely immersed in a complex research study from its start to conclusion.

One year after leaving the Andrus Center, I was now interacting with Powell Lawton, who served as a consultant on the project. His contributions to the research were extremely valuable, particularly his recommendations for a multiple battery of measures to balance out the mutual weaknesses of measures within the second-order construct, "psychological wellbeing." In addition to the epidemiologic data derived from happiness, moral, and psychiatric symptom criteria, we replicated the factor structure of Lawton's Philadelphia Geriatric Scale on our rural population, enhancing understanding of its construct validity across a rural population. Powell offered practical advice regarding construction of measures of the physical and psychosocial environment as well. We later regretted not taking his advice about gathering data on both objective and subjective features of the physical environment; our assessments at that stage were limited to elders' reports of their perceived environments.

Lawton was a clear, analytical conceptualizer and a hard-nosed empiricist. He was gracious, generous, and possessed a prodding dry wit. He had unmatched knowledge of ongoing national and international research, nurtured by his continuing interactions with the many environmental gerontologists who sought him out. He had a well-spring of experience managing datasets, sampling, measurement, and analysis issues, as well as intervention modeling and evaluation. He knew how to do environmental behavioral science and he did it well. Indeed, Powell's deep knowledge of theory, measurement, data interpretation, and application—and the fact that he had published prolifically in *all of these domains*, established him as a premier founder of Environmental Gerontology. Powell was one of the few environmental gerontologists to understand the complexities posed for researchers by *behavior in context*; he was facile with both sides of the B = (f) P, E equation, as well as P × E interactions—a term which he later inserted in his modification of Lewin's equation (Lawton, 1982).

Despite its large sample of elderly residents and communities, this initial collaboration with Windley essentially remains a case study. Our Kansas small-town context represented just one among many possible routes to operationalizing rural environments. However, for the first time, rural gerontology had data illustrating what was *possible*, if not probable, regarding environmental correlates of mental health for elders in tiny towns (2,500 in size and under). To illustrate, our study offered a taxonomy illustrating the diversity of wellbeing profiles (partially engaged, fully engaged, disengaged, and frail) existing among elders in the 18 small towns (Scheidt, 1984). One of the most significant analyses examined differences in psychosocial environmental perceptions as a function of their well-being profile status. Results suggested that older small-town residents resided in distinctly different *perceptual* environments and that these subjective frames of reference may have influenced their receptivity to resources (Scheidt & Windley, 1987). Our modeling of physical environmental, psychosocial, and demographic predictors of mental health for our sample yielded noteworthy similarities as well as differences between older male and female residents (Scheidt & Windley, 1983). Among males, overall activity level, satisfaction with dwelling features, and housing satisfaction were the largest direct predictors of mental health status. Among women, activity level, satisfaction with dwelling features, community satisfaction, and security (safety in home and neighborhood) were the largest direct predictors. Our analysis of living arrangements, including marital status (three-fourths of men versus 44% of women were married) partially explained the finding that men, on the whole, were more content to remain in and around the residence, whereas women sought social stimulation and satisfaction in the wider community. More applied, we constructed service utilization and activity profiles to distinguish service access and use patterns between psychologically vulnerable and well residents across the communities (Windley & Scheidt, 1983). Though we found few differences in frequency of use of everyday services, ease of access for vulnerable elders was highly dependent on the goodwill and transportation provided by indigenous well-elder neighbors and caregivers in local informal social networks.

We took pride in several features of this research. First, in addition to Powell Lawton's contributions, it was well-informed by numerous consultants. Roger Barker, Rudolf Moos, and Richard Lazarus served as formal consultants on this effort as well as a second follow-up effort involving a focus on environmental interactions of elders exhibiting various profiles of psychological wellbeing. Method-wise, it was a model of meticulous planning. We developed and implemented the sampling frame for county-to-town-to elderly residents 6 months before we knew we had secured approval and funding. Our sampling protocol utilized a 3 × 3 sampling matrix composed of three levels of county rurality crossed with three small-town size categories. Our "town panel" approach of using indigenous onsite teams of local residents to represent the project through its duration provides an exemplary protocol for recruiting rural elders (Windley & Scheidt, 1980), including the training and coordination of activities of 10 graduate student interviewers across a 9-month period in one of the worst winters in Kansas history. The management challenges presented by the data-gathering period were immense. The resulting dataset, including hundreds of variables, afforded us invaluable experience in construction of valid second-order variable domains, and the opportunity to use several multivariate statistical applications available at the time. In retrospect, the entire study—from planning to dissemination of results—deserved to be under one cover; we were anxious, however, to publish results more immediately in the professional literature. At the time, the study was viewed as a major contribution to rural aging, with strong implications for Environmental Gerontology.

Relevant to environmental lessons drawn from the project, I offer one more illustration that led to an interesting professional "take-away." During the early analytical phase, Paul and I constructed path models to explore the predictive value of several environmental variables for understanding psychological wellbeing. Two separate regression models—one for the entire sample and another for separate samples of elderly men and women—yielded relatively low R^2 values (ranging from 17%–27%; Scheidt & Windley, 1983; Windley & Scheidt, 1982). I had occasion to present these results at an NIMH grant report conference in Washington, DC. (Scheidt, 1982). I admitted my mild surprise to the research audience that the physical and psychosocial environmental predictors had not explained more variance in subjective wellbeing, citing the "usual method suspects" that might weaken the associations. Afterwards, I had a conversation with Paul Costa, who was developing a research base on the NEO Personality Inventory. He said, "You know, Rick, *happy are those who are happy*." His comment struck home immediately. His research with Robert McCrae was showing that extraversion and neuroticism correlated positively and significantly with positive and negative affect, respectively. He shared his now-familiar view that E and N trait factors may effectively sustain inclinations toward happiness and unhappiness *regardless of the quality one's immediate environment.* Of course, in hindsight, our predictive model was incomplete in this way. A fully informed contextual model must include an array of psychological assessments, including personality. Today, reliable and valid short-form survey measures of these personality traits are available. The Zeitgeist of Environmental Gerontology has shifted in the past three decades, giving greater necessary attention to P-component variables relevant to understanding environmental adaptation and psychological outcomes. Indeed, in a seminal book for our field providing a focus on housing Lawton (1998) lamented that "advances in the environmental knowledge have not been matched by advances in knowledge regarding the person and individual differences in the person-environment transaction" (p. 2). Still of high value, Lawton's chapter presents various "terms of the organism" that he believed must be given serious consideration by theorists in Environmental Gerontology. These include "missing components" of the person such as motivation, cognitive-attentional mechanisms, environmentally linked affect, temperament, preferences, and, of course, personality. Pertinent to our own study, if repeated today, we might well insert these and other psychological constructs, including environmental control, resilience, self-esteem, and place-meaning dimensions.

A COIN IN THE DARKNESS?

In 1982, Carolyn (Lyn) Norris-Baker joined the faculty of the Department of Architecture at K-State. Like Paul, Lyn was trained in architecture as well as behavioral ecology. She earned a B Arch degree at Rice University and a PhD in psychology in environment-behavior studies at the University of Houston. As Paul and I were completing our 18-community project, Lyn began a project working with two small towns in northeastern Kansas, exploring the community involvement, social support, and longitudinal health outcomes among frail older adults. After our completion of these separate projects, the three of us worked together briefly as a team.

In the mid-1980s, a downturn in the rural economy threatened the viability of many small towns under 2,500 in size in the Heartland. At least half of small Kansas towns faced increased unemployment, loss of population, regional outflow of dollars, and loss of business infrastructure, causing challenges to their social and community sustainability. Many elders continued to cling to their residency in these places of their birth. These older adults became the new focus of our interest. We were especially interested in the specific environmental stressors they faced, how they dealt with these, and the associated social and psychological benefits and costs. In 1988, we submitted an NIMH-grant proposal dealing with the effects of rural economic hardship on the wellbeing small-town elders at both aggregate (county) and individual levels across Kansas. The project was not funded, in retrospect for good reasons. The proposed research was viewed as a foray into economic psychology, an arena that stretched us beyond our training and, frankly, our professional comfort zones, even at the time of submission. The rejection of this proposal by NIMH, while disappointing, reinforced my view that interdisciplinary research must draw upon and remain centered within the interests, skill sets, and combined experiential base of the research team.

For me, the result involved a reorientation toward "on-the-ground" field work to understand the phenomenon at hand. In addition to the relatively small amount of explained variance in mental health across elderly residents in our 18-town study, I felt more strongly that the large-scale quantitative survey of environmental variables failed to provide us with the *experiential meanings* these environments held for them. As researchers, we knew that older respondents will graciously answer almost any question we put to them. But were they the *right* questions? Did the methods allow us the opportunity to learn from the older respondent the questions we *should* be asking? The superstructure of our multilayered environmental proposal had taken on a life of its own; we had strayed from "true north"—failing to remain close to the phenomenon at hand. I came to appreciate the story of the researcher who dropped a coin in the darkness but moved under the street lamp several yards away to find it. Lyn and I believed strongly that a valid understanding of the environmental adaptation of older adults in *small declining and dying towns* would not be adequately captured by another large-scale survey. We began talking about adopting a case study paradigm which would allow us to get closer to the coin.

At this juncture, Paul decided to pursue ambitions in upper administration; he became Associate Dean of the College of Architecture and Design at K-State. However, we maintained our professional partnership—largely in writings in Environmental Gerontology. We coedited three books on environment and aging—the last with Hans-Werner Wahl (see Chapter 2). These works focused on housing-related theory (Scheidt & Windley, 1998), a festschrift devoted to Lawton's contributions to physical environments and aging (Scheidt & Windley, 2003) and a volume spearheaded by Wahl focusing on socio-physical environments (Wahl, Scheidt, & Windley, 2003). These coedited works allowed us to interact with talented researchers from the many disciplines within the ecology of aging and afforded us a purview of the activity in the field. Paul left K-State in 1992 to become Dean of Art and Architecture at Idaho State University-Moscow. Our last coauthored work was the chapter on Environmental Gerontology in the *Handbook of the Psychology of Aging* (Scheidt & Windley, 2006). Paul died far too young in January of 2007 of leukemia. Environmental gerontology lost a significant contributor. I remain extremely appreciative of the kindness, mentorship, and professional space so freely shared by this bright, gentle, and humble man.

GHOST TOWNS OF KANSAS

In the late 1980s, Lyn Norris-Baker and I began an in-depth collective case study of four purposively selected small rural Kansas towns experiencing serious decline (in all, we visited 12 small communities in preparation for this field work). This study lasted almost a decade, as we continued to follow two of these communities over time. One exceptional community was followed over a 20-year period, with our last report illustrating its indigenous "place making" efforts to ensure survival (Scheidt, 2010). This "ghost town" study remains the most interesting research experience of my post-PhD career. Our primary intent was to identify the environmental stressors faced by residents in these prototypical communities and to gain an understanding of the adaptive strategies they employed to deal with them. The hardest hit communities were in remote locations, dependent on single land-based industry such as agriculture or oil production, decreasing purchasing power of residents, leakage of retail trade to regional centers, low quality and quantity of services, and inadequate financial resources to repair the towns' infrastructure. In addition, older residents comprised a larger portion of the population of these towns than any other age group. Little information existed regarding the positive or negative impacts of both acute and chronic environmentally induced stress on these communities and upon the mental health of their older residents (Scheidt & Norris-Baker, 1990).

Conceptually, we adopted a fresh contextual view of environmental stress proposed by Aldwin and Stokols (1988). This approach, derived from a transactional paradigm, offered a multilevel, ecologically sensitive view of environmental stress. It assumed that negative environmental events might precipitate diverse *positive as well as negative* outcomes. Residents of these small rural towns were unable to reduce effectively and independently the constant threats to self and community posed by the depressed economic climate. Under these conditions, we believed that traditional homeostatic models of person-environment fit or congruence were ill-suited to provide a full understanding of adaptation that occurs under conditions of constant short- and long-term stress. The transactional paradigm offered a "deviation-amplifying" approach, allowing us to chart specific transactions across inner physical, individual-psychological, socio-cultural, and physical-environmental levels (Scheidt & Norris-Baker, 1990). Our field approach utilized ethnographic interviewing of four dozen older residents, participant observation, archival research, windshield tours, and photo-documentation (Barlett, 1990; Fitchen, 1990). In retrospect, photographs provided a powerful descriptive medium to communicate our work to others. Images afford immediate access to environmental meanings not afforded by narratives or numbers. Our photo documentation of withering and deteriorating storefronts, schools, community centers, services, and residences also allowed objective identification of physical environmental decline. While psychological anthropologists have employed video and photographic data for some time, it is surprising, really, that gerontology researchers have not developed more fully protocols for use of photography as a data-gathering tool that might stand alongside observations and interviews (Ruby, 1996).

These methods generated an immensely interesting and rich array of issues—22 in all—across the four environmental levels. Each issue contained positive and negative behavioral outcomes. We proceeded to "mine" their implications for older residents, targeting community mental health specialists, rural policy makers, and environmental designers and engineers. We coined the term "place therapy" to describe more practical applications of our findings for ameliorating and enriching diverse impacts of place transitions (Scheidt & Norris-Baker, 1999). We discovered a dialectical irony within many of the beneficial and negative outcomes reported by older adults in dying towns. For example, fears that declines in health might necessitate relocation outside of the community led many to monitor their health and health behaviors more carefully. Elders with health issues that would probably marginalize them in more populated towns nonetheless maintained their status as valued contributors to these places. A foreshortened sense of personal and community future was associated with a keen appreciation of the past, with some elders assuming the informal role of local "culture-bearer" or town historian. Loss of formal roles due to the demise of businesses and organizations was offset by the creation of informal roles and "hobby businesses" (such as antique stores). The underpopulated environment led to a sense that one played an important role in serving the community, particularly in understaffed behavior settings. However, several elders—most often women—complained about the role-overload and burn-out associated with fulfilling their volunteer duties. We referred to them as "captives of decline." At a broader level, personal qualities of older adults took on enhanced meaning. Retirees returning to a community following a long career in management, for example, had skill sets put into service of securing outside funding such as grants to aid the town. Crumbling buildings remained untouched, preserved by residents who viewed the ruins as embodiments of personal history. Elders spearheaded the construction of town memorials that validated their existence in shared reminiscence. At the same time, some towns sought to sustain themselves through the creation of new identities beyond their original historic covenant as farm towns. Declining towns attracted "outsiders," new residents seeking cheap housing and wishing to remain "off-radar" (Scheidt, 2010). A signal contribution from our experiences is the accounting of the changing meanings of community for older residents struggling to sustain, reframe, and, in some cases, accept the losses and let go of these environments (Norris-Baker & Scheidt, 2005).

A large degree of the success of this multiyear, mostly self-funded research effort belongs to Lyn Norris-Baker, who is a highly skilled field researcher. She is a natural conceptualizer and methodologist; moreover, she is an excellent, patient observer. She knew how and where to search for "the hiding places of the ego" of older residents in the nooks and crannies of the local environments. Moreover, Lyn has a profound ability to express her observations in writing, providing a lyrical account of the *place struggles* we observed (see Norris-Baker & Scheidt, 1994).

As the "ghost town" project gradually spiraled down, Lyn and I continued to write together on other projects on occasion, despite the fact that she retired to realize her bucket-list dream of owning and operating a Bed-and-Breakfast in New Hampshire. In the wake, I became a bit of an academic Robinson Crusoe. I was rescued from the isolation of my professional island by Dr. Benyamin Schwarz, Professor of the Studio Sequence and Rogers Gallery, at the University of Missouri-Columbia (see Chapter 12). As Editor of *The Journal of Housing for the Elderly*, Ben accepted my idea of coediting a special issue (converted to book format) dedicated to the addressing the title question, *Environmental Gerontology: What Now?* (Scheidt & Schwarz, 2013). This stock-taking effort was very fulfilling. I found Ben to be one of the most unselfish professionals in the field and genuinely concerned about its viability. The volume contains our thoughts and those of several talented researchers regarding the current status and "possible futures" of environmental theory, methods, environmental transformations in community and care settings, and understudied populations and settings. Save for two, I will not reiterate these suggestions for future research here. First, I continue to believe that environmental gerontologists might learn much about the range, processes, and outcomes of environmental adaptations by turning the focus to unique (often understudied) populations, including, for instance, older stigmatized residents of declining small towns, total institutions such as prisons, and purpose-built senior environments (Hrybyk et al., 2013; Scheidt & Norris-Baker, 2013). Second, on a larger scale, we are well aware that Environmental Gerontology has been a global enterprise for several years now. For example, European, Latin American, Asian, and Australian researchers continue to make significant contributions to the ecology of aging (e.g., see Sanchez-Gonzalez & Rodriquez-Rodriquez, 2016). I agree with Wahl's (2016, p. v) presumption that "the context of aging is strongly framed within specific cultures." However, the fundamental nature of the *cultural frame* generates a number of open questions: Under what circumstances does "culture" affect aging in "context?" Specifically, where, how, and for whom does culture—*as an internalized construct* or as a more finely *differentiated socio-environmental component*—affect aging in contexts that vary in type, level, and complexity? Indeed, what might current or future international data contribute to its clearer conceptualization? In an attempt to understand the cultural frame, it would seem useful to pursue collaborative cross-national research efforts dedicated largely to identifying cultural distinctions as well as universals within and between these international contexts for aging.

SOME CLOSING THOUGHTS

Over the past 40 years, advances in theory and research in the ecology of aging have been made by *luminaries*—bright, innovative researchers *lit from within* by their own spark; many are contributors to this volume. As an editor, my contribution has been that of a mirror, reflecting the light they have generated, directing it to wider audiences. It is hoped that our coedited works were successful in this way. In addition to our primary journal publications, I remain proud of our contributions as chapter authors in various edited volumes. In particular, I refer to chapters in the *Handbook of the Psychology of Aging* (Scheidt & Windley, 1985, 2006), Environmental Design Research Association publications (Norris-Baker & Scheidt, 1990, 1992), mental health updates on "at risk" rural elders in the United States (Norris-Baker & Scheidt, 1996; Scheidt, 1985, 1998), and the ethnography of rural place meaning (Norris-Baker & Scheidt, 2005). Included here is our effort to provide environmental gerontologists with a still-relevant survey of the evolution, current status, and future challenges of Lawton and Nahemow's General Ecological Model (Scheidt & Norris-Baker, 2004).

In closing, I find that Environmental Gerontology remains a "good fit" for most of my social environmental interests. I have no regrets or hoped for "do-overs" about my engagements in this wonderful and interesting field. I have been honored to work and to sustain friendships with many of the researchers and scholars in Environmental Gerontology. I hope our efforts to expand understanding of rural elders in particular, especially those who reside in resource-scarce environments, might be viewed as more than archival. We shared their voices and our ideas with policy makers, practitioners, as well as rural researchers at state, national, and international levels (Scheidt, 1997; Scheidt & Windley, 1979). Years hence, I hope our career contributions will be valued for illustrating the diversity of aging in select rural small-town settings across better and worse economic eras, for enhancing understanding of the adaptive challenges of aging-in-place in "at risk" rural environments, and for offering fuller understanding of rural contexts in both variable-oriented and ethnographic research orientations targeting rural elderly populations.

REFERENCES

Aldwin, C., & Stokols, D. (1988). The effects of environmental change on individuals and groups. Some neglected issues in stress research. *Journal of Environmental Psychology*, *8*, 57–75.

Barker, R. (1968). *Ecological psychology: Concepts and methods for studying the environment of human behavior*. Redwood City, CA: Stanford University Press.

Barlett, P. (1990). Qualitative methods in rural studies: Basic principles. *The Rural Sociologist*, *10*(2), 3–14.

Eisdorfer, C., & Lawton, M. P. (Eds.). (1973). *The psychology of adult development and aging*. Washington, DC: American Psychological Association.

Fitchen, J. (1990). "How do you know what to ask if you haven't listened first?" Using anthropological methods to prepare for survey research. *The Rural Sociologist*, *10*(2), 15–22.

Hrybyk, R., Rubinstein, R., Eckert, J. K., Frankowski, A. C., Keimig, L., Nemic, M., et al. (2013). The dark side: Stigma in purpose-built senior environments. In R. Scheidt & B. Schwarz (Eds.), *Environmental gerontology: What now?* (pp. 293–307). New York, NY: Routledge.

Lawton, M. P. (1982). Competence, environmental press, and the adaptation of older people. In M. P. Lawton, P. Windley, & T. O. Byerts (Eds.), *Aging and the environment: Theoretical approaches* (pp. 33–59). New York, NY: Springer Publishing.

Lawton, M. P. (1998). Environment and aging: Theory revisited. In R. Scheidt & P. Windley (Eds.), *Environment and aging theory: A focus on housing* (pp. 1–32). Westport, CT: Greenwood Press.

Lawton, M. P., & Nahemow, L. (1973). Ecology and the aging process. In C. Eisdorfer & M. P. Lawton (Eds.), *The psychology of adult development and aging* (pp. 619–674). Washington, DC: American Psychological Association.

Norris-Baker, C., & Scheidt, R. (1990). Place attachment among older residents of a 'ghost town': A transactional approach. In R. Selby, K. Anthony, J. Choi, & B. Orland (Eds.), *Coming of age* (pp. 333–342). Oklahoma: Environmental Design Research Association.

Norris-Baker, C., & Scheidt, R. (1992). Community covenants: An indicator of sustainable small-town habitats? In E. Arias & M. Gross (Eds.), *Equitable and sustainable habitats* (pp. 30–42). Colorado: Environmental Design Research Association.

Norris-Baker, C., & Scheidt, R. (1994). From 'Our Town' to 'Ghost Town': The changing context of home for rural elders. *International Journal of Aging and Human Development, 38*(3), 181–202.

Norris-Baker, C., & Scheidt, R. (1996). Aging survivors: The mental health of older residents of declining rural communities. In. N. Perrin (Ed.), *Aging and mental health: Aging in the heartland* (pp. 15–33). Blue Springs, MO: Mid-America Congress on Aging.

Norris-Baker, C., & Scheidt, R. (2005). On community as home: Places that endure in rural Kansas. In G. Rowles & H. Chaudhury (Eds.), *Home and identity in late life: International perspectives* (pp. 279–298). New York, NY: Springer Publishing.

Regnier, V. (2003). Powell Lawton's contributions to purpose-built housing design for the elderly. *Journal of Housing for the Elderly, 17*(1–2), 39–53.

Ruby, J. (1996). Visual anthropology. In D. Levinson & M. Ember (Eds.), *Encyclopedia of cultural anthropology, 4*, 1345–1351.

Sanchez-Gonzalez, D., & Rodriquez-Rodriquez, V. (Eds.). (2016). *Environmental gerontology in Europe and Latin America: Policies and perspectives on environment and aging.* New York, NY: Springer Publishing.

Scheidt, R. (1974). Deviance, power, and the occult: A field study. *Journal of Psychology, 87*(1), 21–28.

Scheidt, R. (1982). *Technical assistance workshop for directors: National Institute of Mental Health sponsored Clinical Training Programs in the mental health of the aged.* Invited participant on Research on Aging, Washington, DC.

Scheidt, R. (1984). A taxonomy of well-being for small-town elderly. A case for rural diversity. *The Gerontologist, 24*(1), 84–90.

Scheidt, R. (1985). The mental health of the aged in rural environments. In R. Coward & G. Lee (Eds.), *The elderly in rural society* (pp. 105–127). New York, NY: Springer Publishing.

Scheidt, R. (1997). The ecology of aging: Research illustrations from rural Kansas, USA. *Psychological Journal* (Publication of the Russian Academy of Sciences, Institute of Psychology), *18*, 47–61.

Scheidt, R. (1998). The mental health of elderly in rural environments. In R. Coward & J. Krout (Eds.), *Rural elders: An exploration of the life circumstances and distinctive features of aging in rural America* (pp. 85–104). New York, NY: Springer Publishing.

Scheidt, R. (2010, November). *Place-making interventions and aging-in-place in small dying towns: A report from the Great Plains.* Poster session presented at the meeting of the Gerontological Society of America, New Orleans, LA.

Scheidt, R. (2016). The defense of my aging self: A report from the field. [Special issue]. *The Gerontologist*, *57*(1), 110–115.

Scheidt, R., & Norris-Baker, C. (1990). A transactional approach to environmental stress among older residents of rural communities: Introduction to a special issue. *Journal of Rural Community Psychology*, *11*(1), 5–30.

Scheidt, R., & Norris-Baker, C. (1999). Place therapies for older adults: Conceptual and interventive approaches. *International Journal of Aging and Human Development*, *48*(1), 1–15.

Scheidt, R., & Norris-Baker, C. (2013). Understudied older populations and settings in environmental gerontology: Candidates for future research. In R. Scheidt & B. Schwarz (Eds.), *Environmental gerontology: What now?* (pp. 269–292). New York, NY: Routledge.

Scheidt, R., & Norris-Baker, C. (2004). The general ecological model: Evolution, current status, and future challenges. In H. Wahl, R. Scheidt, & P. Windley (Eds.), *Annual Review of Gerontology and Geriatrics (Vol. 23): Focus on aging in context: Socio-physical environments* (pp. 34–58). New York, NY: Springer Publishing.

Scheidt, R., & Schaie, K. (1978). A taxonomy of situations for an elderly population: Generating situational criteria. *Journal of Gerontology*, 33(6), 848–857.

Scheidt, R., & Schwarz, B. (Eds.). (2013). *Environmental gerontology: What now?* New York, NY: Routledge.

Scheidt, R., & Windley, P. (1979, November). *Environment and mental health of small-town rural elderly.* Invited presentation to the staff of the United States Senate Special Committee on Aging, Washington, DC: U.S. Capitol Building.

Scheidt, R., & Windley, P. (1983). Mental health of small- town elderly residents: An expanded ecological model. *Journal of Gerontology*, 38(4), 472–479.

Scheidt, R., & Windley, P. (1985). The ecology of aging. In J. Birren & K. Warner Schaie (Eds.), *The handbook of the psychology of aging* (pp. 245–260). New York, NY: Van Nostrand.

Scheidt, R., & Windley, P. (1987). Environmental perceptions and patterns of well-being among older Americans in small rural towns. *Comprehensive Gerontology*, *1*(1), 24–29.

Scheidt, R., & Windley, P. (1998). *Environment and aging theory: A focus on housing.* Westport, CT: Greenwood Press.

Scheidt, R., & Windley, P. (Eds.). (2003). *Physical environments and aging: Critical contributions of M. Powell Lawton.* New York, NY: Haworth Press.

Scheidt, R., & Windley, P. (2006). Environmental gerontology: Progress in the post-Lawton era. In K. W. Schaie & J. Birren (Eds.), *The handbook of the psychology of aging* (6th ed., pp. 105–125). New York, NY: Academic Press.

Wahl, H.-W. (2016). Preface. In D. Sanchez-Gonzalez & V. Rodriquez-Rodriquez (Eds.), *Environmental gerontology in Europe and Latin America: Policies and perspectives on environment and aging* (p. v). New York, NY: Springer Publishing.

Wahl, H. W., Scheidt, R., & Windley, P. (Eds.). (2003). *Annual review of gerontology and geriatrics (Vol. 23): Aging in context: Socio-physical environments.* New York, NY: Springer Publishing.

Windley, P., Byerts, T., & Ernst, E. (Eds.). (1975). *Theory development in environment and aging*. Washington, DC: Gerontological Society of America.

Windley, P., & Scheidt, R. (1980). Studying older persons in small rural towns: Environment and well-being. *Educational Gerontology*, *5*, 355–373.

Windley, P., & Scheidt, R. (1982). An ecological model of mental health among small-town rural elderly. *Journal of Gerontology*, *37*(2), 235–242.

Windley, P., & Scheidt, R. (1983). Service utilization and activity participation among psychologically vulnerable and well elderly in rural small towns. *The Gerontologist*, *23*(3), 283–287.

CHAPTER 12

Finding Place

An Intellectual Journey

Benyamin Schwarz

ABSTRACT

Growing up in the multigenerational Israeli community of a kibbutz allowed me a close peek into the lives of individuals of all ages and capabilities who lived their personal dreams in the shadow of this social, collective dream of the twentieth century. As a young architect, I had the opportunity to design several housing complexes for the elderly in communities promising their elderly members social and financial security, appropriate employment to their skills, meaningful participation, and continuous productive lives regardless of their physical or mental abilities. The challenge, which became a central theme of my professional work has been how to create physical environments that sustain older adults and address the fundamental conflict of the human condition: the tension between aspiring spirit and the declining body. Following several years of architectural practice, I went back to school and completed my doctoral studies at the University of Michigan. Three contextual themes have dominated my journey in the field of Environmental Gerontology: (1) the orientation toward applied research and the wish to bring about research-informed practice and practice-aware research; (2) attentiveness to the balance between autonomy and security in long-term care settings; and (3) the significance and meaning of place as people age and become increasingly needy and vulnerable.

http://dx.doi.org/10.1891/0198-8794.38.201

BIOGRAPHICAL NOTES

Neither intellectual histories nor memoirs can be understood apart from the subjective experiences and the social and cultural context of their authors. However, intellectual autobiographies attempt to trace the routes whereby an individual contributes to a particular field of study. Karr (2015) notes that "a fiction writer starts with meaning and then manufactures events to represent it; a memoirist starts with events, then derives meaning from them" (p. xvii). This chapter endeavors to recapture in a short account the pivotal events of my life, and identify the contextual factors that guided my journey through the field of Environmental Gerontology.

Early Childhood

I was born in Czechoslovakia on Christmas day of 1946 to Jewish parents who were the only survivors of the Holocaust in their family. I never knew my grandparents. They were gassed by the Nazis in Auschwitz. My parents were in the process of recovering from the horrors of WWII, trying to forget the past with the intention to remain faithful to life in its present, when the forces of political upheaval and chaos forced them to put their dreams on hold. In the first few months of 1948, with the help of Josef Stalin and his secret police, the Communist Party in Czechoslovakia completed the transformation of the regime into a totalitarian system based on the ideological principles of Marxism-Leninism. The entire cultural and educational system was submitted to a total Communist state control. Planned economy was introduced and private ownership of all means of production eliminated. Czechoslovakia became a satellite state of the Soviet Union and any resistance was eradicated by terror and apprehension. So-called "dissidents" were purged, commonly arrested, and often executed following short show trials.

My parents, who led a comfortable and affluent life, could not adjust to a lifestyle that took away everything they owned and contradicted their essential beliefs. They wanted to immigrate to the United States, but could not secure the necessary documents in order to move to their desired destination. Thus, in the spring of 1949, they packed whatever the Communist authorities allowed them to take with them, and we boarded a train to Italy. After several weeks in Bari, Italy, we embarked on a small ship that took us to the newborn Jewish state of Israel. I was two-and-a-half years old when we arrived at the transition camp for new emigrants near the port of Haifa. Like most of the refugees in the camp, my parents did not speak any Hebrew and were desperate to leave the camp, but they could not function in the Israeli society outside the camp, let alone with an unfamiliar language and culture. So, when my father's cousin came to visit and offered them a chance to live in a kibbutz in the Jordan Valley, they decided to give it a try. We arrived at kibbutz Afikim on a hot day in June 1949. Avoiding communism in Czechoslovakia only to become members of the ultimate Socialist-Zionist experiment of the *Kibbutz* in Israel would prove to be one of the ironies that plagued my parents' lives.

Life in the Kibbutz

Part of the idea of the kibbutz was the wish to create a just and equal society as an alternative to a capitalist society. Thus, kibbutz societies emphasized ideals of collectivity, equality, social solidarity, and mutual responsibility. The common educational goals were to educate the next generation to continue the kibbutz form of life. Consequently, children were raised in children houses within the collective education system which was strictly forced on parents and children. Since all the kibbutz members worked in a position allocated by the "work committee," my father was sent to work in the local plywood factory and my mother was assigned to the children's kitchen where the food for all the kibbutz's children was prepared. All meals for the adults were served in the common dining hall. My parents' dwelling consisted of a small room with no bathroom or running water in a row house that included four more rooms of the same size where our neighbors lived. The communal showers and the bathrooms were situated several minutes' walk from their "room." Since the community provided all basic needs for the members, there were no salaries or other means of compensation. The intention of the system was to practice the slogan "from each according to his or her capacity, to each according to his or her needs." However, the realities of human nature and the rift between perfection and impossibility have always hovered over the utopian ideals of the kibbutz.

Growing up in this multigenerational community allowed a close peek into the lives of many individuals—men, women, children, and elders who lived their personal dreams in the shadow of one of the largest collective dreams of the 20th century. The closeness of life in the kibbutz, in which every person intimately knew everyone else, uncovered for me:

> The core questions that confront all human groups in the consciousness of existence: how one meets death, the meaning of tragedy, the nature of obligation, the character of love—these recurrent questions which are . . . cultural universals, to be found in all societies where [humans] become conscious of the finiteness of existence. (Bell, 1980, p. 333)

In my formative years, I observed day by day kibbutz members aspiring to create a society that elevates community over the individual just to realize that their ideals remain always out of reach. I witnessed the limits posed by human propensities in the efforts to transition from what Ernest Bloch called "abstract utopia" to "concrete utopia." In hindsight, these life experiences influenced my own values, and later my quest for bridging the gap between idealism and realism in communities for elderly people.

I am a "product" of the communal education system of the kibbutz. After completing elementary education in the small school at the kibbutz, I graduated from the vocational, regional high school of the Jordan Valley. Following graduation from high school, I became a member of the kibbutz. After 1 year of serving as a youth-guide in a suburb of Haifa, I began in 1966 my mandatory 3-year service in the Israeli army. During these years I met my wife, Rachel, in the army camp where we both served. We got married 1 week after I was discharged from the army, and we settled in the kibbutz. Our three children, Guy, Mor, and Tom were born in this place. In 1970, I enrolled in the school of architecture at the Technion in Haifa and graduated 5 years later with a degree in architecture and town planning. A year later, while still working for the Kibbutz Planning Department in Tel Aviv, my partner and I opened our architectural office in the kibbutz. We were fortunate to be hired for the design of numerous projects including family housing, educational facilities, offices, industries, cultural venues, and many other buildings for the kibbutzim (plural for a kibbutz) in the vicinity. In 1978, we expanded our office and turned into the Jordan Valley regional department for architectural and planning services. We employed 20 or so architects, engineers, and technicians, and many of the kibbutzim in the Jordan Valley became our clients. These communities were established at the beginning of the 20th century, so in the 1980s, their founding members were older adults who gradually developed needs for special housing and care services. Consequently, we were commissioned to design purposeful housing units for elderly people as well as the regional daycare center for seniors in the Jordan Valley (Figure 12.1). This was my initiation to the field of aging and the environment.

For decades, the kibbutz was considered an ideal community for growing old in Israel. Positive outcomes such as life expectancy, health, and wellbeing of kibbutz members were higher than that of the overall Jewish population in Israel. Because of the total and unconditional responsibility of the kibbutzim to their members and those dependent upon them, elderly people in these closely knit communities enjoyed the social arrangements that responded to their unique physical, social, and emotional needs (Leviatan & Salm, 2007). The communities promised their elderly members inclusive modalities of social security, appropriate employment, cultural integration in community framework, meaningful participation, and continuing productivity regardless of their physical or mental abilities.

The design process of the housing arrangements presented me with opportunities for interaction with many elderly individuals, their families and

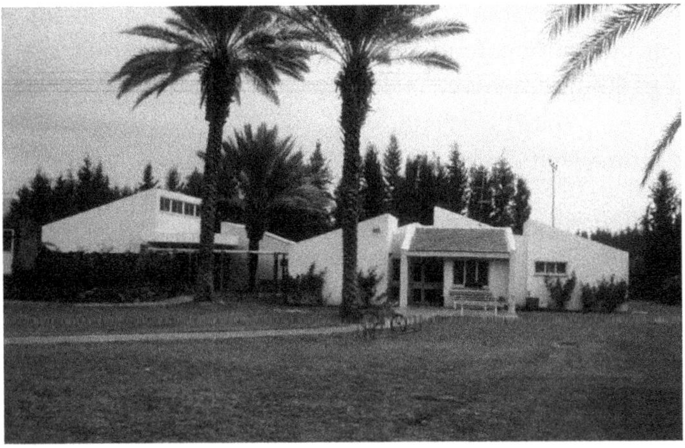

FIGURE 12.1 Regional day-care center for seniors in the Jordan Valley, Israel, 1987.

caregivers. At the same time, it introduced me to the challenges of creating an environment in which a group of older adults with various levels of physical and mental disabilities involuntary live together in an artificial community which compromised the essential conditions of their initial home. It became obvious that many of the physical, social, and metaphysical dimensions of the *home* were not present in the housing and care facilities we designed. We realized that the environmental and emotional detachment that existed between ideal residential life and the unusual situation presented by living in what we called a *supportive old people's home* was difficult to patch up with the physical design. This challenge became a central theme of my line of inquiry.

My chance to go deeper in the field of Environmental Gerontology presented itself in a life-changing hallway conversation. In 1984, I took a leave of absence from the kibbutz and my architectural office to accept a position as an emissary to a Jewish community in the metropolitan area of Detroit, Michigan. We moved our family to the United States and I worked for 3 years in this diplomatic role. As part of my job, I visited the main university campuses in Michigan to present students with study abroad opportunities in Israel. In one of these visits to the University of Michigan, I met Dr. Leon Pastalan in the corridor of the School of Architecture. I recognized his name from the publications I read when I designed housing for the elderly in Israel, and knew he was a renowned scholar in the field of aging and environment. Since the 1970s, he mentored numerous researchers in the field, and his influence on the second generation of knowledge producers in Environmental Gerontology was instrumental. The short visit to Lee's office changed my life. During our discussion, we talked about my professional background and his teaching of aging and the environment, and Lee encouraged me to apply to the doctoral program at the University of Michigan to study Environmental Gerontology. I hesitated to make a commitment, but I took the application forms and after returning to Israel in 1987, I applied and was accepted to the doctoral program. Thus, in the summer of 1988, at the relatively "old" age of 42 I left the kibbutz to begin my PhD studies at the University of Michigan. My wife and two of our children joined me in Ann Arbor a year later. Our oldest son, Guy, stayed in Israel for his mandatory army service.

In his collection of stories, Jorge Luis Borges famously conceived of life as a search through a maze. I was always fascinated by this metaphor. In retrospect, I sometimes wonder what makes us choose a particular branch when we reach a bifurcation in the road of our personal maze. Faced with the opportunities and circumstances of life, I believe that *chance*, rather than calculated decisions put me on the particular path I have followed. To paraphrase Yogi Berra, *we came to the fork in the road, and we took it.*

GATEWAY TO THE FIELD OF ENVIRONMENTAL GERONTOLOGY

My courses at the University of Michigan linked philosophy of science and architectural theories with a special emphasis on environment and behavior studies. These fundamentals guided my intellectual growth. Lee Pastalan became my mentor and dear friend. From him I learned empathy for older people and the psycho-social perspectives on the field of aging and the environment. We had long discussions on the aging process and the environmental vulnerabilities that come with it. We examined the challenges when elderly people are obliged to receive more care services in order to remain in their homes or when they contemplate relocating to more supportive settings. But most of all we contemplated the meaning of places where frail elders reside. I became aware that the meaning of place was no less significant for elders than adequate shelter, food, clothing, and health care.

Two other teachers affected my education in profound ways. Professor Mark Chesler from the School of Sociology introduced me to qualitative research methods. His two-semester intense course was pivotal to the ways I have conducted my own research ever since. His enthusiasm and in-depth understanding of human nature exposed me to social meanings, whereby situations are interpreted and meanings are constructed and shared. Professor Tom Hickey from the School of Public Health opened my eyes to the social, cultural, and economic factors affecting older people in modern society and the delivery of health and related services to the older population in the United States. He made me aware of the diversity of older people, their needs and aspirations, particularly when they develop chronic illnesses. Marked by a loss of physical or mental abilities, these conditions curtail a person's capacity to look after their needs forcing them to move to long-term care (LTC) settings, which became the sites of my research. It was in this class that I was introduced to the intricacies of Alzheimer's disease and other forms of dementia. During that time, I befriended Dr. Uriel Cohen, who shared with me an early version of his book *Holding on to Home,* which he coauthored with Dr. Gerald Weisman. The book's successful translation of research theories into valuable guidelines for practitioners made it a seminal text in my education and teachings.

In September 1992, following 4 years of studies, I successfully defended my dissertation and was awarded the first PhD degree at the School of Architecture in the University of Michigan. Just months later, I traveled to Israel in search for an academic position. My meetings in the School of Architecture at the Technion were encouraging. However, after my return to the United States, I received a letter informing me that the Technion would not have the budget for a faculty position. As a result, in March of 1993, I started searching for an academic position in the United States. To my dismay, I learned that my PhD with an emphasis in environment and behavior studies was not marketable in schools of architecture as architectural education moved away from the psycho-social orientation of the 1970s toward history and theory, and computer-aided design. In contrast, an interior design program in a human sciences college was more welcoming for this line of inquiry. Subsequently, in the summer of 1993, I accepted a position at what became known as the Department of Architectural Studies at the University of Missouri—Columbia. My family and I became American citizens and we built our home in this university town.

Besides teaching architectural theory, design programming, and design studios for undergraduate students, I have mentored a large number of graduate students on site and online. While working with masters and PhD students has been intellectually stimulating and rewarding, the topics of their dissertations have rarely coincided with my interest in Environmental Gerontology. Indeed, the dichotomy between my teachings and research interests has prevented me from teaching courses regarding aging and the environment, but I have strived to sustain my contribution to this field.

An overarching leitmotif underlines my outlook on Environmental Gerontology: the paradoxical nature of aging. As Thomas R. Cole's observed:

> Aging, like illness and death, reveals the most fundamental conflict of the human condition: the tension between infinite ambitions, dreams and desires on the one hand, and vulnerable, limited decaying physical existence on the other—the tragic and ineradicable conflict between spirit and body. (Cole, 1992, p. 239)

Three contextual themes dominated my journey in this field of study. First is my orientation toward applied research and my wish to bring about research-informed practice and practice-aware research. Second is my attentiveness to the balance between autonomy and security in LTC settings; and third is the significance and meaning of place as we age and become needy and vulnerable. These three themes constitute parallel, intertwining threads that bind my intellectual pursuit in Environmental Gerontology. I will briefly discuss these three themes in the following sections.

APPLIED VERSUS BASIC RESEARCH

The question of knowledge at the service of older people versus knowledge as a scholarly goal in its own right, or *basic* versus *applied* research, confronted me when I joined the field of studies in Environmental Gerontology. Early on I realized that the physical environment has limited power to change elders' physical and mental decline. *Places*, on the other hand, have a significant role in older people lives, preventing or allowing them to continue realizing their dreams and remain the authors of their own life stories (Gawande, 2014). Thus, my research has been guided by the attempt to understand how to restore elders' opportunity to exercise environmental control, while maintaining necessary levels of physical and social support. My contribution to the field has concentrated on producing applicable knowledge and helping to disseminate the growing knowledge base in order to affect changes and improve the quality of lives of older people. I became an advocate for translating what we learn "about meaning and significance of place to older people and their wellbeing into concrete recommendations for practice, policy, and design" (Rowles & Bernard, 2013, p. 5).

Because of my architectural background, I came to believe that researchers in Environmental Gerontology share a social mission as well as responsibility to generate knowledge for intervention. However, I recognize that the wicked nature of the relationships between basic knowledge and practice can be challenging, as Lawton (1990) noted:

> Synthesis is rarely a feasible goal in researching an informed design solution because the demand of practical solutions always outstrips the resources of basic science to deliver them. Thus the researcher faces the dilemma of communicating unsatisfying small amounts of knowledge derived from research that meets acceptable methodological standards or, on the other hand, going significantly beyond the data so as to provide concrete design assistance. Either way someone loses, the practitioner in frustration over the limited amount of guidance available from the academic, or the researcher in risking a loss of integrity in going beyond the data. (p. 351)

In a perfect world, basic and applied research can merge and mutually reinforce each other. In reality, however, basic and applied researches differ in purpose, context, and methods. The basic researcher is commonly investigating narrowly focused questions, which enables him or her to concentrate on a single measurement task in a relatively controlled setting. In contrast, a researcher who deals with applicable issues tends to perform her or his investigation in an uncontrolled environment facing multiple ill-constrained, ill-framed questions that often come from real life situations (Schwarz, 2003).

During the years I have been a professor, I have had few opportunities to use research-aware practice in my role as a consultant and an architect. One of the most successful examples came about in 1999 when the owners of a continuing residential care community in St. Louis invited me to consult with their company for developing a 120-bed standalone facility for people with dementia. At that time, the state of Missouri was in the process of developing several facilities in a demonstration project for memory care which aimed at setting benchmarks for innovative environments and care for people with dementia. To assure aging-in-place for the residents, we developed the physical setting to include 3 households, 20 residents in each, who were in the early stages of Alzheimer's, and 60 skilled nursing beds for residents in their late stages of dementia. The memory-care community opened in 2004 and became a testament to the successful collaborative research-informed practice (Figures 12.2 and 12.3).

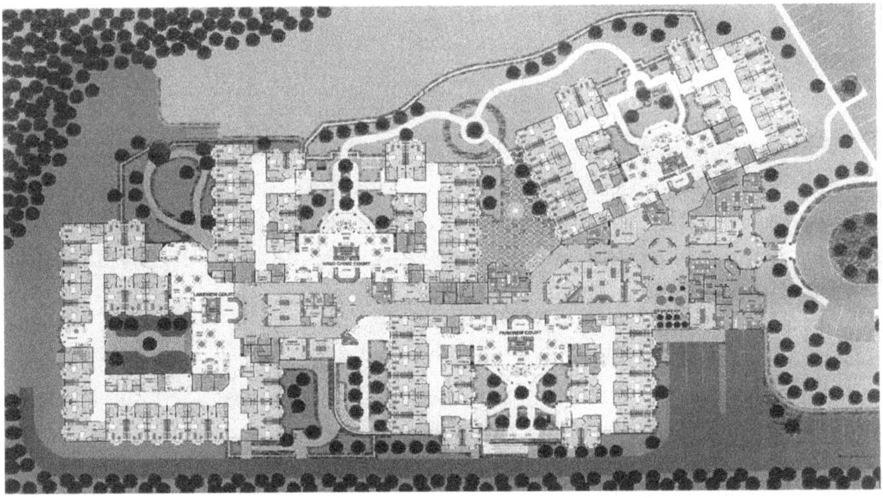

FIGURE 12.2 A 120-bed standalone facility for people with dementia. Site Plan. St. Louis, 2004.

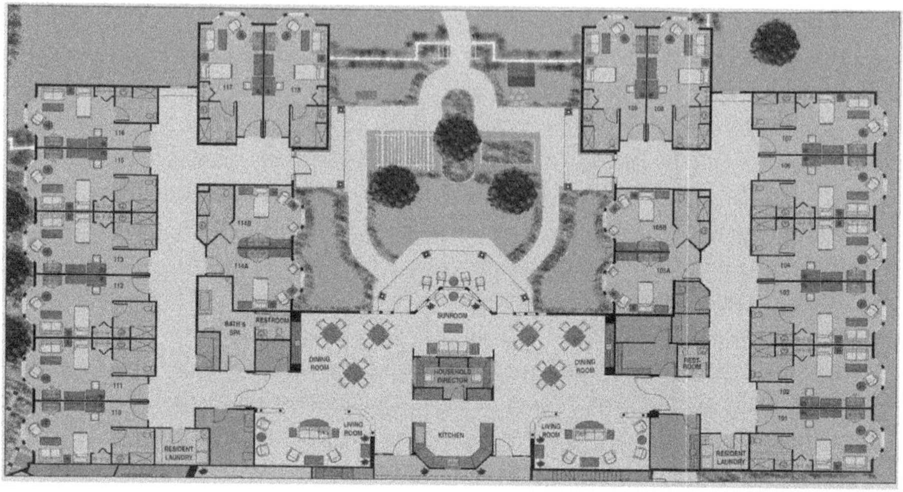

FIGURE 12.3 A 120-bed standalone facility for people with dementia. A residential household. St. Louis, 2004.

During the design and construction process, I recognized (again) that practice is essentially an activity directed toward accomplishing a goal. It deals with real-life problems that require instant decisions, and it involves choice and prioritizing options, which in some cases are based on incomplete knowledge. Basic science cannot provide full answers for practitioners because it is fundamentally incomplete. It consists of no more than the current state of *research* (Gadamer, 1996). Practitioners are required to base their decisions on an imperfect knowledge. Thus, in order to be relevant, Environmental Gerontology should concentrate on the production of practical knowledge that should be driven by actual, everyday practice. "It needs to focus on case studies, precedents, and exemplars that should not be disconnected from their contexts." It needs to generate applicable knowledge that can help to solve particular problems in local situations. And "it must deal with problems as they holistically present themselves in actual situations" (Schwarz, 2013, pp. 19–20).

As a journal editor for over 15 years, I have worked extensively at the intersection of theory and application. In 2000 I became the editor of the *Journal of Housing for the Elderly,* which was conceived by Dr. Leon Pastalan as an academic publication that integrates theoretical and applied research. During my tenure, the journal evolved into an international publication, covering such areas as: identification of salient housing issues that primarily involve the elderly; case studies of successful practitioner experiences regarding the development of better housing facilities for the elderly; refinement of existing methodologies and the development of new ones for evaluating the consequences of diverse residential environments; translation of research findings into usable information for researchers and practitioners alike; and articulation of issues and problems in the development and implementation of housing policies for elderly people. Beside the regular quarterly publications, I benefited from collaborating with guest editors in producing special issues on valuable subjects such as a recent example pertaining to developments of housing for elderly people in Scandinavia (Nord & Schwarz, 2015). Some of the special issues were later printed as edited books (Rodiek & Schwarz, 2005, 2007; Scheidt & Schwarz, 2013). Currently, we are working on a special issue regarding physical environments in age-friendly developments. The journal is perhaps one of the only academic publications dedicated to Environmental Gerontology as its core mission.

AUTONOMY IN LONG-TERM CARE SETTINGS

In the late 1980s, while I was still in graduate school, I learned about assisted living arrangements from Leslie Knight, the Midwest Regional Director for American Association of Homes and Services for the Aging. The success of the pioneering work of Karen Brown Wilson in Oregon and Paul Klaassen's Sunrise communities launched a wave of communities that rapidly spread around the United States and made assisted living one of the most prominent models of LTC. The primary goal of assisted living developments has been to provide LTC services tailored to individual needs in a residential and normalized setting (Schwarz & Brent, 1999a). Assisted living settings have attempted to emulate a *social* rather than a *medical* model of care by including more residential-like attributes and less institutional-like architecture and interior design. In their philosophy of care, assisted living arrangements have tried to eschew the rigid operational regulations of nursing homes and to adapt to changes in conditions of residents by providing individualized care. The program of services has been anticipated to function with the underlying precedence of resident autonomy rather than staff efficiency. In addition to private living spaces, personal decor items from original residences, and smaller groupings of peers, living and care options were adapted to fit the idiosyncratic needs of residents, a stark contrast to the inflexible routines and rules of nursing homes.

The new model was initially a promising alternative to nursing homes. Consequently, in 1995 I organized with Dr. Ruth Brent (Tofle) two symposia in the annual meeting of the Gerontology Society of America in Los Angeles. A year later, we brought together several scholars for a workshop in the Environmental Design Research Association in Salt Lake City under the title *Place Makes a Difference: Advances in Assisted Living*. The symposia attracted researchers and practitioners from social gerontology and environmental design and subsequently led to the publication of the coedited book *Aging Autonomy and Architecture* (Schwarz & Brent, 1999b). The title of the book reflects our shared belief that the architecture of LTC environments affects the freedom of older adults to make decisions and to act on those decisions that touch their lives. We argued that autonomy gives meaning to life and allows elders to control and retain their freedom to shape their lives (Agich, 1993). We recognized that personal autonomy in LTC environments is compromised by the characteristics of other residents, staff conduct, physical settings, available programs, and public policies that govern these facilities. Frail elders who move to LTC settings seek to satisfy, among other needs, security to maximize both their physical safety and peace of mind. However, too often they pay for the perceived security with their personal autonomy (Parmelee & Lawton, 1990).

While some decrease of autonomy is inevitable in advanced old age, a stark loss is imminent for those with terminal dementia. Given the prevalence of dementia with advanced age, applying the concept of autonomy is particularly challenging in this population. Too often we have come to presume that in the care for residents with dementia we have to rule out autonomy. However, both security and autonomy are needed in dementia care. Making places for old people who suffer from mental decline requires imagination and invention beyond the competence of maintaining their safety. Striking a balance between these contradicting demands remains one of the most difficult challenges in the provision of LTC (Schwarz, Chaudhury, & Brent-Tofle, 2004). Dementia care environments will continue to proliferate and improve as the need for these places is growing and because research in Environmental Gerontology "strongly suggests that the physical setting can indeed have a therapeutic role in the care for people with dementia" (Cohen & Weisman, 1991, p. 6). Nevertheless, we recognize that the physical environment, by itself, cannot have direct, deterministic effects on patterns of human physical and mental decline. Thus our role is to develop environments that do not restrain people's choices, in the name of safety and security, but accommodate diverse needs of residents by allowing autonomy and control, in the name of living a meaningful life.

THE SIGNIFICANCE OF PLACE

Central to my dissertation study, *Designing Public Places for Private Lives: A Study of the Design Process of Long-term Care Settings* (Schwarz, 1992) was the significance of *place* and the meaning of all that make up a person's life in a nursing home. Through interviews and observations, I tried to understand the ways social forces and physical design parameters lead participants in the design process to build nursing homes in the United States. I learned that nursing homes were never devised to help people facing dependency in old age, and that in the design of the nursing home environment we have achieved the worst of both worlds: an institutional setting that goes too far while it also does too little for its residents (Schwarz, 1996, 1997). What struck me the most was the overwhelming resentment among residents, their families, and caregivers that the depressing and frightening setting of the nursing home provokes. At the same time, the architects and the design teams I observed in my earlier study kept doing "business as usual," relying on a misguided model, rules, and regulations as if nothing better could be conceived.

We can do better. In fact, I had the pleasure to visit numerous successful models of places for provision of LTC in the United States as well as in northern European countries such as Denmark, Sweden, Finland, and The Netherlands. The qualities and characteristics of the physical environments and programs in these places can inspire architects, care providers, and policy makers to create better places for older people who are forced to leave their home when they can no longer sustain themselves or be sustained by family or social services. We should strive for helping older adults with modest care needs to continue to live independently, preserving their health and wellbeing as long as possible in their homes. Simultaneously, we should enable frail old people with high dependencies to live with dignity and autonomy in LTC settings that make a contribution to their quality of life (Regnier, 1994, 2002).

Few models in recent years have attempted to challenge these difficulties (Thomas, 2004). However any new model will have to simultaneously address the three contradictions that remain at the heart of the efforts to improve LTC settings: (a) the ideal philosophy of care in which residents maintain control of their private lives while they receive care and protection, conflicts too often with the institutional regulations and reimbursement policies; (b) the intent to model the physical environment upon home-like rather than institutional ideas is frequently just a façade behind which institutional patterns refuse to go away; and (c) the effort (or lack of) to integrate housing for elderly people within the community. In reality, integrations into the community are rare and remain simply rhetoric rather than practical solutions.

To advance the practical goals of Environmental Gerontology, we need to challenge the status quo and change the narrative we tell ourselves about the future of LTC. Cosmetic changes to the built environment or care practices constitute a necessary but unsatisfactory incentive for real change. The replacement model should be an embodiment of principles, of which the *normalization* concept is essential (Golant, 2015). In other words, we should emphasize social rather than merely physical care, and make conscious attempts to enhance older adults' opportunities for the exercise of autonomy and prospects for ascribing meaning and significance to their new residential setting.

When this book is published, I will be 70 years old or so. Our adult children gratified us by living their dreams and blessed us with seven grandchildren. Both my parents died when they were still engaged and productive in late life. My mother expired following a short struggle with pneumonia, and my father passed away 13 years earlier while working on a calligraphy project in his study. I do not look forward to coping with the problems of old age and frailty. However, if I had a chance to devise my own environment for growing old, I want to stay at my home and let attention and support modify rather than relocating to a setting dominated by staff. I want to be surrounded by my family and my dogs in the place I built and where my mind touches the world. If the needs arise, I want to be able to schedule needed care around my preferences and wants. I want to be physically and intellectually active, paint in watercolors, read books, and listen to classical and jazz music. I would like to be able to venture out of my home to visit interesting places, enjoy recreational venues, and delight in cultural events. And, I will be looking forward to remaining in my own *place* until the inevitable end.

REFERENCES

Agich, G. (1993). *Autonomy and long-term care*. New York, NY: Oxford University Press.

Bell, D. (1980). The return of the sacred? In D. Bell (Ed.), *The winding passage* (pp. 328–358). Cambridge, MA: ABT Books.

Cohen, U., & Weisman, G. D. (1991). *Holding on to home: Designing environments for people with dementia*. Baltimore, MD: The Johns Hopkins University Press.

Cole, T. R. (1992). *The journey of life: A cultural history of aging in America*. Cambridge, MA: Cambridge University Press.

Gadamer, H.-G. (1996). *The enigma of health: The art of healing in scientific age*. Redwood City, CA: Stanford University Press.

Gawande, A. (2014). *Being mortal: Medicine and what matters in the end*. New York, NY: Metropolitan Books, Henry Holt and Company.

Golant, S. M. (2015). *Aging in the right place*. Baltimore, MD: Health Profession Press.

Karr, M. (2015). *The art of memoir*. New York, NY: Harper.

Lawton, M. P. (1990). An environmental psychologist ages. In I. Altman & K. Christensen (Eds.), *Environment and behaviour studies: Emergent intellectual traditions* (pp. 339–363). New York, NY: Plenum Press.

Leviatan, U., & Salm, C. (2007). Socioeconomic inequality and inequalities in health among kibbutz elderly. In R. Estes (Ed.), *Advancing quality if life in a turbulent world* (pp. 169–190). The Netherlands: Springer Publishing.

Nord, C., & Schwarz, B. (Eds.). (2015). Northern light on housing for older adults. [Special issue]. *Journal of Housing for the Elderly, 29*(1–2), 396–418.

Parmelee, P., & Lawton, M. P. (1990). The design of special environments for the aged. In J. Birren & K. W. Schaie (Eds.), *Handbook of the psychology of aging* (pp. 464–488). New York, NY: Academic Press.

Regnier, V. (1994). *Assisted living housing for elderly: Design innovations from the United States and Europe.* New York, NY: Van Nostrand Reinhold.

Regnier, V. (2002). *Design for assisted living: Guidelines for housing the physically and mentally frail.* New York, NY: Wiley.

Rodiek, S., & Schwarz, B. (Eds.). (2005). *The role of the outdoors in residential environments for aging.* New York, NY: Haworth Press.

Rodiek, S., & Schwarz, B. (Eds.). (2007). *Outdoor environments for people with dementia.* New York, NY: Haworth Press.

Rowles, G. D., & Bernard, M. (2013). The meaning and significance of place in old age. In G. D. Rowles & M. Bernard (Eds.), *Environmental gerontology: Making meaningful places in old age* (pp. 3–24). New York, NY: Springer Publishing.

Scheidt, R., & Schwarz, B. (Eds.). (2013). *Environmental gerontology: What's now?* London, UK: Routledge, Taylor Francis.

Schwarz, B. (1992). *Designing public places for private lives: A study of the design process of long-term care settings* (Doctoral dissertation). Retrieved from ProQuest Dissertations and Theses database. (Accession No. 9308441)

Schwarz, B. (1996). *Nursing home design: Consequences of employing the medical model.* New York, NY: Garland Publishing.

Schwarz, B. (1997). Nursing home design: A misguided architectural model. *Journal of Architectural and Planning Research, 14*(4), 343–359.

Schwarz, B. (2003). M. Powell Lawton's three dilemmas in the field of environment and aging. *Journal of Housing for the Elderly, 17*(1–2), 5–22.

Schwarz, B. (2013). Environmental gerontology: What now? In R. Scheidt & B. Schwarz (Eds.), *Environmental gerontology: What now?* (pp. 19–20). London, UK: Routledge.

Schwarz, B., Chaudhury, H., & Brent-Tofle R. (2004). Effect of design interventions on a dementia care setting. *American Journal of Alzheimer's Disease and Other Dementias, 19*(3), 172–176.

Schwarz, B., & Brent, R. (1999a). Epilogue: Emerging themes, further reflections. In B. Schwarz & R. Brent (Eds.), *Aging, autonomy, and architecture: Advances in assisted living.* Baltimore, MD: The Johns Hopkins University Press.

Schwarz, B., & Brent, R. (Eds.). (1999b). *Aging, autonomy, and architecture: Advances in assisted living.* Baltimore, MD: The Johns Hopkins University Press.

Thomas, W. H. (2004). *What are older people for? How elders will save the world.* Acton, MA: VanderWyk & Burnham.

CHAPTER 13

The Art of Questioning

Margaret P. Calkins

ABSTRACT

The art of questioning—both asking and seeking answers—has been a unifying influence in the career of Dr. Margaret Calkins. From early childhood dinner table discussions to critically framed empirical research questions that seek to deepen our knowledge of how the built environment influences well-being and quality of life for older adults, it is the process of asking and seeking answers to questions that has provided the foundation of her work. High levels of empathy and compassion developed by working in a memory care setting for 5 years, seeing the ways people living with dementia worked to make sense of their surroundings and remain fully engaged in meaningful relationships and their community. She translated this passion into a career that focused on pragmatic solutions though consulting, research, and ultimately academia and philanthropy.

BIOGRAPHICAL NOTES

What's in a Question?

"Should we have a locked unit for our demented [sic] patients?" asked the administrator of a county nursing home, while I was in an environment-behavior studio in 1984 in the master of architecture program at the University of Wisconsin-Milwaukee. As we divided up activities and responsibilities for the project among the students, as luck would have it, I was charged with answering this question. I assumed there would be some research available that would provide a clear

http://dx.doi.org/10.1891/0198-8794.38.217

answer—but there wasn't. The question was too early; there were almost no publications about dementia care settings, except those by the exceptional M. Powell Lawton. The term SCU for "Special Care Units" had not yet been coined. I found the question deeply interesting, though, and intriguing. And since the answer wasn't apparent in the literature, I decided I needed to learn what dementia was, ask my own questions, and then I could make a recommendation for our design. I have never ceased that quest. The key aspect of this story is the power of a question—which is a theme that runs throughout my life. That simple question was powerful enough to launch a career.

As a young child growing up, the act of questioning—both asking and then seeking answers—was central to my family lifestyle. My siblings and I routinely gave "book reportments" at the dinner table talking about what we were reading (for school or pleasure) which was always followed by some probing questions. We had to think deeply about the hidden meanings, not just the surface message. Dad would come home with a word for the night—I particularly remember the discussion about the word *gumption*. Was this a good thing to have (initiative), or does it have downsides (aggressiveness)? The conversation was lively and memorable.

Early Educational Period

My interest in environmental design didn't appear until college, though I was actively doing design work, mostly in the costume department of the theater. I remember my freshman year, after my first day of sewing britches for a production of *The Crucible*, the costume designer gave me a drawing of one of her costume designs and told me to make a pattern for an elegant period dress. I was just beginning to realize that I could look at drawing of a three-dimensional object, and figure out how to draw it out in two dimensions, so it could be created, back in three dimensions. This ability to visually disassemble objects and see how they can be expressed in a different form impacts how I look at environments, supporting my "seeing through the eyes of" different people, especially individuals living with dementia.

At the same time, I was taking a class called the Psychology of Aesthetics, taught by Professor Ron Heyduk, and read an article by Amos Rapoport, "Complexity and Ambiguity in Environmental Design" that really piqued my interest in environmental psychology (Rapoport & Kantor, 1967). The theory suggests that people prefer a moderate amount of complexity in their urban environments: Too simple and straightforward is boring, and too complex is overwhelming and stressful. As a very small school, Kenyon College didn't have many courses in environmental psychology, so I spent 1 year at Harvard University as a visiting student. What a fabulous experience—so many questions to be asked and so many people to ask them to! After college, I decided to take a few years off from school and work. I had a sense I was interested in medical settings of some kind, so I decided to work in a doctors' office to understand how a medical practice works from the inside. I spent 2 years working for a team of eye surgeons. My mother (who has severe glaucoma, along with a lifelong interest in the built environment) had written an article on how the design of the waiting room affected the patient experience. During my 2 years working there, I questioned many of our patients on what they thought about the design of our waiting rooms. Were the oriental rugs nice, or too visually confusing? Was the abstract ink line drawing artwork soothing, or just a blurry mass (mess) to people with vision problems or dilated eyes? Was the light from the lamps restful and comfortable, or insufficient for doing anything to pass the time (people were routinely in the office for 4-7 hours for various tests and procedures). Did they like the music? Did they like to have coffee available (a resounding yes!)? What made them comfortable (a recurring theme in my work now)?

All during this time, I was also asking questions of my brother Peter (who had recently graduated from Harvard's Graduate School of Design) about his approach to design and my interest in environmental psychology. He didn't understand it. I said I wanted to do research (which is all about asking questions) to give architects information to design better buildings, because, frankly, I thought many were designing lousy buildings—from the perspective of the users of the buildings. Peter finally said I'd never get architects to listen to me as a psychologist—I'd have to be an architect to get them to listen to me. He followed this up with a big-brotherly comment of "we all know you can't do that." I marched off to the office of off campus studies, went through the program descriptions for architecture schools, and found that Amos Rapoport was teaching at the School of Architecture and Urban Planning at the University of Wisconsin-Milwaukee (UW-M), and that it had a program called Environment-Behavior Studies. That was it. I didn't even bother to apply anywhere else. In considering this moment in my career, I realize that my brother's statement was really a question: Can someone who isn't a designer sufficiently understand the design process to positively impact it? Is there a role for nondesigners, such as psychologists or physical therapists or speech-language pathologists or medical professionals in the design process? Today, we know the answer is yes, they not only can, but should. But at the time of this conversation, that wasn't as evident. Much of architectural practice was focused on the visual impact of design, particularly the exterior elevation and skin—either postmodernism or deconstructivist approaches—with little focus on the experiences and needs of the users of the setting.

My time in the architecture program at UW-M is when my deep and enduring interest into environments for older adults and people living with dementia developed. For the environment-behavior studio taught by Gerald Weisman and Sherry Ahrentzen that I mentioned at the start of this article, a nearby county nursing home had $40,000 from the county for renovations to their 1926 building, which had been a tuberculosis sanatorium with almost no changes except to eliminate the porches by extending the bedroom walls. The class completed three plans: (a) how to spend $40,000 right away—basically on decorating; (b) how to do the decorating within their annual budget over 5-6 years and use the $40,000 to expand and open the central shared social area; and (c) a blue-sky plan that relocated the nurses station, added an additional "day room" so the residents with dementia could live on one side of the unit within a secure area with two social spaces. I was the person in the class charged with understanding and making recommendations for what people living with dementia needed environmentally. Within weeks, I was hooked! This was the first time Alzheimer's was on the cover of *Time Magazine*. It was just beginning to come out of the closet and be talked about openly. I was the one who suggested we look at creating a separate area for the individuals living with dementia. I was subsequently awarded the American Institute of Architects/American Hospital Association (AIA-AHA) Fellowship in Health Facilities Design, and spent my third year asking lots of questions and writing a design guide for people living with dementia. This was published in 1988 as the first book on dementia design, *Design for Dementia: Planning Environments for the Elderly and Confused* (Calkins, 1988). I certainly wouldn't use those terms ("The Elderly and Confused") now, which is a sign of how far we have come. By the way, the nursing home liked our blue-sky plan, and the county subsequently approved $400,000 for the project, at which point the administrator had the funds to hire a licensed architect to work on the project. I am still in contact with that administrator today.

This period—my second 2 years of the master's program at UW-M—represented an amazing collision of fortuitous factors that focused my attention: the right studio project (with the right questions), the beginning of open discussion about Alzheimer's disease, and the AIA/AHA fellowship opportunity.

I came to UW-M when the environment-behavior program was relatively new, and rare in schools of architecture or design. When I first learned about Lawton's Competence-Press Model (Lawton & Nahemow, 1973), it made immediate sense, because it was built on the same principles as Rapaport's complexity theory—only it was more dynamic in that it also accommodated people with different sets and levels of competencies. Working with this model, I focused on the experience of the person in the environment—specifically individuals living with the symptoms of Alzheimer's or dementia. What are the most salient characteristics (e.g., competencies) of these individuals that impacts how they perceive and function in the world, and how do you translate these into design guidance (to regulate the amount and type of environmental press)? Working with Dr. Gerry Weisman, I started to develop a set of therapeutic goals that would become a driving force to my work and publications, and to the work of others. Always, I was asking myself questions: What are the needs and desires of the users of a building? How does the design of the built environment support and enable achievement of those goals? How might the goals, needs, preferences of the individual living with dementia be different from those of families, or of direct care staff, or administrators and owners? Good design will integrate all these different goals into a cohesive whole that meets the needs of people and program alike. This issue gets to the very heart of the nature of "environment" and the work of Lewin (1951) and Bronfenbrenner (1976). Understanding the layers (micro, meso, exo, macro) at which the environments around us exists and impacts everything we do, which are also indelibly intertwined by our own individual characteristics and personal experiences, social network and environment, (organizational, or cultural) all of which take place within a built and natural physical environment—was something I grappled with for a long time. This framework has guided my work for many years, allowing me pose questions from so many different perspectives that there is never an end to them.

I can't leave this period without mentioning that my first Environmental Design Research Association conference was in 1984 in San Luis Opisbo, where I met M. Powell Lawton—who would have a profound effect on my career. Powell was probably the most gifted, intellectually generous, humble person I will ever have the privilege to know. I would often consult with him when I had questions that I didn't know how to address, and his insights always provided a direction for my work. I still miss him and his amazing contributions to the field of Environmental Gerontology.

DOING APPLIED RESEARCH FROM WITHIN

After graduating from the architecture program in Milwaukee, I had a wonderful opportunity to work on the design, operation and evaluation of an early model assisted living residence for people living with dementia, which was another important formative period in my career. The Corinne Dolan Alzheimer Center was designed by Stephen Nemtin of Taliesin Associated Architects, and Chari Weber was the administrator. The building and program were very advanced for the time: It had 2 living areas of 12 residents, each with a kitchen, dining room, and family room, and the 2 households shared a living room and other support spaces. We were committed to doing environmental research, which was a primary reason why I was interested in working on this project. We were very specific about articulating our environmental hypotheses—a very early example of an evidence-based design practice, well before the term *evidence-based design* was even coined. We conducted eight studies, and here I'll describe two that had significant impact on the field: personal items at bedroom entrance and highly visible toilet rooms.

The Dolan Center was the first dementia care project that incorporated a display case at the bedroom entrance to help residents independently identify their bedrooms. Most people have never lived in a house with 12 (or 18 or 30) identical bedroom doorways and the literature was replete with anecdotes of how residents living with dementia couldn't find their own room and were going into their neighbors' rooms, which might escalate and cause tension. It also took a lot of staff time to direct people to their own rooms. Therefore, I hypothesized that having resident's own personal belongings, displayed in a case outside the bedroom entrance, would help people identify their own rooms. Residents acted as their own control in the research, having both personal items and, separately, unique but nonpersonal items in their display cases. Each day a research assistant would ask each resident to show them where their room was. The results were positive: people were more successful and finding their rooms and/or taking less time to successfully identify their room with the personalized items in the display care (Namazi, Rosner, & Rechlin, 1991). But the real story here isn't the research results—it was that care communities started adopting and incorporating bedroom display cases even before the research was completed and published. This was an environmental element that just made sense to care providers, and it is now one of the most pervasive elements in dementia care settings around the world. In fact, we didn't conduct the research as I had originally conceptualized it—which was to compare two-dimensional cues with three-dimensional cues. While we were the first to incorporate three-dimensional display cases, other communities had been putting photos by residents' rooms, though with mixed success as a wayfinding cue. To me, the question was whether real, three-dimensional artifacts—trophies, china shoe collections, dolls, or other memorabilia—were more effective than two-dimensional representations (typically photos). This is information that helps designers know how to design a building, whereas knowing whether "personal" or "unique but nonpersonal" items is more effective doesn't tell the designer how to design. This was what my brother meant when he said I'd "have to be an architect" to be effective. There is a difference between "environmental" research and "design" research. Environmental research, in my view, is research that helps us understand person-environment interactions, but not necessarily in a way that is actionable in the design process. Knowing that "personally meaningful items" (which were both two and three dimensional) are better than nonpersonally meaningful items doesn't tell a designer how or what to design. Design research (studying whether three-dimensional items are more effective than two-dimensional representations) gives explicit information about the design of the built environment. These display cases were expensive to install—were they worth it? Unfortunately, we still don't have a good research-based answer to that question. Subsequent research by others has look at various types of cues (Nolan, Mathews, Truesdell-Todd, & VanDorp, 2002) but no one has explicitly compared two- versus three-dimensional objects of equal salience to the individual as a wayfinding cue.

The second research project was impactful for a different reason. Incontinence is a huge issue both for the individual living with dementia and for caregivers. Thus, designing the environment to compensate for cognitive and physical/visual changes to enable people to maintain independence in managing continence longer was an important goal of the design. The bedrooms, all private, had a sink and a toilet on the outside wall, with partial walls and a curtain for visual privacy. The floor and walls were dark red, while the toilet was white. My hypothesis was that having direct visual access to a highly visible toilet would enhance the ability of residents to maintain continence. For 2 weeks, half the residents had their curtains closed so they had to go behind the curtain to find the toilet, while the other half had their curtains in an open position so the toilet was highly visible; then the conditions were switched. The results were very strong—when the curtains were closed, the toilets were used 37 times, while over the same period, the toilets were used 285 times when the curtain was open and the toilet was visible—this is an eight-fold increase (Namazi & Johnson, 1991). Interestingly, there were several residents who were offended by having the toilet so visible in the open curtain condition, and tried to find ways to pull the curtain closed so they didn't have to see it all the time. I asked myself, why? Apparently, their sense of privacy had not been sufficiently eroded by the disease process. Next question: Is there a way to design the room so the bathroom can be as visible as an individual needs it to be, without it being overly visible? The answer is yes—sliding doors (often just one but I have used two that come together to form a corner) allow greater visibility. But the toilet still needs to be directly visible from the bed, and there needs to be sufficient contrast so that the toilet stands out visually from the adjacent walls and floor (see Figure 13.1).

These studies represent an early example of what we now refer to as evidence-based design and as design research. Hamilton (2003) developed a system for categorizing the quality of evidence-based design practice, which moves from articulating specific design hypotheses to conducting research and publicly disseminating the results. We very specifically looked at the evidence, such as it was, prior to designing the building and created specific hypotheses about how

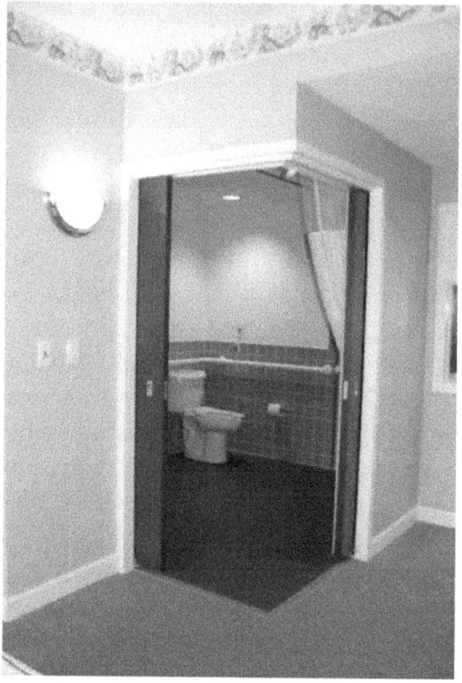

FIGURE 13.1 Ohio Eastern Star bathroom. Architect: Neokler and Hull.

the building would impact the residents' functioning. Not only did we then conduct research to test our hypotheses, but we made accommodations in the design to support the research (a step beyond Hamilton's framework). For example, best practice information would have suggested that the two sides of the building be different-visually, spatially, or in terms of interior design treatment-to help residents orient themselves to which part of the building they were in. However, if one side of the building included articulated columns to define the kitchen area and the other side didn't, residents might come to learn that their bedroom was across from the kitchen with columns, and be using that as a cue instead of the mementos in their display case. So, since any differences in the design might potentially lead to a difference in a study outcome, we designed to two sides to be identical. The eight research studies were published in two issues of *The American Journal of Alzheimer's Care and Related Disorders & Research*. This research experience convinced me that I wanted to pursue a career in research, and for that, I needed a PhD degree. I went back to UW-M, this time as senior fellow at the Institute on Aging and Environment at the School of Architecture and Urban Planning, generously funded by the Helen Bader Foundation.

Going back for my PhD opened a whole new world of opportunities and questions. SCUs for people living with dementia were rapidly developing, and often the costs were higher than "regular" units. The government was interested in knowing whether SCUs were effective as a treatment, and what facets of design, operations, staff, training, and so forth made them more or less effective. The National Institute on Aging funded a series of research projects to evaluate SCUs (Alzheimer's Disease & Associated Disorders, 1994), and Gerry Weisman and I were brought in, with support from The Retirement Research Foundation, as consultants to assist the researchers in assessing the physical environment. Dr. Phil Sloane had developed the Therapeutic Environments Screen Scale as a tool for measuring the physical environment of nursing home environments, but it was new and hadn't been well validated; moreover, there was no other existing tool to validate it against. Working with Powell Lawton and Phil Sloane, we developed and validated the Professional Environmental Assessment Protocol (Lawton et al., 2000). This was an amazing opportunity to work with some of the best and brightest minds in the dementia care arena. The conversations and question at the heart of our discussions were incredible and stretched my mind even further. Through this and other related work, we developed a set of Therapeutic Goals that could be used as a guide for not only understanding and developing supportive congregate living settings, but evaluating them. These goals included: maximize awareness and orientation, enhance continuity of self, opportunities for personal control, facilitation of social contact, provision of privacy, regulation and quality of stimulation, support functional abilities, and maximize safety and security. At the time these were directed at dementia care settings, but that was about to change.

THE IDEAS YEARS

And this opened the door to what would be a cornerstone of the next phase of my career of conducting and dissemination applied research, developing resources that would help care providers understand what constitutes a good care setting—a place where people want to live, not a place of last resort where one goes to live the last days of life and die (which is largely how nursing homes were thought of, and unfortunately which some still are). For many years, it had largely been assumed that once someone had a diagnosis of Alzheimer 's disease or another dementia, they were incapable of almost anything: They couldn't learn, they couldn't make decisions, they needed help with everything. In short, they were considered incompetent and dependent. But I knew that people living with dementia have many residual abilities, regardless of where in the course of the disease they were. I had seen it at the Corinne Dolan Center and other care communities I began to work with. They not only have abilities but also have rights. The right to be treated with dignity and respect, the right to comfort and a sense of belonging, deep and meaningful relationships with people who can work around your communication challenges, with opportunities to live life the way you choose and not have someone else make every decision for you.

I increasingly realized that what I had been working on for individuals living with dementia was equally applicable to any and everyone who needs the support that a nursing home or assisted-living community provides. The concept of "person-centered care" had been gaining momentum through the early 1990s, and was embodied by the work of the National Citizens Coalition for Nursing Home Reform (now Consumer Voice), Pioneer Network, and Planetree. People with dementia are people first, with the same basic needs and desires as everyone else. Translating person-centered values into the design of real settings is not always easy (especially with earlier versions of building and life-safety codes). Over the years, I've come to the opinion that the building or physical environment is only about 30% of what makes for a supportive care setting. Moving away from the staff-centric, institutional (in Irving Goffman's [1960] use of the term) approach to care is much more difficult. Changing the institutional core values and beliefs, changing decades of how care was provided, has been and continues to be the industry's biggest challenge.

I had incorporated IDEAS: Innovative Designs in Environments for an Aging Society in 1991 as a consulting firm when I went back for my PhD. As I hired staff, I kept in mind the value that a multidisciplinary team perspective brings to projects, so I hired occupational therapists, a speech language pathologist, a sociologist, a medical anthropologist, and several additional designers. From the mid-1990s through 2010, I and my colleagues developed a number of resources (e.g., Briller, Proffitt, Perez, & Calkins, 2001; Briller, Proffitt, Perez, Calkins & Marsden, 2001; Brush, Calkins, Bruce, & Sanford, 2012; Marsden, Briller, Calkins, & Proffitt, 2001; Perez, Proffitt, & Calkins, 2001) presented at hundreds of conferences (cf. Calkins, 2002, 2004, 2006, 2008), and wrote prolifically for both trade/professional publications and peer-reviewed journals (e.g., Calkins, 2007; Calkins & Keane, 2008; Calkins & Weisman, 1999; Day & Calkins, 2002), extolling the values and virtues of dementia-supportive environments and person-centered care. In 1998, I set up IDEAS Institute, an independent, nonprofit research institute through which we could conduct empirical design research. Together, through these two organizations, we were able to engage in a broad array of activities, from consulting to resources development to more traditional applied research, and build a body of work that has shaped how environments for older adults are created. Over the years, we obtained over $6.5 million dollars in grants, much it from the National Institute on Aging. The independent (nonuniversity or government affiliated) nature allowed us to be nimble to respond to different challenges and opportunities that presented themselves. There were times when a foundation didn't understand what this type of free-standing (nonuniversity affiliated) research organization was, and wouldn't fund us.

It was during this time that I met Dr. Robert N. Mayer, President of The Hulda B. & Maurice L. Rothschild Foundation. I put Rob in the same category as Powell Lawton, dedicated, passionate, humble, and awe-inspiring. The foundation was the only national philanthropy dedicating to improving quality of life for residents in long-term care, following the values and practices of person-centered care. Rob, who passed away in 2015, had an amazing ability to ask the tough questions (Sound familiar? No wonder we got along so well.) and bring the right people together to find answers. He asked, "What are the barriers to adopting person-centered care?" Early on, the response he got most often was "Regulations." But, people said regulations are regulations, and you can't change them. There was almost nothing Rob loved more than a good challenge, so we set about finding a way to change the regulations. We started with the National Fire Protection Association's Life Safety Code (LSC). This code, which is designed to make buildings safer, especially from fires, is specifically referenced by the federal government, and thus applies to almost every nursing home in the country. We had a goal of making the LSC more accommodating of person-centered values. For example, people who are living in a nursing home should have access to a kitchen where they can bake cookies or make a meal if they desire. But kitchens were not allowed in areas where residents lived or slept. At that time (around 2010), the government, through the Centers for Medicare & Medicaid Services (CMS), was referencing the 2000 edition of LSC. I chaired the Rothschild/Pioneer Network Life Safety Code Task Force and we convened a group of about 30 stakeholders, and developed a long list of regulations that were considered barriers. We found that many items had already been changed in the 2003, 2006, and 2009 editions of the code, but very few people knew about the changes because most states (though by no means all) continued to reference what CMS referenced. We ultimately developed four proposals for changes to the code, which became known as the "Culture Change Proposals." These were related to residential style kitchens open to corridors and sleeping compartments, use of gas fireplaces, the amount of personalized, nonflame retardant-treated decorations allowed, and furniture in the corridor so residents could stop and rest, and thus not have to rely on a wheelchair for mobility.

A few people on the committee had years of experience with the code development process. Doug Erickson, CEO of the Facilities Guidelines Institute was one, and when he heard what we were trying to get passed, he said it would take us 20 years to get kitchens allowed in nursing home living areas. This was just the kind of challenge Rob and I loved. We set to work (with a steering committee of the Task Force) and made our arguments so persuasive that we were ultimately successful in getting all four proposals approved and adopted into the 2012 LSC. But since CMS still referenced the 2000 edition of the LSC, this set of changes didn't make much of a difference. We continued to push CMS to mandate these codes, and in 2012 CMS officially stated that they would offer categorical waivers to any care community that wanted to build to the 2012 standards, *just for these four topics* (CMS, 2012). In July 2014, when CMS decided it would take steps to adopt the 2012 LSC in its entirety, I was told that it was, in large part, due to the kitchen proposal we had submitted. This was such a significant change from previous editions (which had mostly been incremental changes from their previous editions), and captured the evolving person-centered care movement that was taking place in the long-term care industry, that it was time to adopt the latest version of the LSC. This was a real victory.

However, the LSC is separate and distinct from the building codes, which are mostly promulgated by the International Code Council. One of the other barriers Rob and I heard about was the conflicts between the different sets of regulations. So, we set off with the goal of reducing disparities and conflicts between at least some of the different codes and regulations that impact long-term care communities. The four "Culture Change Proposals" were proposed to the International Code Council, and adopted in 2014 with very similar language. I have stayed involved in the code process ever since, continuing to make changes that support long-term care communities becoming less institutional and more like a home, which is where people want to live.

During this time, I was working on a variety of other projects—both consulting and research. One of the most interesting was a cost-value analysis of private versus shared rooms in nursing homes. Funded by The Commonwealth Fund, this project looked at psychosocial, clinical, operational, and cost factors related to offering private rooms to residents in nursing homes. Residents and families expressed a strong preference for private rooms, as did staff who said there was significantly more resident-to-resident tension when people were sharing a bedroom, especially a traditional side-by-side (hospital-style) room. There were a few examples of alternatives design of shared rooms, generally called "enhanced shared rooms," where everyone has their own defined territory, their own window, and equal access to the bathroom without having to trespass through the roommate's territory (Figure 13.2). While the sample of these rooms was small, the consensus was that the "enhanced shared rooms" felt more like a private room than a traditional shared room (Calkins

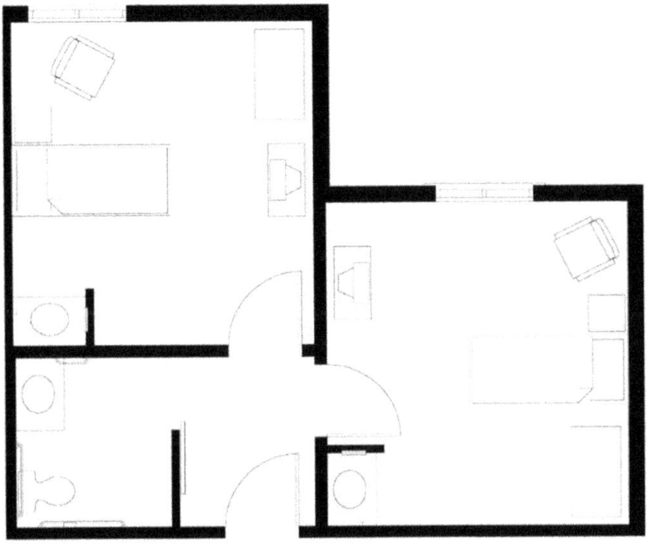

FIGURE 13.2 Enhanced shared room, Air Force Village. Designer: Gaius Nelson, Nelson Tremain Architects P.A.

& Casella, 2007). Note that I do not call those semiprivate rooms; having a piece of fabric to separate the living space of two individuals should in no way be considered even partially private. The most interesting result of this study was the cost analysis. Having worked as a consultant for over 20 years, I had seen how the construction budget often dictated design decisions. But first time construction/capital costs (land, construction, and fees) are only about 6% of the life-cycle cost of a health-care setting, with consumables, such as energy and building maintenance between 11% and 16%, and staffing costs comprising 77% to 88%, based on a 40-year life-cycle costing model (Perkins Eastman, 2013). So a design feature that has a positive impact on staffing, and thus maybe reduce turnover (which is a significant ongoing operational cost for nursing homes) would have a positive impact on the life cycle or total costs of the project. Also, a first-time construction cost approach does not consider alternative revenue options. So that is the approach I took in doing this research. Not surprisingly, the analysis showed that it costs more to build private rooms with their own bathroom than to construct shared rooms. However, when we added the life-cycle costs and revenues of private rooms, which generally are associated with slightly higher revenue rates, the results were more interesting. Nationally, the rate for private rooms was an average of $23 per day higher than for shared rooms (no data were available on enhanced shared rooms). When we look at this cost differential, the difference in construction costs can be recouped in less than 2 years (per person, so 4 years total) if the rooms are fully occupied, and in less than 4 months if 1 bed remains unoccupied because it is a shared room (lost revenue is the full room rate, not $23 per day). Given an average debt service of 30 years, the care community gets more revenue by building all (or a majority) of private rooms. Some have argued that for some residents or state Medicaid budgets (which pays for a significant portion of nursing homes costs), this $23 per day difference is unaffordable. Carrying the analysis out further, the data suggest that the construction cost differential comes to about $2.50 per person per day (2007 estimates). This marginal construction cost increase needs to be weighed with reference to the positive outcomes of private rooms that include increased resident, family, and staff satisfaction, and improved clinical outcomes, especially related to iatrogenic infections, and operations costs such as potential reduced staff turnover from staff being less stressed.

Several of my projects were more applied in nature, such as developing an assistive wardrobe (Calkins, 2012). Having spent significant time in care communities, I was aware of so many ways in which the environment was not supporting the needs and abilities of residents, especially those living with dementia. Many care communities continue to value staff efficiency over supporting residents' independence, which translates into doing *for* the resident, not doing *with* or helping the resident *to do*. In a traditional care-giving practice, staff would automatically help residents get dressed in the morning instead of supporting their autonomous dressing, which can take more time. It appeared that decisional aspects of dressing were particularly difficult for residents living with dementia; selecting a complete outfit from overcrammed closets or tiny wardrobes (often only 24 inches wide) and getting the necessary items together (undergarments, socks, top, and slacks), and knowing in what order to don clothes was challenging. We developed "The Assistive Wardrobe" (now sold by Claflin Contract Furnishings) which had numerous features designed to support all residents: grab bars for postural/balance support when accessing clothing, a hook to hang items on which getting other items out, a light that turns on automatically, easily accessible storage bins on the doors for frequently used items, a hanging bar that easily pulls out to reduce reach distance, drawers with clear fronts so people can see what is inside the drawer, a full length mirror, and more (Figure 13.3).

I also consulted with many design firms and care communities to create new buildings, the majority of which were designed to serve individuals living with dementia. One very successful project was the Memory Care Assisted Living at Cypress Cove, designed by SFCS. The 2-story plan includes 4 households for 11 residents each in private rooms and 3-fixture bathrooms, with the kitchen

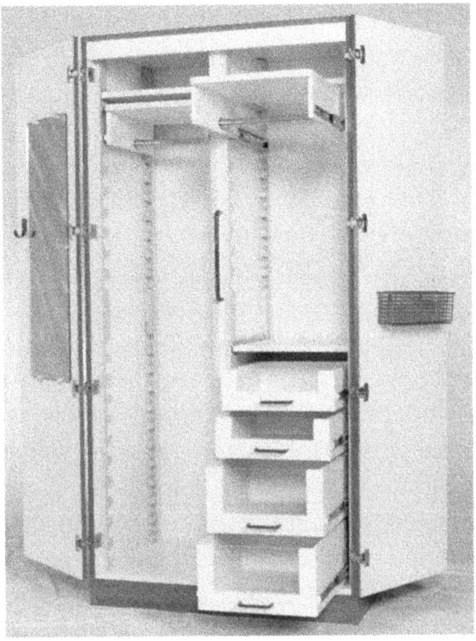

FIGURE 13.3 Assistive wardrobe.

and dining room facing a small but wonderfully creative courtyard filled with interesting things to do and watch. There is an elevator that directly connects the upper level households to the courtyard, so that residents can go outside whenever they want without having to wait to be accompanied by staff. The layout allows for some residents' bedrooms to be slightly more private while some are situated to maximize visibility and orientation. We worked with Dr. Mariana Figueiro of Renselier Polytech Institute to create circadian pattern lighting (bluer mid-day and warmer in the morning and evening) to help the residents maintain appropriate circadian rhythms.

This focus on applied research has been a constant theme throughout my career. I am less interested in advancing our theoretical understanding of Environmental Gerontology as I am fundamentally pragmatic. When I see a problem, I want to develop a solution that will have immediate impact. I have always been a problem solver—ask a question and look for an answer. I have wondered if I might have addressed different issues had I worked in a long-term care setting beyond the 5 years I was at the Corinne Dolan Center. Instead, I spent much of my career consulting on projects for a variety of clients and different architectural teams, and in this way, I have had the opportunity to raise the awareness design sensitivity of numerous providers and practitioners.

MOVING INTO ACADEMIA

In 2010, I began to explore a deeper commitment to academia, adjunct teaching first at The Erickson School at University of Maryland Baltimore County in the Management of Aging Services program, under Dr. Ronch, and then at Kent State University College of Architecture and Environmental Design. In 2014, I took a full-time position at Kent State University. While I only stayed full-time for 2 years, it was an exciting excursion in my career. The opportunity to work with a cohort of students (as opposed to working with individual graduate students, which I had done off and on since completing with my PhD) and instill in them an appreciation for the importance of always considering the perspectives of the users of the setting—the residents or patients, their family or chosen care partners, the staff—was wonderful. My most innovative class is one called Designing for Patient Populations Across the Lifespan. We start with birthing centers and neonatal intensive care units, moved through inpatient, ambulatory and specialty services (such as oncology), and end with nursing homes and hospice settings. Each class is co-taught by a designer, clinician, and patient or patient-advocate. So, the students are consistently learning about the different settings, from the perspective of different users and designers. They learn how to ask questions (my favorite approach to anything!).

As I considered this move into part-time and then full-time academia from my successful consulting career, I was reminded of some advice my father gave to my brother Andy, who was considering a job change that was somewhat risky, but with potential high rewards in terms of impact on the educational system. My father, who was probably around 70 at the time, said that as you age and reflect on your life, you seldom regret opportunities taken that didn't work out as you hoped, but are more likely to regret opportunities or challenges not taken. Better to have tried and not succeeded than not to have tried.

So, when I was asked in 2014 whether I would come to Kent full-time to be the program coordinator of the Elliot Program in Health Care Design, which offers both a Graduate Certificate in Health Care Facilities and a post-professional Master's in Health Care Design, I said yes. Moving to academia full-time represented a significant change in my career. This is an online program, so we had students from as far away as Brazil. Learning how to create a sense of community in an online environment is a different kind of challenge, but one I enjoyed. My learning curve was steep, as health-care design is substantially different from senior living design, although there are some consistencies. Patient-centered care is becoming as strong as the person-centered movement is.

THE PRESENT

In 2016, I changed course again and became the executive director of The Mayer-Rothschild Foundation, a family foundation based in Chicago, which is dedicated to improving quality of life for elders in long-term care by supporting person-centered care practices. Founded in honor of the late Dr. Robert N. Mayer, with whom I had been working since 2002 on multiple projects (such as the Rothschild Regulatory Task Forces described above), The Mayer-Rothschild Foundation is dedicated to empowering long-term care communities to serve all elders with dignity and respect and to honor their life choices. The Foundation is focused on activities that will lead to systemic change—such as revising codes and guidelines, developing state-based initiatives that educate providers and regulators and make it easier for care communities to listen to the voices of the residents, and creating programs that will celebrate those communities that are deeply adopting person-centered values and practices. This is different from the consulting work I did for much of my career, which mostly had impact on an individual project, with some of the knowledge carried forward by the design team to their other projects, or by others seeing or learning about the project through conference presentations, publications, or site visits. The Foundation will work on some research projects, especially when they are focused on issues or strategies that will have systemic or policy-level implications. For the more applied research, I turn that over to the many younger researchers who have come into this field over the past two decades. Your work is important as we continue to need to understand how to create settings that support the bio-psycho-social-emotional wellbeing of older adults, regardless of where they live. There are so many people who are entering their third phase of life, with much more diversity, that the work will never end. But each project does make a difference.

In turning my efforts to systemic level changes, I hope I can have broader and deeper impact on the long-term care industry. These are exciting times, in part because CMS has recently revised their rules for how they will survey nursing homes with a much deeper focus on person-centered care values. Similar to the work we did on the LSC in 2010, this will have a much greater industry impact because it sets a new standard that all nursing communities will have to adopt. It won't be an easy shift for some care communities. However, the new rules very much aligned with values and practices—programmatic, organizational, and environmental—that I have been advocating since the mid-1980s.

REFLECTIONS ON THE PAST AND PRESENT

The question posed 30 years ago—"Should we have a locked unit for our demented [sic] patients?"—has shaped my career, starting with a focus on environments specifically for individual living with dementia, which led to a recognition that the underlying principles and values for that group was equally applicable to all individuals who live in long-term care settings. If I were to answer that question now, I would say probably not. Segregating individuals who are living with dementia perpetuates the stigma that "they" are different from "us," and by implication somehow less than "us." I agree with Dr. Al Power (2014, 2017) that we need to be more accepting and inclusive and find solutions that meet everyone's needs.

I hope the applied nature of my research has helped pique the interest of subsequent generations of researchers and care providers—they see that research can have an immediate practical application and add to our theoretical understanding of how and why things work the way they do. As ubiquitous as display cases are at bedroom entrances now, I smile when someone takes the time to stop and tell me why they have them and how they work—if only they knew I originally came up with this idea!

Working in a nursing home for 5 years also had a tremendous impact on my thinking—and is something I would highly recommend. When I consulted with care communities or considered the utility of the information a given applied research project might generate, I could draw on my understanding of what a specialized memory care program was really like. It kept me out of the "white tower of academia" and grounded my work in a very real sense. I would highly recommend this approach: if you are going to focus on a particular type of setting, getting to know it deeply by working in it for several years will be time well spent.

I not only asked questions, but I learned from others: Powell Lawton, Gerry Weisman, Amos Rapaport, Uriel Cohen, Robert Harr, my parents, and brother Peter, and too many others to name. Most of the lessons were positive, showing me a path I wanted to follow, but some of the lessons were of how not to do things. I'm proud to be able to say that most everyone who has worked with and for me over the years would say it was a great work experience. Creating opportunities for others to grow and learn, develop their career paths by publishing and presenting at conferences, such that even when they left IDEAS or IDEAS Institute it was always on good terms, is important for me. Several of my former colleagues/employees have pursued academic careers and are chairs of their departments, heading programs, or, in one case, a college president. Others have launched their own successful consulting careers. I hope I have been to them what my many mentors were to me.

LOOKING FORWARD: THE FUTURE

There is still so much more work to be done. The quality of much of the environmental research being conducted continues to be modest—low sample sizes, single site, and insufficient methods for measuring environmental conditions are all too common. My hope is that through the work of The Mayer-Rothschild Foundation we can support high quality environmental research which has practical application. For example, what are the measurable impacts of enhanced-shared rooms over traditional side-by-side shared rooms? This includes clinical outcomes of differential nosocomial infection rates, impact on sleep hygiene and falls, as well as impact on staff and resident stress and satisfaction. And if the evidence is sufficiently strong, then we'll use it to change the regulations, disallowing construction of the traditional side-by-side shared rooms in long-term care. After all, they aren't allowed in hospitals anymore, and that change was based almost exclusively on nosocomial infection data.

Given the aging demographics in the United States (and indeed almost everywhere worldwide) I think the field also needs to be serious about taking on the challenge of the massive amount of housing stock that is not supportive of elders as they age—houses that have steps and other features that can become almost total barriers to independence, and indeed are the cause of accidents that lead to increased morbidity and mortality. It amazes me that the principles of Universal Design (UD) are still not more widely adopted in housing construction (Calkins, Sanford, & Proffitt, 2001). There is virtually no downside to UD. And on an urban design scale, the design of neighborhoods (if you can still call them that) that necessitate being able to drive a car to get almost anywhere combined with poor public transportation infrastructure is going to isolate so many people in the future. There is growing interest in age and dementia-friendly communities and the village-to-village movement, although these efforts are still in their infancy. The promises of advanced technology and the internet of things (IOT) is intriguing, but can it really replace the role of the person as care partner? I both doubt it and hope not. While the "smart home" can and does exist now, it is only affordable by a relatively small minority of individuals. There are tremendous challenges ahead, which create a virtually unlimited set of opportunities for people to find ways to have a positive impact.

CLOSING THOUGHTS

Over my career, I have shifted my focus from working with care communities and practicing designers on individual projects to research that has broader application to policy, and regulatory work impacting every nursing home in the country. I'm proud to be considered a leader in the movement that recognizes the inherent worth, dignity and right to a higher quality of life for individuals who can no longer live at home and need the support of shared residential long-term residences. There is a lot of work yet to be done, and I'm ready to accept the challenge to keep improving the systems, until we get it right. Are you with me?

REFERENCES

Alzheimer's Disease & Associated Disorders. (1994). Official publication of the world federation of neurology. *Dementia Research Group, 8*, S1.

Briller, S., Proffitt, M., Perez, K., & Calkins, M. (2001). *Creating successful dementia care settings: Understanding the environment through aging senses* (Vol. 1). Towson, MD: Health Professions Press.

Briller, S., Proffitt, M., Perez, K., Calkins, M., & Marsden, J. (2001). *Creating successful dementia care settings: Maximizing cognitive and functional abilities* (Vol. 2). Towson, MD: Health Professions Press.

Bronfenbrenner, U. (1976). The experimental ecology of education. *Teachers College Record, 78*(2), 157–178.

Brush, J., Calkins, M., Bruce, C., & Sanford, J. (2012). *Environment & communication assessment toolkit for dementia care.* Towson, MD: Health Professional Press.

Calkins, M. (1988). *Design for dementia: Planning environments for the elderly and confused.* Bethesda, MD: National Health Publishing.

Calkins M. (2002, October). *Environment, design, and architecture in dementia.* Keynote plenary at the 18th International Conference of Alzheimer's Disease International, Barcelona, Spain.

Calkins, M. (2004, October). *Living environment and quality of care.* Invited workshop keynote at Alzheimer's Disease International 25th Annual Conference, Kyoto, Japan.

Calkins, M. (2006). *Promoting self-directed care: Creating a sense of home.* Invited keynote address at Alzheimer Society of Manitoba Annual Conference, Winnipeg, Canada.

Calkins, M. (2007). *Creating home in the nursing home: Fantasy or reality* [White paper]. Retrieved from https://www.pioneernetwork.net/?s=fantasy

Calkins, M. (2008, June). *Evidence based design for people with dementia.* Invited plenary session, Pan-Asian Alzheimer's Disease International Conference, Taipei, Taiwan.

Calkins, M. (2012, June). *Using the environment to support dressing and continence: Results from recent research.* Presentation at Leading Age Pennsylvania, Hershey, PA.

Calkins, M., & Cassella, C. (2007). Exploring the cost and value of private versus shared bedrooms in nursing homes. *The Gerontologist, 47*(2), 169–183.

Calkins, M., & Keane, W. (2008). Tomorrows assisted living and nursing homes: The converging worlds of residential long-term care. In S. Golant & J. Hyde (Eds.), *The assisted living residence: A vision for the future* (pp. 86–118). Baltimore, MD: Johns Hopkins University Press.

Calkins, M. P., Sanford, J., & Proffitt, M. (2001). Design for dementia: Challenges and lessons learned for universal design. In W. Preiser & A. Churchman (Eds.), *Universal design handbook* (22.1–22.24). New York, NY: McGraw-Hill Publishers.

Calkins, M. P., & Weisman, G. D. (1999). Models for environmental assessment. In R. Brent & B. Schwarz (Eds.), *Aging, autonomy and architecture: Advances in assisted living* (pp. 130–140). Baltimore, MD: Johns Hopkins University Press.

Centers for Medicare & Medicaid Services. (2012). *Survey & Certification Letter* [S&C-12-21-LSC]. Washington, DC. Retrieved from https://www.cms.gov/Medicare/Provider-Enrollment-and-Certification/SurveyCertificationGenInfo/Downloads/SCLetter12_21-.pdf

Day, K., & Calkins, M. P. (2002). Design and dementia. In R. Bechtel & A. Churchman (Eds.), *Handbook of environmental psychology* (pp. 2–53). Hoboken, NJ: John Wiley & Sons.

Goffman, E. (1960). *Asylums: Essays on the social situation of mental patients and other inmates*. New York, NY: Doubleday.

Hamilton, D. K. (2003). Four levels of evidence-based practice. *Healthcare Design*, 3, 18–26.

Lawton, M. P., & Nahemow, L. (1973). Ecology and the aging process. In C. Eisdorfer & M. P. Lawton (Eds.), *The psychology of adult development and aging* (pp. 619–674). Washington, DC: American Psychological Association.

Lawton M. P., Weisman G. D., Sloane, P., Norris-Baker, C., Calkins, M., & Zimmerman, S. I. (2000). Professional environmental assessment procedure for special care units for elders with dementing illness and its relationship to the therapeutic environment screening schedule. *Alzheimer Disease & Associated Disorders, 14*(1), 28–38.

Lewin, K. (1951). *Field theory in social science*. New York, NY: Harper & Row.

Marsden, J., Briller, S., Calkins, M., & Proffitt, M. (2001). *Creating successful dementia care settings: Enhancing identity and sense of home* (Vol. 4). Baltimore, MD: Health Professions Press.

Namazi, K., & Johnson, B. D. (1991). Environmental effects on incontinence problems in Alzheimer's disease patients. *The American Journal of Alzheimer's Care and Related Disorders & Research, 6*(6), 16–21.

Namazi, K., Rosner, T., & Rechlin, L. (1991). Long-term memory cuing to reduce visuo-spatial disorientation in Alzheimer's disease patients in a special care unit. *The American Journal of Alzheimer's Care and Related Disorders & Research, 6*(6), 3–9.

Nolan, B., Mathews, R., Truesdell-Todd, G., & VanDorp, A. (2002). Evaluation of the effect of orientation cues on wayfinding in persons with dementia. *Alzheimer's Care Quarterly, 3*(1), 46–49.

Perez, K., Proffitt, M., & Calkins, M. (2001). *Creating successful dementia care settings: minimizing disruptive behaviors* (Vol. 3). Baltimore, MD: Health Professions Press.

Perkins Eastman, B. (2013). *Building type basics for senior living*. Hoboken, NJ: Wiley Press.

Power, A. (2014). *Dementia beyond disease: Enhancing well-being*. Baltimore, MD: Health Professions Press.

Power, A. (2017). *Dementia beyond drugs: Changing the culture of care*. Baltimore, MD: Health Professions Press.

Rapoport, A., & Kantor, R. (1967). Complexity and ambiguity in environmental design. *Journal of the American Institute of Planners, 33*(4), 210–221.

CHAPTER 14

A Compelling Societal Problem Makes for a Good Professional Life

Victor Regnier

ABSTRACT

A desire to combine a passion for design with the social commitment of helping older people have a better and more independent life in appropriate and supportive housing, summarizes the broadest motivation for my career. The medium I chose to accomplish this was through university-based teaching and research. The topics I selected and the investigations I pursued were often identified by interactions with designers and frail older people but they almost always focused on real-world problems that affected the quality of life. The primary motivation for publishing my work was to share it with others who might find insights from my work helpful in creating better environments for cognitively and physically frail older people. I quickly discovered that design and management were equally important in creating a satisfying outcome. Like the design of an automobile, the environment was created to be manipulated not just admired. Also that not just architecture, but plant materials, location criteria, interior design features, families, friends, and caregivers all had an important influence on the "environment." My interests in aesthetics and theory were never far away but they were just not as satisfying as knowing my work or my ideas had made an older person happier or more able to live a better life.

http://dx.doi.org/10.1891/0198-8794.38.239

BIOGRAPHICAL NOTES

If there were a continuum of theoretical to applied research to categorize the careers of the researchers in this volume—I would be on the end nearest to application. I consider myself an architect and researcher who has been trained in a multidisciplinary context. In fact, I would say that my research profile, which consists mainly of evidence-based research explorations, has always been motivated by squeezing utility from research investigations. This is a result of my interest in environmental design and the desire to inform decision making at the drafting board (or today on the computer). I have always been interested in "making" architecture with my hands or later directing its production by others. Another important aspect of my profile is the desire to share my experiences with the academic and practice community. I have done this through teaching, consulting, and producing books and monographs that chronicle my academic and professional experiences. My early family life nurtured a strong work ethic and my training stimulated a process of thinking about problems from many different perspectives. I am a big thinker, but realize it is the details of an implemented idea that make it noteworthy.

My career path has been directed, but like most, has resulted more from opportunities than a well-articulated master plan. In Jim Birren's guided autobiography guidebook (Birren & Cochran, 2001), he describes a process of inspecting life experiences in a way that reveals overlaps with other individuals and favorable circumstances. The impact of major events (attending college, first jobs, marriage, etc.) creates decision points where life can quickly change direction. Jim Birren was fond of describing it as a fork in the road. At these important junctures, one's future is often impacted by a choice or an interaction with a significant colleague. These experiences close some doors while opening others. How you nurture or exploit these new opportunities and how you close the door on previous ones, accounts for the evolution of your professional and personal life. The purpose of this edited volume is to understand, like a jigsaw puzzle, how the professional experiences of each researcher filled out the gestalt picture of Environmental Gerontology.

What makes life fun and interesting is its unpredictability. Some major events like our date of death are completely unknown. Not knowing it makes the adventure of living life more robust. So it has been with my career. Like landing a slithering fish in a boat you have some control, but there is always the possibility that you will lose it. Starting from the beginning is maybe as good as any method to tell this story, which weaves personal interests and professional experiences together with the outcomes of my academic and professional work.

EARLY EXPERIENCES

I was born in a Kansas City suburb to a contractor/developer father and a mother who gave up being a librarian to manage the books for the family business. Dad was always working and as soon as my brother and I reached our pre-teenage years, we were presented with a framing hammer and a request to join the family enterprise. My sister experienced a less directed life when she was young, but later became an important influence in the family business. Everyone in my family was exposed to an "extreme work ethic"—something akin to what it was like growing up on a farm. We all had tasks that contributed to the greater good. Also, our personal and work lives frequently blended together. My grandparents lived with us in a three-generation household so I was exposed at an early age to their wisdom and affection.

My interest in architecture was triggered by the observations of my fourth grade teacher who told my parents based on school artwork that I should consider a creative field like architecture. My father liked that idea, because in his growing business he needed someone to carry out those kinds of tasks. So I became the budding architect while my brother was assigned the finance/banker role. While in high school, I had the opportunity to design commercial and residential projects for my father and later during college, I took responsibility for the construction management of several commercial projects. All the while learning by watching skilled laborers and professionals do their jobs. During this time, I had my first life-changing experience working in the office of Uri Seiden, a well-known Kansas City structural engineer and architect. I wanted to be just like him and he encouraged me to pursue architectural engineering at the regional land grant college, Kansas State University (KSU).

When I got to K-State, it became increasingly clear that my true interest lied in design and during my third year of college, I added an additional degree, architecture, which lengthened my stay to 6.5 years. The timing was helpful during the active recruitment period for the Vietnam conflict. My academic exposure to both architecture and engineering made it difficult for me to reconcile the competing demands of both these professions. Architecture won out but my engineering exposure nurtured an interest in numbers and rationality, which later became useful as my interest in research evolved. In Manhattan Kansas, work opportunities in an architect's office were minimal. Bill Eidson, considered one of the best local architects, hired me part-time based on my experience and immediately assigned me to a new project in the office. It was one of the first Housing and Urban Development (HUD)-subsided high-rise, elderly housing projects commissioned in the late 1960s. Asked to research the architectural program, I was amazed to find little information about social considerations and how a project such as this could support the needs of older residents. In the late 1960s, architects were reluctant to discuss these issues partly because little was known about them.

I was interested in graduate studies in large-scale planning and decided to apply to several well-known programs. I was accepted to the Architecture Association in London but had no way to finance the program costs. While searching the bulletin board in the architecture and regional planning office at KSU, I came across an advertisement for a master's program in architecture and gerontology at the University of Southern California (USC). After further investigation, the program appeared relevant to those unanswered programming questions I had encountered in the local HUD project. It also solved my financing dilemma because tuition costs were covered by a federal training grant. I applied and was accepted by the Program's Director Eric Pawley, to begin the 2-year program in the fall of 1971.

USC ANDRUS GERONTOLOGY CENTER

The program was amazing. It was interdisciplinary and addressed planning and architecture issues, but also exposed me to the work of other aging researchers including accomplished scholars like James Birren (Psychology), Tuck Finch (Biology), Vern Bengtsen (Sociology), and Paul Kerschner (Social Policy). Jim Birren who directed the Andrus Gerontology Center had an interest and positive attitude toward planned housing for older people. His enthusiasm was nurtured by evaluation work he initiated and coordinated at Leisure World, one of the first large scale active adult communities in the United States. In fact, Ross Cortese, the developer of Leisure World was one of the first donors to offer funding for the aging program at USC. Later, the American Association of Retired Persons (AARP) funded the new building and named it after Ethel Percy Andrus, their founder. In the mid-1980s, I worked with Cortese to conceptualize an international collection of communities that would have allowed retirees to live in communities across the globe for short periods of time. This was an extension of his interest in combining travel with living abroad in communities that were custom-fitted to the interests of recent retirees. Unfortunately, he died suddenly before this vision could be implemented.

Student colleagues Tom Byerts, Dick Eribes, and Hal Kendig were part of the program and Bob Newcomer was the preceptor of urban planning. During my training, I had a second life-changing experience when I met Powell Lawton. Powell came for a 3-day visit and talked about his national study of public housing, which was multidimensional and formed the basis for his book, *Planning and*

Managing Housing for the Elderly (Lawton, 1974). I was amazed by his knowledge and research acumen. He found my work interesting and I acquired my first nonrelated father figure. Powell continued to be a fount of ideas, theories, and experience and we stayed as close friends for 30 years, until his death in 2001. My thesis dealt with the use of cognitive mapping in defining the neighborhoods of older people in two public housing projects in San Francisco. My interest was in reconciling the definition and extent of the neighborhood through hand-drawn maps and an inventory of retail and service use patterns in two very different areas of the city.

Anxious to start a practice and become licensed as an architect, I joined Lou Gelwicks as his Director of Planning at Gerontological Planning Associates in Santa Monica, CA. Using survey and focus group techniques, I created architectural programs for several elderly housing complexes.

I immediately started teaching part-time at USC and 15 months later was recruited full time to administer the last year of the Administration on Aging (AoA) training grant, which had supported me as a student. My tenure there extended for 7 years at which time I was the Laboratory Chief of Environmental Studies. USC Gerontology in the mid-1970s was extraordinary with Warner Schaie, Eileen Crimmins, David Cutler, and Phoebe Liebig as colleagues.

At this time I started working with psychologist David Walsh on a National Institute of Mental Health-funded project and an AoA Title IV community research analysis project. Both projects focused on how neighborhoods worked as support systems for older residents. We used cognitive mapping techniques and diaries to map use patterns in four Los Angeles neighborhoods. I also met psychologist Rick Scheldt (see Chapter 11, A "Good Fit": Professionally Aging in Small Kansas Towns) when he was a postdoc at USC and encouraged him to consider developing similar analysis techniques with Paul Windley at KSU.

I became involved with Tom Byerts as an executive board member for his Gerontological Society-based project on environments and aging. It was there that I got to know Lee Pastalan, Sandra Howell, Joe Koncelik, and Paul Windley. I was the youngest member of the group and greatly enjoyed the mentoring and advice it provided. This was an important time for interacting with a variety of new colleagues through conference presentations, subcontracts, and a jointly edited book project. These included Edward Steinfeld, Graham Rowles, John Zeisel, Jerry Weisman, Uriel Cohen, Steve Golant, Lori Hiatt, and Ben Schwarz. Later, Margaret Calkins and Michael Hunt were added to this list (see Chapter 3, The Meaning of Place in Environmental Gerontology; Chapter 4, Intellectual Origins of Residential Normalcy Theory; Chapter 6, Weisman title; Chapter 13, Calkins title; Chapter 12, Finding Place: An Intellectual Journey; Chapter 16, A Career

Outside the Mainstream). My first edited book (Regnier, 1979) brought together a series of essays from students who took a graduate research studio examining planning analysis techniques we were developing for our Administration on Aging Title IV research grant.

UNIVERSITY OF ILLINOIS

In 1979, I was recruited to the University of Illinois, Champaign-Urbana for a tenured position. It was a joint appointment between the Program of Housing Research and Development and the Graduate Program in Housing Design in the School of Architecture. There, Bob Katz and Sue Weidemann became important colleagues and collaborators. While there, I expanded my interest in site design by writing a National Endowment for the Arts research grant looking at the use of outdoor spaces around housing projects for the elderly. This examination sparked an interest in landscape architecture. There were developments on a personal level during that time. In 1980, I married Judith Gonda, a post-doc at USC and had two children, Jennifer (landscape architect) and Heather (screenwriter and producer). Being a father was a great privilege as well as a big responsibility.

I started a second book at Illinois, which satisfied my interest in examining the important findings of 15 noteworthy studies. These were amazing studies that were relevant to architects but had not been formulated to communicate their findings to this important audience. I coauthored with the contributor of each chapter conclusions in the form of Design Directives, which also provided a rationale for implementation. This pushed the work to reveal its practical influence on design decision making. The book's coauthor, Jon Pynoos, did the same for policy implications. This book (Figure 14.1; Regnier & Pynoos, 1987) connected me with the work and the personalities of people like Fran Carp, Galen Cranz, Bob Herman, Rudy Moos, and Ray Struyk.

One of the most positive experiences during my time at Illinois was teaching and getting to know a graduate student named David Hoglund. His creative work on Woodside Place, Copper Ridge, NewBridge, and more than 5,000 elderly housing units throughout the world is a testament to the impact and influence his work and thinking has had on the field. To this day, we continue to lecture and work together on various projects.

USC ARCHITECTURE AND GERONTOLOGY

In 1983, Jim Birren and Bob Harris (the respective Deans of the Schools of Gerontology and Architecture at USC) recruited me back to USC for a joint

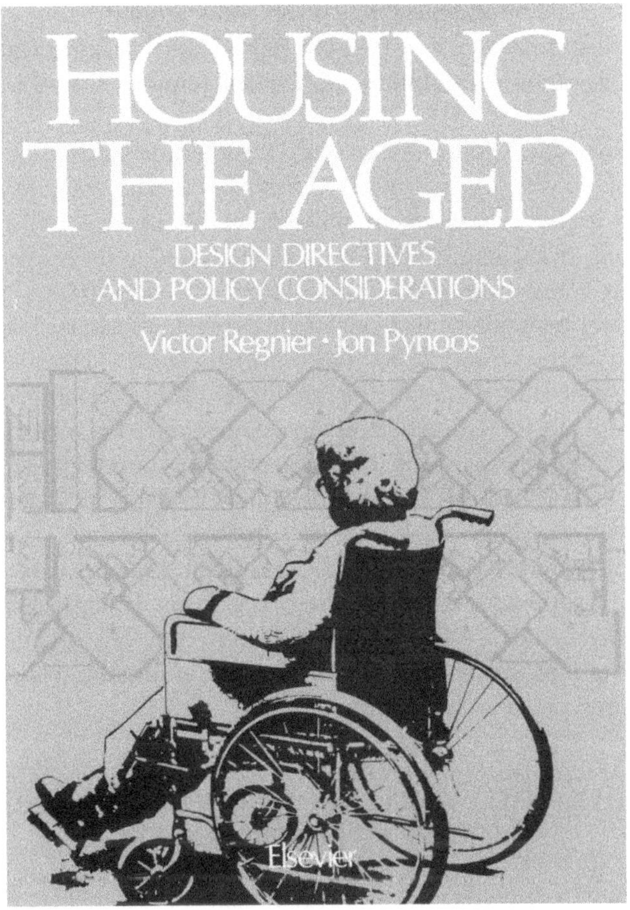

FIGURE 14.1 *Housing the Aged* re-examined the work of 15 environmental design researchers seeking specific Design Directives and Policy Considerations from noteworthy research projects they had previously authored. The conclusions to each chapter were co-authored between the researcher and Regnier/Pynoos to seek an accurate, explicit and comparable set of conclusions.
Source: Regnier and Pynoos (1987).

appointment between both schools. I broadened my focus and became more immersed in research outside of aging, including environments for people with handicaps, the homeless, and children. In the next 7 years, I continued my interest in bridge building between research and practice through nearly a hundred consultations with architects and sponsors of elderly housing projects and community centers. During that time, I noticed that many professionals interested in this knowledge read books, but rarely were aware of published research articles. It was clear that if I wanted to have an impact on the field of architecture, I needed to focus on books and monographs that could be shared with architects and sponsors.

Jon Pynoos and I continued to work together on research projects as well as jointly teaching classes at USC. We partitioned our research territory into purpose-built housing and home modifications/falls so we could work together more effectively. In the late 1980s, I became interested in the burgeoning area of assisted living. Many of these projects were remakes of board and care housing with a stronger, professional focus on personal care and higher quality standards.

An important grant from the Chicago-based Retirement Research Foundation started with identifying architects and sponsors of noteworthy projects throughout the United States. In this research, I was fascinated by the design approaches, management strategies, and financing approaches that were being tested. I published this research (Regnier, Hamilton, & Yatabe, 1995) as a Columbia University Press book with two graduate students. This book examined the philosophy, physical form and operational strategies that characterized this emerging building type. During these interviews, I met Paul Klaassen, the CEO of Sunrise Senior Living, who had a strong interest in Dutch models of housing for the frail. In the mid-1990s, I would eventually work with him to develop a prototype for assisted living.

FULBRIGHT AND EXPOSURE TO NORTHERN EUROPEAN MODELS OF LTC

Working on a research project that was jointly ventured with the UCLA medical school, I met John Beck, MD, from the Department of Geriatrics. Beck was the first to suggest that I study northern European housing projects for frail older people. In 1991, I received a Fulbright grant entitled the Western Regional Research Award. This allowed me to visit 100 projects in five northern European countries (Finland, Sweden, Denmark, Norway, and Netherlands). When there, I studied their systems and approaches to caring for frail older people. These countries had an especially strong focus on residential settings as well as staying at home. It opened my eyes to many ideas that were not present in the United States. The northern European approach to housing and service support was more user-centered and would have ironically violated many regulations in the United States that were in place to protect older people. These countries were also more committed to keeping older frail people out of institutions. Facility staff was better trained and the architecture of the buildings was far more beautiful and thoughtful. The differences and similarities in approaches taken in these five countries also reflected their history and culture. The spirit of respect and competition they shared also raised the bar as they sought to learn from one another.

The result of this research was a Van Nostrand book (Figure 14.2; Regnier, 1994), which contrasted European and U.S. exemplar projects. It won the Progressive Architecture Research Award in 1994. The book focused on case studies and described how these projects were advancing the field. It typically used evidence-based methods such as case studies that involved face-to-face interviews and evaluations of each visited building. I was able to discern

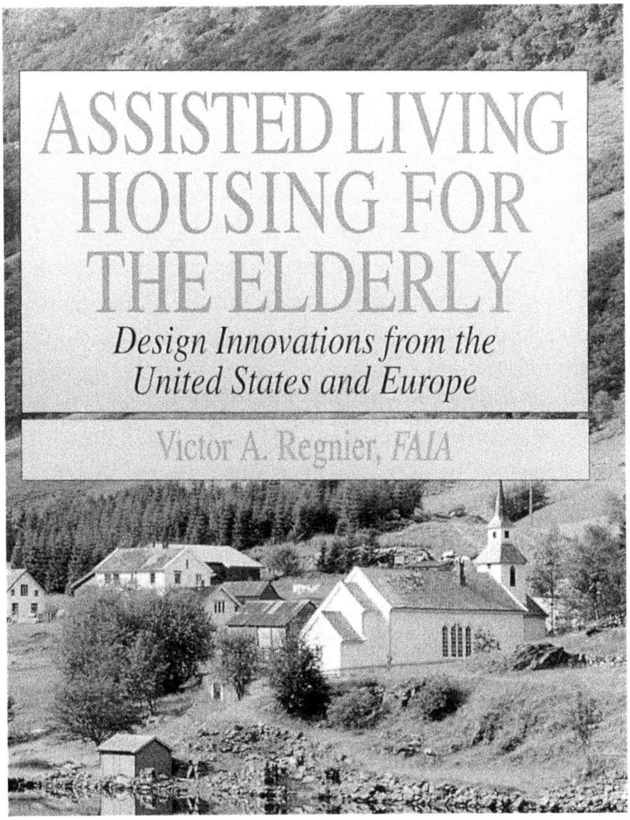

FIGURE 14.2 *Assisted Living Housing for the Aged* used site visits that employed multi-dimensional sources to examine 100 housing and service projects for mentally and physically frail older people in Finland, Sweden, Denmark, Norway, the Netherlands and the US. Six chapters sought to define the emerging building type of assisted living and 10 case studies detailed information about how design, operation and site placement helped older people live a more independent life.
Source: Regnier (1994).

differences in practice and outcome between each of these countries as well as between the United States and northern Europe.

In 1992, I became involved in the USC School of Architecture leadership. I was appointed interim Dean of architecture. As it turned out, an initial 1-year appointment stretched out to 3.5 years. While I was in the process of restarting my research in 1996, Sunrise Senior Living and my old colleague Paul Klaassen approached me to design and advise on the production of their assisted living prototype. I had earlier worked with Marriott on their new prototypical design. As a career academic I was interested in staying at the university. USC and the School of Architecture supported the goal of continuing my practice exposure to the field by reducing my tenured appointment to 50%.

From 1996 to 2008 I worked on hundreds of projects in 32 U.S. states, the UK, Canada, and Germany for Sunrise Senior Living. This enabled me to become more involved in management while understanding more precisely how a philosophy of care was affected by the design of the building. Working with 9 different architects in the United States and internationally, I interpreted the prototype design for every project while developing new insights from 8 to 10 evidence-based Post Occupancy Evaluations (POEs) each year. The experience helped me to identify the most important design considerations addressed by the architects while learning more about the realities of large-scale international development.

In 2000, my father died of a brain tumor. My mother, who died later, in 2004, had acquired dementia in the mid-90s. My time with both of them (they shared a nursing home room) was invaluable both personally and professionally. It enhanced my ability to understand at a much deeper level the problems of aging in an institution. Having a physically and mentally frail parent was both a heavy family responsibility as well as an emotional learning experience. Between 1994 and 2000, thanks to a heavy travel schedule, I was able to visit them every month, even though they were 1,500 miles away. After 2000, I had additional family business responsibilities, but also had the opportunity to establish with my siblings a charitable foundation—centered on education and children.

INTEREST IN APARTMENTS/CONDOS FOR LIFE

In 2002, I returned to northern Europe to visit and investigate another 100 residential care homes. Visiting the same countries 10 years later allowed me to monitor progress and changes in practice. This work culminated in another book (Figure 14.3; Regnier, 2002) that used case studies, but also summarized important priorities through a description of 100 important ideas/insights I had gleaned from my research and practice experiences. These topics, subdivided into 10 categories, were complimented with photos and short essays. My focus

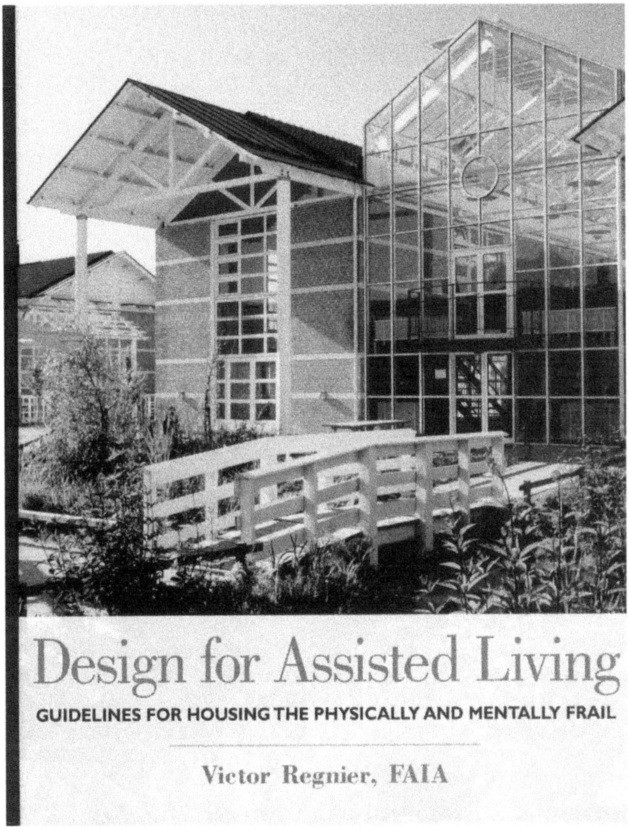

FIGURE 14.3 *Design for Assisted Living* involved examinations of 100 different housing and service projects a decade after *Assisted Living Housing for the Aged* was published. Findings were organized around chapters that 1) refined the definition of Assisted Living, 2) identified 100 critical design considerations, 3) explored in detail 15 case studies from northern Europe and the US, and 4) sought unifying trends and design considerations. Special care was taken to identify the role of culture, lifestyle and policy considerations present in different countries that led to an emphasis on autonomy.
Source: Regnier, (2002).

also broadened to interior design, landscaping, site selection, dementia design, and attributes like staff satisfaction and resident happiness.

During the research, I was introduced to the Apartment for Life building type in Rotterdam. I became a proponent of this building type and have monitored progress at the initial project, Humanitas Bergweg, through site visits every 3 to 5 years, primarily examining its evolution over time. In 2006, I began work on another book that involved boomer preferences. In 2011, I visited another

50 projects primarily in Denmark, Sweden, Netherlands, and Finland. Because of the recession and the focus on keeping people in their own homes there were fewer new projects.

Between 2009 and 2012, I initiated a broad based continuing education program that centered on the USC School of Architecture. I also became the Vice Dean of External Relations—involving alumni and practicing professionals in school-related activities. During this time, my interest in the Apartment for Life prototype continued through the offering of graduate studio classes that centered on this building type. Spring studios (Figure 14.4; Regnier, 2010, 2013, 2014)

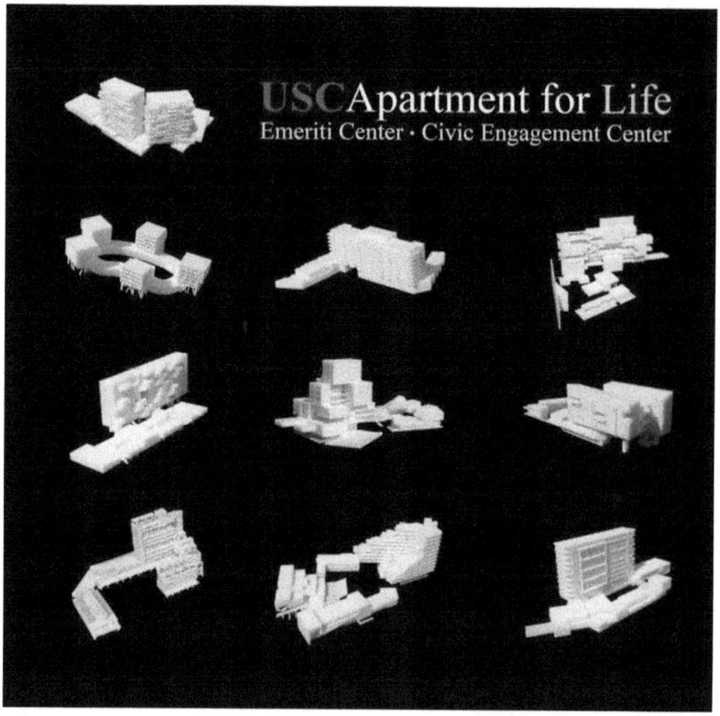

FIGURE 14.4 *USC Apartment for Life* chronicled 10 student design projects that resulted from a USC Graduate Studio. The purpose was to apply the Dutch Apartment for Life prototype to a site on the University of Southern California campus. Programs that extended the interests of the Emeriti Center and the Civic Engagement Center were combined with 60 housing units for retired faculty and staff. The publication identified in detail four noteworthy student solutions and described how the mixed-use projects addressed 10 important design, program and urban considerations.
Source: Regnier (2013).

explored the building type in several different contexts. Self-published monographs were written that documented the student work.

In 2014, I received a second Fulbright which was based on research and teaching in Portugal. I consulted with a studio taught at the Catholic University. Working with Antonio Carvalho, who had recently completed his dissertation on housing for the older frail in Portugal, I lectured on aging topics at several local universities and worked with design students to explore their thesis interests. My experiences in Portugal were a major contrast to what I had experienced in northern Europe. Older people were more likely to stay at home and age in the community. This peaked my interest in the age-friendly cities movement and the idea of helping older people in place. It became clear to me that helping older people stay in their homes (or purpose-built independent housing) in familiar neighborhoods was the single most effective solution we could explore. It is not without irony that my thinking circled back to my neighborhood research in the early 1970s. After visiting projects for the frail elderly in Portugal I began writing a final book, which has taken a broader perspective on the issue of housing in a long-lived society (Regnier, n.d.).

Working on this book, I saw the need to redefine assisted living from a facility-based setting to an investigation of how the oldest-old can deal with the problem of frailty and housing. I became convinced that a two-tier approach of helping the older frail was necessary. A home-care-based system was needed to help frail elders stay in normal housing or purpose built dwellings in the community. Also a major reconceptualization of the nursing home for end-of-life care was required. Building on northern European models, we need to replace substandard shared nursing homes with larger private units within smaller, more intimate clusters. These are tried and tested models that have operated in Scandinavia for decades and have only recently become recognized in decentralized small cluster models in the United States.

Also community-based care systems are becoming far more important as a source of support for dual eligible recipients (Medicare/Medicaid). Current work explores themes like advanced electro-mechanical/communications technology, the sharing economy, biophilia (the love of living systems—mostly applied to plants) and programs like PACE (Program of All-Inclusive Care for the Elderly), the Village movement (Beacon Hill Village) and more widely available home-care delivered services. Assisted living has promise, but the costs of care and the limitations in the amount of medical support that can be provided has limited the utility of this facility type. Assisted living has been characterized by its focus on delivering a product/service that was consumer-driven. However, some assisted living companies, like many proprietary nursing home chains, are becoming more profit motivated.

CONCLUSIONS

In the competing world of prices and risk, even nonprofit organizations now increasingly act more like big corporations. The regulations that are considered necessary to guarantee safety and quality are often not effective in producing a final outcome that is an improvement. In northern Europe, there seems to be more respect for the aged and jobs associated with care giving are still considered important and honorable. In the United States, those jobs—especially at the lowest compensation levels—compete with fast food chains and seem to have lost their value to society.

Artificial intelligence and robotics appear to be transitioning to practical future modalities for care giving. Hopefully they will allow the older person more freedom and choices rather than limiting their lives further. The increase in the numbers of the oldest-old population (especially those with dementia) and the reduction in the number of younger people available and motivated to work with older people will continue to be a concern in the future.

SIX IMPORTANT HIGHLIGHTS

1. The Four Notable Phases of My Academic/Research Career

(i) Planning analysis work at the neighborhood scale (1973–1979). How do older people use neighborhoods? What are their perceptions about safety? What specific attributes should they contain? How can we stimulate more social exchange at this scale? What new mixed-use prototypes are helpful to explore?

(ii) Translating research into practice (1979–1990). How can we identify aspects of the environment that are critical to satisfaction and facilitate environmental use?

(iii) Interest in a range of residential alternatives to long-term care (1990–present).

(iv) Interest in the idea of Apartments for Life (1996–present). This allows older people to stay at home or in an adaptable purpose-built residential context where long-term care services are delivered.

2. Key Scientific/Creative Contributions

(i) Bridge between design and research: Testing ideas in the field that could make a qualitative difference in the lives of older people. Also dealing with the architect's predisposition to be creative and original without careful analysis of the impact design decisions have on the older person.

(ii) Key contributor to assisted living prototype development: The Sunrise Senior Living assisted living/dementia model was replicated and improved over 12 years in hundreds of projects seeking to integrate care and design. These consecutive projects were scrutinized through dozens of POEs. The model and attributes of the model became useful exemplars for others to follow and improve.

(iii) Explored innovative ideas from northern European: These included buildings and services for the mentally and physically frail and their differences and similarities to U.S. practice. These were illustrated in three books.

(iv) Advocated for the idea of allowing older people to age in place in purpose built housing: Studied the approach to peripatetic, home-care-based services that avoided institutionalization—a practice that is common in Scandinavia.

(v) Methodically developed evidence-based research techniques for assessing best practices in design for older people: Techniques like this have become popular in many professional disciplines because they do not attempt the difficult task of identifying underlying factors, but simply evaluate methods, products, and protocols.

3. Evolution of Research Over Time

(i) Started with multidisciplinary research involving psychologists and policy analysts (1974–1980).

(ii) Developed methods using site visits, interview techniques, and behavioral mapping for uncovering the impact of the environment on older residents (1980–1994).

(iii) Discovered the impact of landscape and interior design on residents and their lifestyles. Learning about the therapeutic impacts buildings have on people piqued my interest in exercise, social exchange, and socially friendly spaces (1994–present).

4. Potential Implications

(i) Examined how to help older people become more independent in the community through the development of purpose-built models of housing with services.

5. Research/Practice Topics I Plan to Work On

(i) Apartments/Condos for Life: These are housing and service combinations that demonstrate methods for delivering services to older people and thus allowing them to stay independent in normal housing.

(ii) Models of family friendly design and policies that encourage multigenerational exchange.

(iii) Evolution of new technologies: Especially technologies that make it easier for an older person to maintain their independence in the community.

6. Open Questions and Emergent Challenges

(i) How will planned housing deal with the increasing number of oldest-old? What are the best methods to allow these individuals to live a free, safe, and independent life outside of an institution?
(ii) How will people with dementia be served in less institutional settings in the future? Is making them small (less than 12 residents) the best answer? Should individual unit designs be larger? Today's approach is to accommodate older people in a single-occupancy 250-275 SF unit. Is that really adequate?
(iii) How can technology contribute to making older people more capable of carrying out activities of daily living or instrumental activities of daily living (ADL/IADL's) and maintaining their independence in normal housing?
(iv) What new devices will be introduced to move people out of their bed and into the bathroom? How do we get people safely into a wheelchair or mobility device?
(v) How can we contribute to the testing of these ideas? How can we adjust or relax regulations and other impediments that block us from testing new solutions. Does our tendency to establish rules and protocols lock us into specific solutions that have little flexibility—not to mention room for innovation?

FINAL THOUGHTS

A little more than 45 years ago, I started studying the topic of housing and services for older people. A lot of good work and careful thinking has characterized our current knowledge about how to help older people live happier and more independent lives in the community and in housing with services. We have come to recognize that there is no single answer to the complex problem of living a well-supported life in old age. Models from other countries have helped us inspect our solutions and question our assumptions. New technologies have made it easier to communicate and continue to make it easier to live with goods and services delivered just in time. On the horizon new medical treatments are likely to extend life and diseases like cancer and dementia appear to be more understood than ever before. We have made a dent in the assumptions about what defines the need for institutionalization and have helped people to avoid it. Our standards for nursing homes are still deplorably low and our compassion for medicaid nursing home recipients (older, low-income females) are an embarrassment to our long-term care system. So much is yet to be done.

As I reach my seventh decade, those interesting questions now seem increasingly personal. It is also much clearer that regardless of what I think or want, I will join the ages when my time is up. But much like my past mentors and professional heroes, I feel like it has been a well-lived professional life that has helped all of us to better understand an evolving and compelling societal issue.

REFERENCES

Birren, J. E., & Cochran, K. (2001). *Telling stories of life through guided autobiography groups*. Baltimore, MD: The John Hopkins Press.

Lawton, M. P. (1975). *Planning and managing housing for the elderly*. New York, NY: John Wiley and Sons.

Regnier, V. (Ed.). (1979). *Planning for the elderly: Alternative community analysis techniques*. Los Angeles, CA: USC Press.

Regnier, V. (1994). *Assisted living housing for the elderly: Design innovations from the United States and Europe*. New York, NY: John Wiley and Sons.

Regnier, V. (2002). *Design for assisted living: Guidelines for housing the physically and mentally frail*. New York, NY: John Wiley and Sons.

Regnier, V. (2010). *USC emeriti center: A vision for the future*. San Francisco, CA: Blurb, Inc.

Regnier, V. (2013). *USC apartment for life: Emeriti center, civic + engagement center*. San Francisco, CA: Blurb, Inc.

Regnier, V. (2014). *MPTF apartment for life: Motion picture and television fund campus*. San Francisco, CA: Blurb, Inc.

Regnier, V. (n.d.). *Housing design for an increasingly older population* [Manuscript in preparation]. New York, NY: John Wiley and Sons.

Regnier, V., Hamilton, J., & Yatabe, S. (1995). *Assisted living for the aged and frail: Innovations in design, management and financing*. New York, NY: Columbia University Press.

Regnier, V., & Pynoos, J. (Eds.). (1987). *Housing the aged: Design directives and policy considerations*. New York, NY: Elsevier.

CHAPTER 15

Discovering Environment–Behavior Studies

A Personal Adventure

John Zeisel

ABSTRACT

This chapter presents a personal intellectual and professional adventure of discovery. Starting with natural curiosity and a penchant to observe the world as it is (empirically) John Zeisel was privileged to be a member of a group of lively minds who uncovered the field of Environment–Behavior (E-B) and its application to gerontology. The chapter describes the steps he climbed studying the Domestic Peace Core in the "hollers" of Eastern Kentucky, becoming academically involved with social science research, and seeking a way to apply that knowledge in design through working side-by-side with architecture students and practicing designers of all sorts. The result—discovering the common research and design development spiral some call the Zeiral. Building on this common process, he merged research and design in an applied consulting practice and in an organization—Hearthstone Alzheimer Care—that manages residential treatment for persons with dementia. The chapter describes breakthroughs including how the physical environment improves the lives of persons living with dementia, how the neurosciences help E-B practitioners and designers understand the way the physical environment affects our brains and mental processes, and how the term "ecopsychosocial" best expresses the phenomena otherwise called "nonpharmacological"—because it includes the physical environment ("eco"). The chapter

http://dx.doi.org/10.1891/0198-8794.38.257

explains how Zeisel's two seminal books are critical in the development of E-B as a field: "Inquiry by Design" exploring the link between design and research in an early form of "evidence-based design" and "I'm Still Here" in changing the way professionals and everyday people view dementia—as a stage in life that can be influenced for the better through ecopsychosocial approaches—a message of hope.

BIOGRAPHICAL NOTES

My professional and intellectual lives have always been one. I followed, or so it seems, I followed my interests and ended up creating a professional life that reflected those interests. I was never told I had to work or earn a living—not even when cousins who were better off were working summer jobs selling fruits and vegetables. I was always attracted to and involved in theater—local theater groups as a child, then summer stock bit parts and tearing down sets, then acting and stage managing off-Broadway before there was an official off-Broadway. Theater prepared me for lecturing and teaching—something I was drawn to, enjoyed, and thrived on since I started working, and still do.

I never was drawn to a profession like being a doctor, lawyer, or businessman; since the beginning, education for me was an exploration into different realms. Before going to university, I studied languages, I learned to write a précis of books, I read—although it was not something I did for leisure; I played competitive tennis, but never had the killer instinct to win the big matches. Above all, I learned to observe the world around me and appreciate how interesting it all was. This interest—*observing as I did*—I now believe was the root of my interest in E-B or Environment–Behavior studies.

E-B to me boils down to seeing the world around us and all its connections as one—not environments that house behaviors; not settings separate from perceptions of, attitudes toward, and beliefs about environments—but all together. Doing this requires observing without bias, without artificial distinctions and theory—empirically. That's what empirical means—observing without theory—letting what we see and hear be the basis for how we interpret the world around us rather than depending on how we think the world ought to be organized to guide our observations.

Not reading a great deal, I didn't have a lot of models for seeing the world—no architectural mind, ecological mind, or psychological mind. I ended up in college (at Columbia University) studying Chinese language, oriental studies (history and philosophy and literature), and comparative literature.

Sociology became my focus in graduate school (School of Graduate Studies at Columbia University) because a graduate degree was just something members of my family pursued—it was expected. In addition to being a second-generation sociologist, it was the time of the Vietnam War and an academic deferment was automatic for graduate school students. When I started my courses in sociology and started to sink my teeth into the approaches of social science, I felt comfortable, completely at home. We were taught theoretical models—structural functionalism (Merton, 1948, 1968), exchange theory (Blau, 1964; Homans, 1958), and symbolic interactionism (Goffman, 1956)—none to the exclusion of the others. We were taught methods and methodology (surveys, focused interviewing, observing) as ways to explore the world around us. We had practical research experience. My first major research study was as a field worker at Columbia's Bureau of Applied Social Research evaluating the work of the first year of Domestic Peace Corps volunteers; my focus was on those volunteers in the "hollers" of South Eastern Kentucky. The environment and how it influenced the lives of the mostly unemployed Kentucky coal miners was striking. The closed coal mines caused unemployment. The "hollers" they lived in—a "holler" is a creek with no water that don't go nowhere—caused isolation. And the rickety wood houses they lived in reinforced their poverty. This was my first confrontation with E-B.

All this education and experience led me to my first significant professional question and eventual decision—"How can I make my learning and thinking useful?" I was committed to applying my knowledge, not just thinking about it or teaching—although teaching was one of the routes I took to applying the sociology I had absorbed. I did not teach sociologists, rather those who might use these approaches—architects.

I fell upon what later became my part of the field of E-B while still at university, working on a school project with my then partner and later brother-in-law Brent Brolin. We carefully analyzed the life of the Italian working class residents of Boston's West End as described by sociologist Herbert Gans in his insightful study *The Urban Villagers* (Gans, 1962). Using his book as source material, we identified the way men and women used their kitchens and living rooms; the way young men used the street corners and local shops; and the way their entire lives were centered on the street. Employing an analytic approach pioneered by architect Christopher Alexander in his groundbreaking *Notes on the Synthesis of Form* (Alexander, 1964), we organized the analysis into 20 user-needs "requirements." These formed the basis for Brent's design of a set of buildings for the West End site that—had they been built instead of the high rise urban renewal buildings that were eventually constructed—would have reflected, respected, and met the needs of this group of users. We ended up translating *The Urban Villagers* into an architectural and urban design response to the needs of Boston's Italian West Enders (see Figure 15.1).

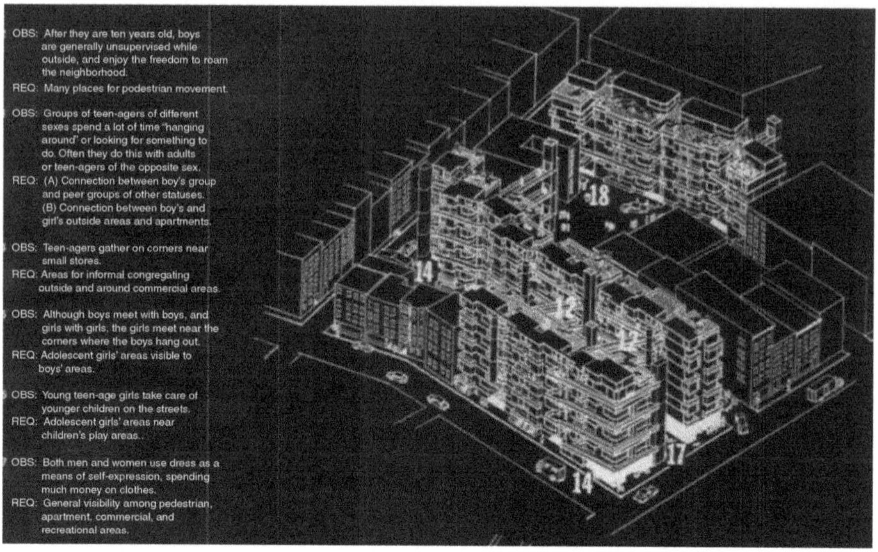

FIGURE 15.1 West End user responsive building with "observations" and "requirements."
Source: Brolin and Zeisel (1968).

My part of this project, which eventually became central to my life's work, centered on applying social facts and knowledge in the design professions. The result of this collaboration was my first publication—*Mass Housing: Social Research and Design* (Brolin & Zeisel, 1968). Brent had brought to my attention Alexander's approach of breaking down social observations into concise "mouthfuls" or "bites" useful to designers—the central thesis of his *Notes on the Synthesis of Form.* Although Chris later moved on from *Notes*—see his *The City is Not a Tree* (Alexander, 1965)—the bits that underlay the formulations on *Notes*—which Brent and I defined as design requirements—developed later into Alexander's "patterns"—the root of his iconic *Pattern Language* (Alexander, Silverstein, & Ishikawa, 1977)—still an important resource for E-Bers and designers alike.

Brent was an architecture student at Yale and I a sociology graduate student at Columbia; we worked together whenever we could. He submitted his project as a studio submission and I later used parts of the work in my PhD thesis. In 1968 we submitted the project for presentation at the First International Design Methods Group conference at the Massachusetts Institute of Technology (MIT) in Cambridge, Massachusetts. To this day I consider that conference the "pre-EDRA" conference, since such EDRA luminaries as Michael Brill, Gary Moore, and John Eberhard attended the MIT conference and the Environmental Design Research Association (EDRA) held its first official conference the following year.

Our presentation which suggested that social research could be used to inform and even direct design decisions engendered much discussion and debate, even raised voices. We were definitely on to something.

We had also submitted the project as an article to what I was told (at that time, I didn't know much about the field of architecture or design) was a prestigious architecture journal—*Architectural Forum*. We were advised not to have high hopes of being published because *Forum* "didn't publish student work." We heard nothing for months until one day we decided to call them—on the principle that the *creaky wheel receives the grease*. Ellen Berkeley, a *Forum* editor, called us back a few days later and said that they decided to publish the article and would we please come into her office.

Extremely excited by the fact that public acknowledgment was just around the corner for what we felt was a new way to create evidence-based design—although this term was not in use at that time—we made an appointment and showed up. Ellen offered us two pages for the article. We said we needed four because the drawings themselves would take up two pages. The article "Mass Housing: Social Research and Design" (Brolin & Zeisel, 1968) eventually was published on six pages with three pages of drawings. We asked Ellen why they took so long to decide and why they now decided to publish us. Ellen explained that one of their long-distance editors—Roger Montgomery, Professor of Urban Planning at University of California-Berkeley, had been the deciding factor for publication and he had just recently gotten back to them. We were obviously in his debt. Finally, Ellen asked us if $195 would be acceptable. It was obviously worth more than that to have the article published so we readily agreed. Then Ellen stopped us. "I am talking about paying you for the article not you paying us. If there is one thing you learn from this situation," she continued "it is that ideas are worth something—worth getting paid for."

Later, I was instrumental in establishing, with journalist Ann Ferebee, a relatively short-lived magazine called *Design and Environment* which sent me to conferences and to interview experts for stories. One of these was a conference in San Francisco where I had the opportunity to visit Roger Montgomery, later a good friend, at nearby Berkeley. I arrived in my eastern three-piece suit and he told me he was correcting his class's final exam and would I please remove my jacket, vest, and tie and sit down. Once I did, Roger handed me one of the exam papers he was correcting to read. The test question was one sentence: "Read Brolin & Zeisel's *Urban Villager's Design* article and comment."

That article was a turning point in my professional life because—like other publications since—it led to a significant new institutional connection. A student at Harvard University's department of architecture, Tony Pangaro, was so interested in the article he suggested that Brent and I be invited to a final housing studio design jury at Harvard—which we attended. I remember Jose Luis Sert, then dean of the Graduate School of Design (GSD), came in with an impressive retinue of professors and made insightful and biting comments to the students. A few months later I received a phone call from the acting chair of the department at Harvard, Tom Stifter, asking me if I would like to receive a Loeb Fellowship in Environmental Design at Harvard—flying in 2 days a week for the school year. What did I need to do? "Just say yes," Tom said. The Loeb Fellowship was brand new and there were no formal requirements. I took a breath, thought a little, and said yes, although I had recently accepted a teaching position at McGill University in Montreal. I ended up traveling weekly between Montreal (3 days), Cambridge, MA (2 days), and NYC on weekends.

I stayed at Harvard for another 8 years with research funding from the Kaplan Foundation and an Assistant Professor position—until a new chair of the department realized that they wanted to focus on big-"D" design instead of social objectives of design. That was all for me at Harvard—at that time. While there, however, I founded *Harvard's Architecture Research Office* and started to publish a series of coauthored white-covered books with black sans serif titles linking research to design—which I then continued to publish after leaving Harvard: the first was an evaluation of a nearby family housing project, *Charlesview Housing* (Zeisel & Griffin, 1975), the second, a summary of research on family housing design, *Housing Designed for Families* (Zeisel & Welch, 1981). When I left, I started my own consulting firm and made my first inroads to Environmental Gerontology, carrying out research on and publishing three new volumes: *Low-Rise Elderly Housing for Older People* (Zeisel, Welch, Epp, & Demos, 1978), *Mid-Rise Housing for Older people* (Zeisel, Welch, Epp, & Demos 1981), and *Congregate Housing for Older People* (Zeisel, Welch, & Parker, 1984). Each was the result of something applied: a research project, a design competition, and a design contract.

In the mean time, I had received another fellowship, this time at the Netherlands Institute for Advanced Study in Wassenaar, Holland, where I wrote most of my first major book, *Inquiry by Design* (Zeisel, 1984), focused on research and design theory and methods. The theory dealt with the processes of design and research and how the two can enrich each other. The methods part focused on what research methods are particularly useful in gathering data on E-B topics and how they need to be organized to do so: observations of behavior, observations of the physical environment, surveys, focused interviews, analysis of records, and analysis of architectural plans. It became a major textbook in courses that taught "environmental psychology" as many people called the growing field. Until this time, my assistant professorship at Harvard's GSD served as my calling card among academics and professionals in both sociology and architecture.

Before publication of *Inquiry by Design* I was often referred to as the socially oriented "architect" at Harvard's GSD. At conferences people seemed interested in what I had to say, but I did not represent a cohesive theory or doctrine. After the book's publication I was sought after by other schools and professional groups more because of the publication and the approach to research and design it represented than because of my Harvard position. This was not only positive for me personally but also, as it turned out, necessary. A new school dean and a new department chair were moving Harvard's Architecture Department away from social science and toward computer technologies. My approach to design was no longer valued in that setting. It was time for me to move on.

The publication of *Inquiry by Design* (1984) seemed to give me an independent foothold that no longer needed a set academic base to be recognized. I started my own research and design consulting company—Zeisel Research and later Building Diagnostics Inc, focusing more on applied research than teaching. In addition to consulting on building projects with individual architects and their clients (Zeisel & Maxwell, 1993), I received contracts to write guidelines for predesign programming from the U.S. General Services Administration, for housing for older people from the National Institute on Aging, and design programming for hospitals from the Canadian Government (Zeisel & Harvey, 1993). I did not stop teaching altogether—I just did not search out permanent academic employment. I had already been on the faculty at Yale University and McGill University, and after Harvard I continued as a visiting professor at the University of Minnesota, flying to Minneapolis every other week for a year, and later at Salford University (UK), where I remain a visiting professor, I also lectured annually in courses at the University of Quebec at Montreal and at the Sorbonne (Paris), although my primary work was outside of the academy—carrying out research, writing user-specific design guidebooks, and programming and evaluating major building projects.

Since 1993, I have been in business running Hearthstone Alzheimer Care, an organization which manages Assisted Living Residences for persons living with dementia—at one time as many as seven in New York and Massachusetts—trains care partners nationally and internationally in the approach I developed called *I'm Still Here*, and through the affiliated I'm Still Here Foundation develops art and cultural engagement programs for persons living with dementia both within assisted living communities and at home. Hearthstone Assisted Living Residences all are designed according to eight basic design criteria described later in this chapter that have been the keystone of my evidence-based design approach to dementia settings.

As a result of my work with people living with dementia, I was invited by my mentor, colleague, and friend John Eberhard, to be on the inaugural board of the Academy of Neuroscience for Architecture (ANFA). After all, dementia is foremost a condition of the brain. I spent 5 years reading neuroscience, developing a perspective that included the neurosciences in E-B studies, a dimension omitted in the original version of *Inquiry by Design*. In 2006, the revised edition of the book added chapters on how the neurosciences can greatly extend our understanding of E-B theory and methods—as well as adding case studies from my own and the research and design work of other close friends and thinkers from whom I have learned so much—among them Clare Cooper-Marcus, Jacqueline Vischer, Henry Sanoff, and Wolf Preiser.

The subtitle of the book reflects this change: *Environment-Behavior-Neuroscience for Architecture, Interiors, Landscape, and Planning.*

Based on my Hearthstone experience, I wrote a second major book—*I'm Still Here: A Breakthrough Approach to Caring for People Living With Dementia* (Zeisel, 2009). The book describes how persons with dementia are actually more present to the world around them than the popular myth that they lose a sense of self and their short-term memories. It goes on to draw on my E-B background to demonstrate how an appropriately designed and planned physical environment can serve as a cognitive "prosthetic" to help those with dementia find their way, develop a sense of self, act meaningfully, and generally support each person's "personhood." It goes on to provide guidance for engaging persons with dementia through the visual arts, dramatic arts, and environment.

KEY SCIENTIFIC CONTRIBUTIONS

Contributions in science can be made in the form of theory, empirical findings, studies that prove or disprove hypotheses, and even innovative ways of displaying information. Among my contributions in these areas are the following—each named and briefly described.

The Basic Eight Design Criteria for Supportive Dementia Treatment

My research efforts—other than applied predesign programming and postoccupancy evaluation projects—have primarily aimed at uncovering how the physical designed environment can employ the capacities in the brains of persons with dementia to overcome and substitute for the evident losses these persons experience over time living with dementia. A major research effort in this area resulted in an article with a team of others (Zeisel et al., 2003) that identifies how the following eight criteria correlate with reductions in agitation, depression, social isolation, and other dementia "symptoms" among those living in Special Care Units in nursing homes.

- Exit control
- Walking paths
- Privacy and personalization
- Common spaces
- Outdoor access
- Residential quality
- Support for independence
- Sensory comprehension

Since identifying these criteria in 1994 (Zeisel, Hyde, & Levkoff, 1994) and carrying out the research to demonstrate their correlation with reduced challenging behaviors in 2004, I and others have designed many assisted living neighborhoods meeting these criteria. These eight criteria remain central to design of assisted living settings for persons living with Alzheimer's.

The Zeiral

Observing designers and researchers at work in Harvard design studios, when consulting with architects, interior designers, and landscape architects, and reading the literature on developmental processes, I arrived at a simple formulation of both research and design development—one that leads naturally to defining how research and design can be easily connected. Each cycle of the Zeiral-spiral comprises three distinct yet linked creative efforts: *imaging, presenting, and testing* (see Figure 15.2). The first is the mental effort of foreseeing a not-yet-realized final project. Second is the physical effort of expressing the future object or hypothesis in words or pictures. The third step requires stepping back to compare image

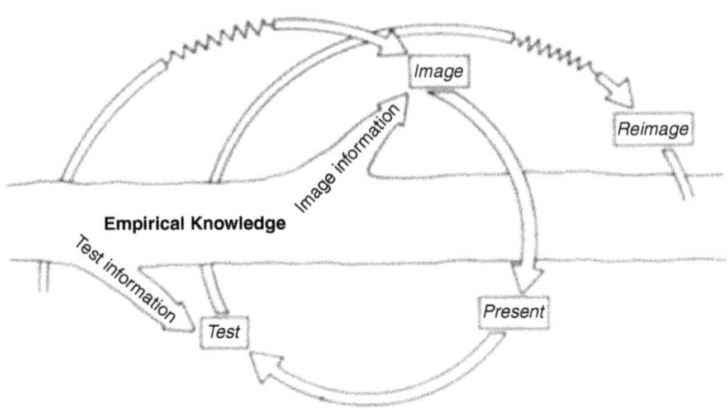

FIGURE 15.2 The "Zeiral" Design & Research Development Spiral from *Inquiry by Design*. *Source:* Zeisel (1984).

and presentation to determine how to refine both image and presentation so that they better fit the goals of the project.

Repeating this *image-presentation-test* (I-P-T) process several times, maybe six or seven, brings the inventor, architect, or researcher increasingly closer to where the I-P-T components are all close enough to each other to represent a final resolution to the design, the research, the evolutionary object (see Figure 15.3).

At each step, the researcher or designer draws on existing knowledge available at the time to inform decisions. The I-P-T diagram and the *Zeiral Developmental Spiral* can be applied equally well to a research as to a design process. In this way they seamlessly link to each other. Both have been a central part of E-B literature, theory, and practice since the early 1980s.

Triangulation of Methods in E-B Studies

I strongly believe in using several methods at the same time to study a single subject—called triangulation. My background in both qualitative and quantitative methods in the social sciences introduced me to a broad range of methods and methodologies. The basic six were: observing the physical environment for

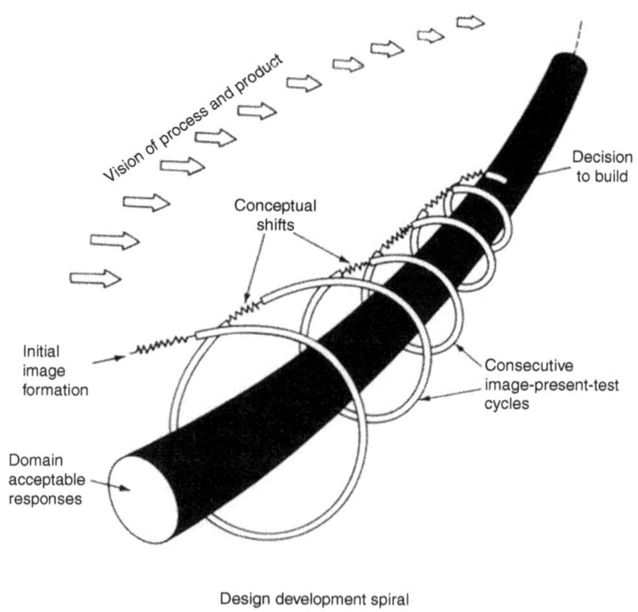

FIGURE 15.3 Present–test and design and research cycle from *Inquiry by Design*.
Source: Zeisel (1984).

cues of use and meaning; observing behavior to determine actual use and also symbolic meanings of things; constructing and conducting large social surveys; conducting focused interviews; analyzing data previously collected for other purposes; and reading plans for their meaning and intent. In *Inquiry by Design* I draw on the qualities of each of these methods, identifying how each can enlighten essential subject matter of E-B studies: on the one hand, persons' behavior in, perceptions of, and attitudes toward the physical environment in which they live, work, and play; on the other hand, the built environment in all its scales and wherever in the life of the environment it happens to be. Methods and data can be applied to environments in design, as completed plans, or as lived in environments available for evaluation—postoccupancy evaluation (POE). The book emphasizes how the six main research methods can be employed simultaneously to triangulate on E-B topics. It makes them readily available to designers and design students in straightforward language with simple examples drawn from E-B studies, as well as to social scientists who generally are not accustomed to studying physical environments. The book also stresses the need to use both qualitative and quantitative methodologies in equal proportion at different stages of research.

Design Annotation as a Method of Communicating the Link Between Design Research and Design Decisions

Researchers tend to communicate their work in words, graphs, tables, and articles. Designers tend to communicate their work in plans, drawings, sketches, and models. In E-B studies, even when both groups intend to communicate a link between behavioral or social goals and design decisions, the form of their communication stands as a barrier. Annotated plans in which research is written in words next to the relevant design decisions on actual plans is an extremely useful linking method—whether in the beginning of a project describing intended research objectives, in the middle of a project to express hypothetical ways to meet those objectives, or after completion to identify elements ripe for postoccupancy evaluation. This approach has been incorporated into design education and practice wherever instructors or practitioners intend to employ research to inform design.

The Role of Physical Environment in Mental Processes: Cueing, Remembering, Learning, Way Finding, and More

Between 2000 and 2006 I read almost exclusively the work of neuroscientists—researchers, practitioners, and theoreticians. In the revised edition of *Inquiry by Design* (Zeisel, 2006) I included new chapters on the neurosciences and the role they can play in E-B studies. This revised edition built on my previous work which included guidelines for designing for persons living with dementia based on understanding the way persons with Alzheimer's mentally process their environments (Zeisel, 2001; Zeisel & Raia, 2000). At the same time, as a founding board member of the ANFA in San Diego, I helped establish and promoted the link from the direction of architecture. By making this link official—introducing the neurosciences and the design professions to each other—and helping to create the neurosciences as an integral part of and a new E-B specialty, I believe I added to this important step forward in the science of E-B (see Figure 15.4).

What does this link include? First, we now know that our brains interpret and filter environmental and sensory inputs, resulting in neurotransmitters (like adrenaline, dopamine, cortisol, and oxytocin) flooding our bodies and influencing how we feel and behave. The simplest example is the *flight or fight* response triggered by our hypothalamus in response to environmental stimuli. This awareness leads to employing E-B methods aimed at identifying these neurotransmitter reactions—such as saliva tests to determine cortisol levels. Second, by understanding how our brains interpret the environment, we gain insight into "*why*" people respond to environments the way they do in addition to the behavioral data we already gather that tells us "*how*" they respond. Third, we know and can study in further detail the way our brains use the physical and social environments around us to improve memory, learning, way finding, and even behavior appropriate to specific settings. Amazingly, the environment around us is not only a setting within which we act individually and collectively, but it also plays an integral role in mental processes—at the cellular level. For example, every cell in our hippocampus (an organ in our brains) stamps each experience we have with both the time and place of its occurrence—enabling us to recall experiences using environmental cues.

Rusty gage
Salk Institute Neuroscientist

- *The brain controls our behavior*
- *Genes control the blueprint for design & structure of the brain*
- *The environment can modulate the function of genes & ultimately the structure of our brain*
- *Changes in the environment change our brains & therfore our behavior*
- *Architecture changes our brains & our behavior*

FIGURE 15.4 The connection between neuroscience and the built environment.
Source: Zeisel (2006).

Design for Aging

Through the Harvard Architectural Research Office, which I founded, as well as through my own consultancy after leaving Harvard, I helped establish the field of design for aging as a legitimate field of research and research translation. I was not alone in doing this—Clare Cooper-Marcus, Sandra Howell, Powell Lawton, Margaret Calkins, Uriel Cohen, and Gerald Weisman among many others played an equally important role. However, my three books: *Low-Rise Housing for Older People: Behavioral Criteria for Design* (Zeisel, Welch, Epp, & Demos, 1978); *Mid-Rise Housing for Older People: Behavioral Criteria for Design*; and *Independence through Interdependence: Congregate Housing for Older People* (Zeisel, Welch, Epp, & Demos, 1981) set the stage for architecture and interior design students as well as practitioners to study and design housing particularly suited to the needs of older residents. These books indicate, among other things, the need for housing that is small and thus affordable and manageable, that contain all the amenities of full living units no matter how small, and that include socially and individually supportive interior and exterior common spaces. The books draw examples of each evidence-based criterion from actual designs (among these architectural submissions for design competitions) with annotations indicating the trade-offs the designers made. The books make the point, by inference from the alternative "solutions" offered, that employing evidence does not mean a particular design is determined, but rather, high quality design requires sensitivity on the part of a design team in making trade-offs between the ways multiple objectives are met. An early article on the eight basic criteria for dementia design—building on the significant work of earlier researchers—helped develop a framework for designing for dementia more or less as a fourth volume in this series (Zeisel, Hyde, & Levkoff, 1994).

Design for Dementia—A Nonpharmacological "Treatment"

As my work advanced, I switched research and practice interests from all "older persons" to those living with dementia/Alzheimer's. This group of users are more dependent on the physical environment as a behavioral, perceptual, and attitudinal prosthesis—relying more on the environment than other elders for cues to appropriate behaviors, way-finding abilities, a sense of self, lower anxiety—as well as to help them remember. If design for dementia influences the person so profoundly and if appropriate design reduces the need for pharmacological agents—such as antianxiety medications, antipsychotics, antidepressants, and so on—the environment is actually a "treatment" for dementia. From the start of my work on residential design to support persons with dementia I have made this point in articles (Zeisel & Raia, 2000; Zeisel &

Tyson, 1999) and in linking the effects of design to identifiable neuroscience mechanisms. While the term "treatment" is seen by some as too referential to a medical approach, my use of this term has been a conscious attempt to include environmental modifications in what is referred to as medical "treatments"—both pharmaceutical and nonpharmacological interventions. In *I'm Still Here* I promote employing nonpharmacological approaches before turning to pharmaceutical ones to influence behaviors of persons with dementia—and point out that this two-phase approach is what is employed by the medical profession to treat most if not all medical problems and situations from obesity to childbirth, from insomnia to a broken leg. For example, rather than immediately prescribing an antidepressant to overcome a person's depression, one can prescribe a walk outside in the sun or show that person photographs of successful times in their life and talk about those times. In order to reduce aggressive behavior, rather than prescribe antipsychotics, one can find the trigger for that aggressive behavior—possibly a locked door preventing the person from going outdoors to a safe garden, and change that environment—unlock the door. This shift in the definition of design from merely a setting for behavior ("behavior setting") to a medical treatment is potentially another major contribution.

I'm Still Here—A Positive "Hope" Approach to Dementia

The major public face of dementia is *despair*, seen and promoted as an inevitable downward spiral toward the loss of personhood and death, once a person receives a diagnosis of "dementia of the Alzheimer's type." With this overarching negative stigma attached, it is difficult for care partners and even members of the medical profession to promote any "treatments" or "therapies" at all. Why waste time and money if it will do no good! The public narrative (Ganz, 2011) of despair that is promoted by major Alzheimer's organizations looking for funding for themselves and for drug research (despair sells!) leads to inaction on the one hand and a search for a quick-fix medication on the other. HOPE in dementia, defined as YCMAD (Ganz's term) "You Can Make a Difference"—is based on understanding the many skills and abilities the neurosciences inform us people with dementia maintain. YCMAD means that nonpharmacological interventions that draw on these hard-wired and acquired abilities and skills can positively affect the lives of persons with dementia. Examples of this include the brain's natural curiosity that enables persons with dementia to learn procedurally even when their episodic memory is challenged; that when persons with dementia are engaged in helping others their hard-wired caring capacities come to the fore; and that when visual art perception and music—hard wired developmental abilities—are elicited, persons with dementia are positively engaged even until the end of their lives. My work changing the public narrative of despair to one of HOPE points to the efficacy of greater research efforts into nonpharmacological interventions (see Figure 15.5).

Ecopsychosocial—Relabeling the Term "Nonpharmacological"

The term "nonpharmacological" refers to everything that is not a medical drug—a class of objects that exists but is too amorphous to have any meaning. Greater specificity is required to be able to compare characteristics of different members of the object class and to carry out research on comparative effects on the same outcome category. We use very few terms, if any, in this way: we do not say "not hate" when we mean love; we do not say "not furniture" when we mean cooking appliances; and we do not use the term "not cooking" for eating. This is obviously silly, yet the field of dementia care as well as the care of many other illnesses and conditions have been using this term for quite some time. In a jointly authored article (Zeisel, Reisberg, Whitehouse, Woods, & Verheul, 2016) my coauthors and I reason and argue for employing the term "ecopsychosocial" to replace "nonpharmacological" in the literature and in practice. This term includes environmental interventions as well as those that affect the individual directly and his or her social context. *Eco* means "home" in Greek—the physical setting—thus ecopsychosocial includes environmental design interventions from architecture, to interiors, to landscape, and even urban planning. *Psycho* refers to all interventions that effect the person directly

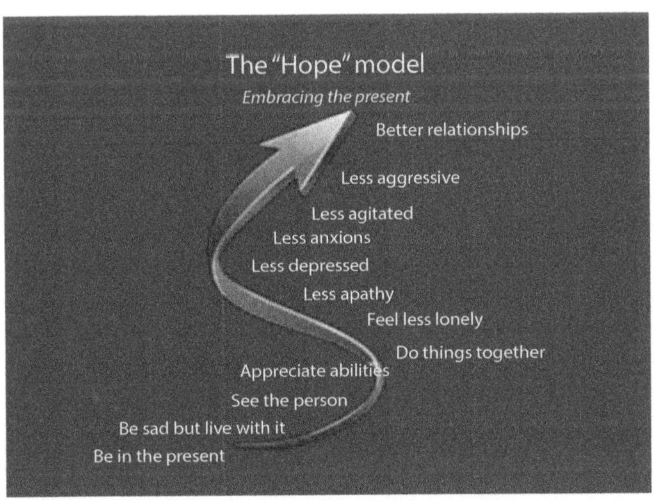

FIGURE 15.5 The Zeisel destigmatized HOPE model for dementia.

such as training the individual or light therapy for the individual. *Socio* refers to all actions that modify or otherwise affect the social environment such as creating a club or school where someone participates as a group member. The term is particularly important for the field of E-B because it makes direct reference to "environment" as a nonpharmacological intervention. This epistemological contribution has been planted as a seed in the literature with an invitation to the scientific community to raise issues, comment, and employ the new term. In turn, our hope is that the term engenders increased research funding, more comparative studies, and greater use of multiple ecopsychosocial interventions in an additive manner.

POTENTIAL IMPLICATIONS OF SCHOLARLY AND APPLIED RESEARCH CONTRIBUTIONS

Some of the implications of key conceptual, methodological, research, and applied contributions to Environmental Gerontology and the aging society at large have been included in previous sections. Here I summarize the major ones.

Environmental gerontology is a subspecialty in E-B studies based on the understanding that the physical environment is integrally connected to the ability of all of us as we age to do so with minimum handicap, greatest ability to exploit our own abilities, and greatest joy. All of my work, from the *Zeiral* that gave others the tools to seamlessly link research and design to establishing design guidelines for older housing residents and those with dementia contribute to this specialty.

One implication that can be drawn is that in meeting the needs of those who are old today, we should use the tools and methods available to study the needs of future generations and plan housing and communities that meet emerging needs—rather than merely thinking that images from the 1940s and 1950s will be relevant to future generations of older people.

Another implication is that by making design needs and processes explicit—annotated plans is just an example—older persons with less design training can fully participate in the creation of environments appropriate for their own needs. Designers and researchers have the means to effectively engage in a participatory design process and include older users in those design processes rather than merely treating them as *subjects* of research.

I expect that the major contribution I will have been seen to have made to both Environmental Gerontology and to the larger aging society lie in the area of dementia care and dementia design. First, my work has contributed to the way people think and feel about those with dementia—from a feeling of despair at dementia being a lost cause to seeing those living with dementia as a social user group like any other. In Environmental Gerontology, my work—carried out with colleagues from the beginning of my career Polly Welch, Gayle Epp, Stephen Demos, Joan Hyde, and Powell Lawton and more recently with colleagues at Hearthstone including Sue Blackler, Sharon Johnson, Dan Colucci, Mike Skrajner, and Gregg Gorzelle—serve as the basis for extensive hypotheses that we and others are building into physical environmental designs and that others will test through postoccupancy evaluations.

In the larger societal picture, my work has contributed directly to reducing the stigma associated with dementia—a stigma accepted not only by the greater society but also by care partners and persons living with dementia. Their self-worth is damaged by the implicit despair narrative society embraces. One example of this change is the movement for guided tours of museums pioneered through the *I'm Still Here* Foundation. Originally a small initiative funded by our foundation and developed by us at the Museum of Modern Art, this program has grown to worldwide proportions; almost every country in Europe, Australia, as well as some in the Far East have such programs in museums, enabling and encouraging persons with dementia to join the larger society—in this case in museums. An even more vibrant social approach with the same goals and objectives but in many other venues is the program called *It Takes a Village* where events are held weekly not only in museums, but in venues including yoga studios, parks, historical sites, restaurants, art galleries, movie theaters, and libraries. This program is also geared to opening up our social settings to those with dementia presently staying home and in "facilities."

A major implication of this work is in the arena of "human rights"—establishing in society that all persons, including those with dementia who might have difficulty remembering things or putting tasks in the correct order—have the right to be full members of society and take part in all "citizens" locations and services.

FOCUS IN THE COMING YEARS

- Presently and in the near future my focus is first on developing "ecopsychosocial" interventions as accepted and evidence-based modalities of treatment for dementia.
- Second, when "ecopsychosocial" modalities are accepted as a positive epistemological class, my research will focus on the linkages and overlaps between ecopsychosocial, pharmaceutical, and basic science approaches to dementia and to mild cognitive impairment and dementia of the Alzheimer's type.

- Third, I am concentrating increasingly on the role of community in dementia care—an outgrowth of the human rights agenda. Defining community and figuring out how to create dementia-capable and friendly communities, is a growing focus.

Broader Perspectives in the Field of Environmental Gerontology for the Upcoming Years

- Societies are all getting older—not only as cultures but as a percentage of the population. When you ride in the subway or metro, when you go to a restaurant, when you walk in a park you see many more younger people than older people. Where are they? Why are older people not out and about in our cities, in our public spaces, in our cultural venues? Perhaps it is because those places are not hospitable and welcoming to older members of society. Perhaps older persons are increasingly retreating to "senior ghettos" where other older persons provide familiarity and security. Perhaps they are holding up in their homes and apartments because they feel their physical and mental frailty are handicaps. A great and inviting open question for the field of Environmental Gerontology that needs to be addressed is understanding this phenomenon better and creating public places that are welcoming to all—including elders and those with dementia—where generations can be together without fear of the unknown and fear of emotional or physical assault.
- Conceptual/methodological/empirical tasks—the greatest need we have as a field of study and practice is professional agreement, perhaps "standardization," of methods and methodologies. Without those, we are merely a group of individuals each with her or his own unique tools and no common objects to apply those tools to. It is as if each of us has designed our own screwdriver tip and therefore none of us can use the same screws to build a building. More developed sciences and professions adopt practical agreements where eventually they all share the same tools—not always the best tool but at least those agreed to—and thus they can create a critical mass of knowledge and practice respected by others. Many great minds in our field have contributed ideas, concepts, empirical approaches, and methodologies—but very few have been consensually adopted. Doing so is to me the greatest challenge we need to deal with so that we can develop a community of shared approaches, so that conceptual/methodological/and empirical efforts can be connected and a critical mass of data, findings, and relevant information developed.

IN SUM

Each of us has paths we follow—personal, emotional, spiritual, intellectual, academic, professional. Some of our paths seem preordained by location, birth, family history—"every man in my family has been a doctor, so me too." My professional path has been driven by interest and passion and has not wavered from the goals of discovering something new and improving the world in some way for others. I never stayed in a job because I was in it. I searched out new adventures because they were more interesting than another option. Duckworth has called this continual passion and perseverance—Grit (Duckworth, 2016). The grit that has driven me has continually led me to delve further into the relationship between women, men, and their environments. To me this direction seems self-evident—what else is there but ourselves, our social environments, and our physical context?

That path is mine. Each reader of this autobiographical journey has his or her own path to create. I hope that in my story is the seed of yours—an idea or a process or a way that sparks your imagination and engages your grit. There are always new ideas to have, new concepts to develop, and new ways of thinking to discover in E-B studies and in Environmental Gerontology.

REFERENCES

Alexander, C. (1964). *Notes on the synthesis of form*. Cambridge, MA: Harvard University Press.

Alexander, C. (1965). City is not a tree. *Architectural Forum, 122*(1), 58–62.

Alexander, C., Silverstein, M., & Ishikawa, S. (1977). *A pattern language*. New York, NY: Oxford University Press.

Blau, P. (1964). *Exchange and power in social life*. New York, NY: Wiley.

Brolin, B. C., & Zeisel, J. (1968). Mass housing: Social research and design. *The Architectural Forum*, 66–71.

Duckworth, A. (2016). *Grit: the power of passion and perseverance*. New York, NY: Scribner.

Gans, H. J. (1962). *The urban villagers*. New York, NY: The Free Press.

Ganz, M. (2011). Public narrative, collective action, and power. In S. Odugbemi & T. Lee (Eds.), *Accountability through public opinion: From inertia to public action* (pp. 273–290). Washington, DC: World Bank eLibrary.

Goffman, E. (1956). *The presentation of self in everyday life*. New York, NY: Random House.

Homans, C. (1958). Social behavior as exchange. *American Journal of Sociology, 62*, 597–606.

Merton, R. K. (1948, 1968). *Social theory and social structure*. New York, NY: The Free Press.

Zeisel, J. (1984). *Inquiry by design: Tools for environment-behavior research*. New York, NY: Cambridge University Press.

Zeisel, J. (2001). Universal design to support the brain and its development. In P. Wolfgang & E. Ostroff (Eds.), *Universal design handbook*. New York, NY: McGraw-Hill.

Zeisel, J. (2006). *Inquiry by design: Environment/behavior/neuroscience in architecture, interiors, landscape and planning* (Revised Edition). New York, NY: W. W. Norton.

Zeisel, J. (2009). *I'm still here: A breakthrough approach to understanding someone living with Alzheimer's*. New York, NY: Penguin/Avery Books.

Zeisel, J. & Griffin, M. (1975). *Charlesview housing: A diagnostic evaluation*. Cambridge, MA: Architecture Research Office, Graduate School of Design, Harvard University.

Zeisel, J., & Harvey, J. (1993). The Canadian hospital program: Towards a POE paradigm. In M. Conan & C. Zimring (Eds.), *Towards a Critical Practice of Architecture* Paris, France: Centre Scientifique et Technique de Batiment.

Zeisel, J., Hyde, J., & Levkoff, S. (1994). Best practices: An environment-behavior (E-B) model for Alzheimer special care units. *American Journal of Alzheimer's Care & Research, 9*(2), 4–21.

Zeisel, J., & Maxwell, M. (1993). Functional reprogramming: The H-E-B case study. In P. Wolfgang (Ed.), *Professional practice in facility programming* (pp. 153–184). New York, NY: Van Nostrand Reinhold.

Zeisel, J., & Raia, P. (2000). Non-pharmacological treatment for Alzheimer's disease: A mind-brain approach. *American Journal of Alzheimer's Disease and Other Dementias, 15*(6), 331–340.

Zeisel, J., Reisberg, B., Whitehouse, P., Woods, R., & Verheul, A. (2016). Ecopsychosocial interventions in cognitive decline and dementia: A new terminology and a new paradigm. *American Journal of Alzheimer's Disease & Other Dementias*, 1–6.

Zeisel, J., & Tyson, M. (1999). Alzheimer's treatment gardens. In C. Cooper Marcus & M. Barnes (Eds.), *Healing gardens: Therapeutic benefits and design recommendations*. New York, NY: John Wiley & Sons.

Zeisel, J., & Welch, P. (1981). *Housing designed for families: A summary of research*. Cambridge, MA: Joint Center for Urban Studies for MIT and Harvard.

Zeisel, J., Welch, P., Epp, G., & Demos, S. (1978). *Low-rise housing for older people: Behavioral criteria for design*. Washington, DC: U.S. Government Printing Office.

Zeisel, J., Welch, P., Epp, G., & Demos, S. (1981). *Mid-rise elevator housing for older people: Behavioral criteria for design*. Washington, DC: U.S. Government Printing Office.

Zeisel, J., Welch, P., & Parker, V. (1984). *Independence through interdependence: Congregate housing for older people*. Boston, MA: Massachusetts Department of Elder Affairs.

Zeisel, J., Silverstein N. M., Hyde, J., Levkoff, S., Lawton, M. P., & Holmes, W. (2003). Environmental correlates to behavioral outcomes in Alzheimer's special care units. *The Gerontologist*, 43(5), 697–711.

CHAPTER 16

A Career Outside the Mainstream

Edward Steinfeld

ABSTRACT

Edward Steinfeld first started studying aging at the Department of Architecture and Institute of Gerontology at the University of Michigan, with his mentor, Lee Pastalan. His work departed from what became mainstream Environmental Gerontology as he focused on design of the broader community environment as opposed to environments purpose-built for an aging population. While holding a joint appointment at the All-University Gerontology Center and the School of Architecture at Syracuse University, he conducted a landmark research study that led to a major expansion and revision of a consensus standard used in the design of built environments in the United States. This research also underlies, to this day, the requirements of federal accessibility laws, including the Americans with Disabilities Act Standards. At the University at Buffalo, SUNY School of Architecture and Planning, he founded the center for Inclusive Design and Environmental Access. Over the last 30 years, the Center has conducted research and development activities, consulting services, educational initiatives, and knowledge dissemination in universal design and accessibility. It seeks to advance design of communities to accommodate all citizens throughout their lifespans by enhancing usability, health, and social participation.

BIOGRAPHICAL NOTES

I grew up in a working-class neighborhood in Boston. When I was 10, I moved to a small rural town that was just starting to transform into a bedroom suburb. My

http://dx.doi.org/10.1891/0198-8794.38.277

parents were committed to social justice and there was a constant critical discussion at our dining table about social relations, world events, and politics. They also raised me to respect the older generation, a part of our Jewish heritage. In fact, we shared a house with my maternal grandparents until I was 10, and for 3 years of that time, we lived in the same apartment. The men on my mother's side of the family were all in the building trades, as was my father. I became interested in buildings, machines and technology. Inspired by a book by Frank Lloyd Wright I found in my local library, I decided to be an architect by the time I was in the 10th grade.

EDUCATION

I started undergraduate school in Architecture at Carnegie Mellon University (CMU) in 1963. Three undergraduate experiences stand out as important influences in shaping my career. In my sophomore year, I moved off campus to live in a "bohemian" community, the Greenwich Village of Pittsburgh. I socialized with a diverse group of people, learned how to take risks and explored a counterculture lifestyle. I also met my life-long love, Ellen, who was an art student at the time and is now a successful professional artist. They say that much of one's formative education happens outside the classroom and that was certainly the case with me during those years. Although there was a lot of angst and alienation all around me, my focus on gaining professional knowledge and skills gave me a sense of purpose. Although I was very concerned about the same issues, angry protest and dropping out were not part of my mental schema.

For the most part, architecture students in those days didn't question what they learned or how it was taught and had a clear sense of their future career as practitioners. But one summer, I had a work study job under the supervision of Troy West, a faculty member who was just starting to develop a way to practice architecture by working directly with low-income neighborhood groups, what we now call community design centers. Troy showed me how architecture could be a form of social action and professional education could be enhanced through service learning (e.g., Hardin, Eribas, & Poster, 2006). I started to be critical of how architecture was practiced. It seemed to me that, in the public realm, the profession was primarily concerned with helping those with a lot of money make more money and in the residential realm, promoting status achievement through conspicuous consumption (Veblen, 1912). A social action approach to the profession resonated with my strong desire to do something with my life that made the world a better place.

Then, Charles Eastman, who had just finished his PhD work at Berkeley came to teach at CMU in my fifth year. His first course, which I took, was called "Introduction to Environmental Design Research." This opened my eyes to another way of thinking about architecture. In general, design was and is taught by reference to precedent and learning from people with more experience. But Eastman's course was about generating architectural knowledge through systematic *research*. I was particularly interested in the work of Ed Hall and the Gestalt psychologists, because, by then, I was wondering if architects really knew what they were doing. There were so many inhospitable buildings around that I wondered if they had the knowledge to do their work well. I was also interested in the everyday decisions architects make. How could we predict how people would respond to buildings and how could we find out what was best for building inhabitants? I was happy to learn that someone was actually studying these questions and I decided to join them if I could. It is noteworthy that Gerald Weisman, a noted environmental gerontologist, was a classmate and close friend of mine and I think he took this course with me as well.

I applied to several graduate schools expressing my interests and one day received a call from Lee Pastalan at the University of Michigan (UM), who offered me a fellowship to study gerontology. Lee is a sociologist and gerontologist who was a faculty member in the Department of Architecture and associated with the Institute of Gerontology. By this time, I was married, so a fellowship sounded good, but I had no idea what gerontology meant! Lee explained that it was the study of aging and that it was part of a multidisciplinary program. I knew Michigan's School of Architecture was pioneering in architectural research and studying aging only meant good things to me, given my family background, so I jumped at the opportunity and entered graduate school in the fall of 1968. I had the Gerontology Fellowship from that year through 1972.

Graduate school was an incredible experience for me. At CMU, the library was very small and heavily engineering and science oriented. At Michigan, I could spend days in the stacks finding new books of interest in the social sciences. Although the classes I took were very good, browsing the stacks was also a very important form of education equivalent to surfing the Internet today. The gerontology fellows were all funded by the administration on aging to educate a new cadre of experts in aging that could be ready to meet the challenges of the anticipated demographic trends. There was a shared mission and sense of purpose among us, in contrast to the alienation and rootlessness among many students and young people at the time. Multidisciplinary education was the paradigm, encouraged by the architecture faculty as well as the social gerontologists. I also took many courses in the urban planning department and in natural resources that provided me intellectual tools for understanding urbanism and ways of thinking about the future.

After I finished a 1-year Master of Architecture degree, the School of Architecture started a doctorate program in architecture. I applied for the program and was accepted in the first class of five students. This was a formative experience. It was, I believe, the first doctorate program in architecture to welcome students with interests other than architectural history or criticism. We were exposed to a wide range of research topics in the field—computing, sustainability, professional practice, building technology, and human behavior. I continued to be funded by the Institute of Gerontology and work with Lee, who was an inspiring and supportive mentor. I also learned much from Steve Paraskevopoulos and Ted Larsen, both architects who had unusual careers. They were insiders but also very critical of how architecture was practiced, and they were strong advocates of applying knowledge from science and technology to address social issues. The faculty were very supportive of independent creative thinking. Graduate students were not viewed as disciples of the masters but rather junior associates who were working together with the faculty to initiate new threads of research and practice.

In the summer of 1968, inner city riots spread across the country after the assassinations of Martin Luther King and Bobby Kennedy. The riots in Detroit, 40 miles from Ann Arbor, were some of the worst. Ellen and I were in Europe all summer. I had received a fellowship at CMU that enabled us to travel for almost 4 months between undergraduate and graduate programs. Although I did not have the contacts or knowledge to explore design for aging in Europe at the time, I was impressed with the vibrant urban culture of European cities and especially with the emphasis on design for human function that we found in Scandinavia. A day-long "Life Seeing" tour sponsored by the Danish tourism organization gave us a peek into the inner workings of a social democracy including visits to a senior center and a day-care center. We also spent 10 days in the middle of the 1968 student rebellion in Paris and witnessed the despair of Italians when Robert Kennedy was assassinated back in the United States.

My first assistantship at UM was to help a faculty member in the Center of Conflict Resolution develop and manage a course designed to study the causes of the rioting and the City of Detroit's response. I was offered this position because of my previous experience with Troy West. It helped me obtain a better understanding of the social causes and experience of poverty and sparked an interest in policy, which became a major aspect of my scholarly career. It also brought home the importance of urban planning in shaping cities and how neglect of basic human needs can be poisonous to society.

My interests in planning and urbanism led to my doctoral dissertation research which focused on an important policy issue at the time, age segregation. In the early years of social gerontology, there was a debate about age segregation. The research showed that living in a location with a high density of older people promoted continued social engagement (Rosow, 1967). Early research, later confirmed, showed that age-segregated housing environments for older people have many benefits for residents. Morale and life satisfaction improves; residents feel less alone and isolated; they can manage independently longer; and they benefit from better delivery of services and mutual assistance (Carp, 1975; Golant, 2015). I was curious, however, about whether age segregation was cutting off residents from broader community engagement. I asked older people what level of density and control over contact with younger people (specifically, children under 5 and their families) they preferred (see Figure 16.1). I discovered that the people I surveyed preferred a high density of older people but most did not want to be isolated from young people, and, they wanted control over the nature of their interaction rather than being forced to interact (Steinfeld, 1973).

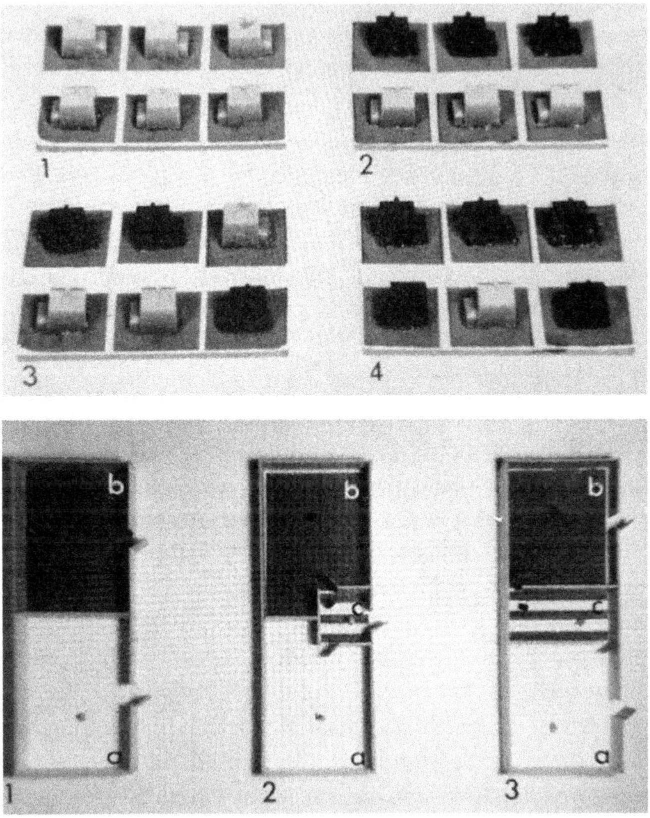

FIGURE 16.1 Models used to assess the preferences of older people for degrees of age integration. Toy houses with different colors represented different types of integration of older people and families with young children in neighborhoods. Models of different circulation plans for a community center with both a child-care center and a senior center elicited preferences for control over interaction with young children.

Rather than focusing my future work on environments designed specifically for aging, I became interested in how the general environment could be designed to facilitate aging as well as other groups often marginalized by designers. I picked up on this interest in the study of accessibility, new community planning, residential repair and renovation programs, senior centers, pedestrian environments, visitable housing, life-span housing design, transportation, and product design. All my interests came together in the second half of my career through the concept of universal design.

EMPLOYMENT

In 1971, I left Ann Arbor. I took a research position in the Architectural Research Section of the Center for Building Technology, at the National Bureau of Standards (NBS; now called the National Institute for Science and Technology), which is part of the Department of Commerce. I was following in the footsteps of my future colleagues, the late Michael Brill and John Archea. In fact, John Eberhard, the founding dean of the SUNY/Buffalo School of Architecture and Planning, directed the Center for Building Technology before becoming dean.

At NBS, I learned about the importance of building standards in shaping the built environment, gained insight into innovation in the building industry, was exposed to building economics, and was indoctrinated on the performance concept. Although I didn't stay there long, the job provided me an opportunity that changed the trajectory of my career. Our section chief was asked to recommend a staff member to be the Department of Commerce's representative to a subcommittee of the President's Committee on Employment of the Physically Handicapped (which later morphed into the Office of Disability Employment Policy in the Department of Labor) called the Barrier Free Design Committee. By virtue of my gerontology background I was the only one on the staff who knew anything about design for people with disabilities. So, he asked if I wanted to do it and I agreed.

From that point on, my career diverged significantly from that of other environmental gerontologists. I learned that the standards at the time were not adequately addressing the needs and that the research on the topic was extremely limited. In fact, the existing standards were based on the abilities of a small group of young wheelchair users, almost all of whom were athletes. And, the findings of that work were not even documented in the literature. Further, the growing Independent Living Movement fueled the rise of a disability rights advocacy effort led by people with disabilities themselves. The existing standards had been developed by rehabilitation professionals with the assistance of architects who were experienced in design of rehabilitation hospitals and other health-care settings. Their work was primarily for young people, not older populations. I quickly learned that the advocates had many serious concerns about the ineffectiveness of the standards and regulations and the lack of attention to accessibility to housing. The fact that accessibility was mandated by law intrigued me because improving building standards could put teeth into the application of research results.

I left NBS in 1973 to take a joint appointment at Syracuse University (SU). Warren Beatty, Dean of the School of Social Work at SU, obtained a similar grant like the one that had funded me at Michigan, to set up a multidisciplinary gerontology center. I was hired to do research and education at the All University Gerontology Center and be a tenured track faculty member at the School of Architecture—clearly the perfect fit for someone with my education. The Gerontological Society of America (GSA) had a grant focused on developing research and teaching in Environmental Gerontology at this time and I participated in their activities. The late Tom Byerts, an architect who had studied gerontology at USC, also on a gerontology fellowship, directed that grant. The first sponsored project I obtained was a small subgrant from the GSA to research and develop a self-instructional learning module called Barrier Free Design for the Elderly (Steinfeld & Schroeder, 1976).

Still participating in the Barrier Free Design Committee, I advocated for completing empirical research to support improved standards. Advocates around the country were convincing government agencies to improve the existing accessibility standards. There was no empirical evidence base for new requirements so they were based on anecdotal experience of the most vocal advocates. Different requirements were cropping up all over the country which was causing a problem for practitioners and led to suboptimal standards in some cases and questionable requirements in others. The leaders of the committee convinced the U.S. Department of Housing and Urban Development (HUD) to fund a research effort to update the existing standard on accessibility. I competed and received a grant that was quite large for the time. A 2-year project turned into a 6-year project. The "New ANSI[1] Standard Project," established the main thread of my research career. It was the first and only comprehensive study of accessibility, incorporating research methods from human factors, social science, economics, and design (Steinfeld, 1977).

At Syracuse, I assembled a multidisciplinary team including Steve Schroeder, an architect and former student assistant on the GSA project,

[1]The American National Standards Institute (ANSI) is a not-for-profit organization that oversees the development of voluntary standards. The first accessibility standard in the U.S. was *ANSI A117.1 Making Buildings and Facilities Accessible to the Physically Handicapped*. That standard has been revised many times since this project. The Secretariat of the Committee is now the International Code Council and the standard is called *ICC/ANSI A117.1 Accessible and Usable Buildings and Facilities*.

Marilyn Bishop, an occupational therapist, the late Rolf Faste, a professor in the Industrial Design Department at SU, James Duncan and James Aiello, graduate students in geography, Deborah Chollet, a graduate student in economics, and many architecture students who assisted with data collection and did most of our drafting. I also became the secretary of the ANSI A117 standards committee and the main author and editor of the standard, which turned out to be on-the-job training in knowledge translation and the process of innovation diffusion. Both of these skills benefited me throughout my career. We recruited a diverse sample of research participants with many types of disabilities, oversampling older people because of the association of disability and age. We also had extensive interaction with the fledgling disability rights community, engaging many advocates in our standards development activities. Figure 16.2 shows part of the apparatus we used in our human factors research.

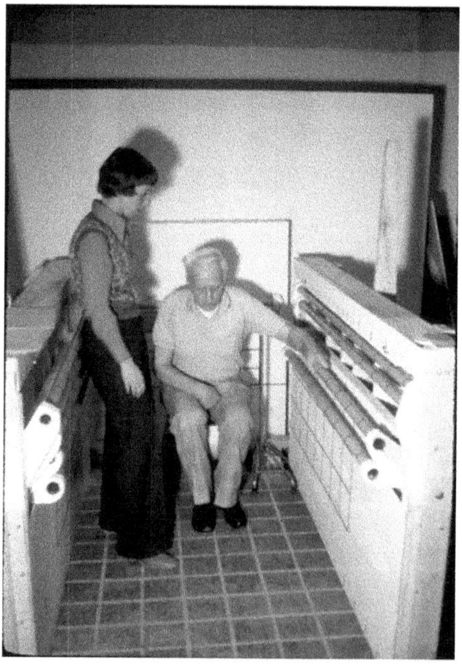

FIGURE 16.2 Apparatus used to study the design of toilet stalls in the New ANSI Standards Project. The walls and grab bars were adjusted through a series of fitting trials to identify the minimum width needed and where individuals preferred to use grab bars.

ACHIEVEMENTS

The New ANSI Standard Project was so successful that the basic guidelines for accessible design we developed were adopted by all 50 states and incorporated into the ADA Accessibility Guidelines and in other accessibility standards in the United States and other countries. They remain a part of the ADA 2010 Standards and the current ICC/ANSI A117.1 standard for accessible design that is referenced by the International Building Code, which is the major model building code in the United States. The project had a huge impact on the shape of the built environment in North America. Although this research was not strictly in the field of gerontology, the results have an impact on every older person today who visits a public building or has an accessible apartment. The project won a Progressive Architecture Research Award and a Research Recognition Award from the National Endowment for the Arts. To improve knowledge of the new standards in the profession, I wrote a series of five articles explaining the standards and the research results that supported them for the leading American architecture journal, *Architectural Record* (Steinfeld, 1979a, 1979b, 1979c, 1979d, 1980a, 1980b). Several years later, I contributed a chapter on adaptable housing to Jon Pynoos and Victor Regnier's book, *Housing the Aged: Policy Directives and Policy Considerations* (1987), which brought this research to the attention to the gerontology community. The work had another impact on Environmental Gerontology. As part of the design research work, our team developed the "Enabler" concept, which inspired Susanne Iwarsson to develop the *Housing Enabler* (see Chapter 8, From Occupational Therapy to Environmental Gerontology).

Although the idea of building dwellings that could be adjusted to the needs of the residents originated in Sweden with the Focus Society, the concept of adaptable housing we developed was tailored for mass application to all housing in the U.S. context. This concept underlies both the Fair Housing Accessibility Guidelines, which now apply to all multifamily housing in the United States, and the concept of "visitability" for single family housing. The concept of adaptable housing addresses the fact that not all people with disabilities have the same needs or preferences and that it is often impossible to find an accessible dwelling when needed. Adaptable housing is particularly relevant to older people because it is an important enabling element of successful aging in place.

Nevertheless, the SU architecture faculty did not appreciate the importance of this work and I was viewed as marginal to the school, although valued by the Gerontology Center. Since the Architecture Department controlled my promotion and tenure, in 1978, I moved down the NY State Thruway to SUNY/Buffalo to take a position in architecture that was advertised with an explicit focus on social issues. The Architecture Department was newly reorganized based on the foundation of an experimental, but nonaccredited degree program. I was one of the first groups of faculty members in the newly configured department and had the opportunity to help shape its future. At Buffalo, I established the Center for Inclusive Design and Environmental Access (IDeA) and steadily built a research program focusing at first on the human factors of accessibility with funding primarily from the United States. Access Board and HUD, but later expanding to other issues.

In the late 1980s, I started collaborated with William Mann and his colleague, Joseph Lane, in the Department of Occupational Therapy (OT) at Buffalo. This work included participation in a grant called the Rehabilitation Engineering Research Center (RERC) on Technology for Successful Aging, which brought my interests in gerontology and disability together but also expanded my interests from architecture and planning to assistive technology, transportation, and product design. The affiliation with the OT Department also enabled me to develop an earlier interest in home modifications for older people (Steinfeld, 1981) into a service program. RERCs are center of excellence grants funded by the National Institute for Disability, Independent Living and Rehabilitation Research (NIDILRR), U.S. Department of Health and Human Services. My late colleague Scott Danford and I also worked with Carl Granger, the developer of the Functional Independence Measure, on another NIDILRR center grant through which we developed scales to measure the influence of the built environment on rehabilitation outcomes and identify the causes of problems people encounter while interacting with the environment (see Figure 16.3). Those scales have been used by both IDeA Center researchers in numerous projects (Steinfeld & Danford, 1997) and by other researchers as well, notably by a research group

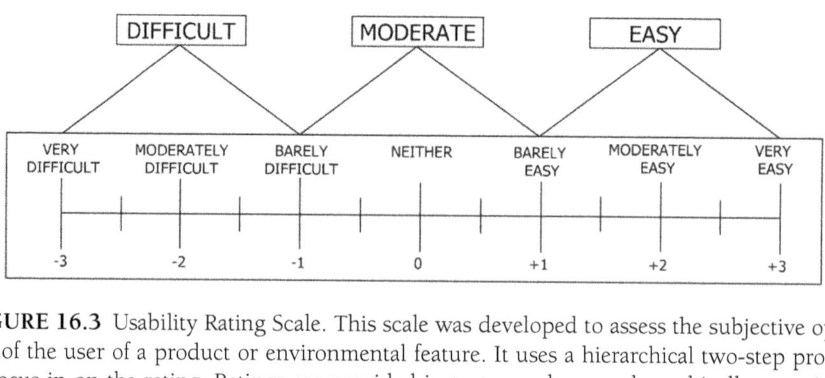

FIGURE 16.3 Usability Rating Scale. This scale was developed to assess the subjective opinion of the user of a product or environmental feature. It uses a hierarchical two-step process to focus in on the rating. Ratings are provided in text, numbers, and graphically to assist in understanding.
Source: Steinfeld & Danford (1999).

at Case Western University that studies functional electrical stimulation (Bieri, Triolo, Danford, & Steinfeld, 2000).

For the last 20 years or so, I have invested most of my time and effort in the field of universal design. Universal design, by our definition, is "a process that enables and empowers a diverse population by improving human performance, health and wellness, and social participation" (Steinfeld & Maisel, 2012, p. 29). Figure 16.4 illustrates the scope of universal design. Architect Ron Mace is credited by many sources as the originator of the term (Mace, 1985). He and I became friends and colleagues when we were both members of the Barrier Free Design Committee. My former colleague, Abir Mullick, and I worked with Ron and his team in the mid-1990s to develop the seminal *Principles of Universal Design* which have been translated into many languages and helped to clarify the concept for a wide audience (Story, 1998).

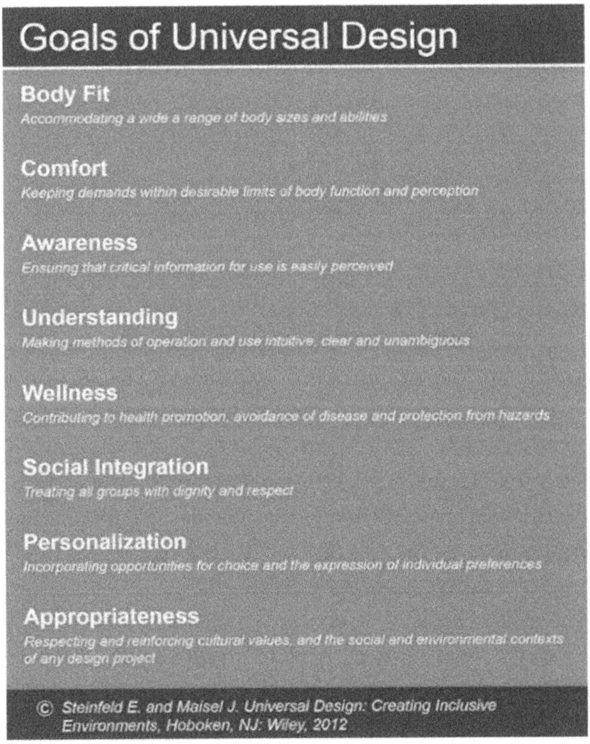
Goals of Universal Design
Body Fit
Accommodating a wide a range of body sizes and abilities
Comfort
Keeping demands within desirable limits of body function and perception
Awareness
Ensuring that critical information for use is easily perceived
Understanding
Making methods of operation and use intuitive, clear and unambiguous
Wellness
Contributing to health promotion, avoidance of disease and protection from hazards
Social Integration
Treating all groups with dignity and respect
Personalization
Incorporating opportunities for choice and the expression of individual preferences
Appropriateness
Respecting and reinforcing cultural values, and the social and environmental contexts of any design project
© Steinfeld E. and Maisel J. Universal Design: Creating Inclusive Environments, Hoboken, NJ: Wiley, 2012

FIGURE 16.4 The goals of universal design. The goals are conceived as outcomes of design related to usability (Goals 1–4), health and wellness (Goal 5), and social participation (Goals 6-8). Examples of universal design in a variety of design fields can be found in Steinfeld and Maisel (2012).

To me, it is critical that we do not address aging out of context. No one is defined by her or his age alone. Our identities are mostly formed when we are young so designing environments for aging reduces the complexity of design for people to only one factor in the formation of identity. The idea that there should be "environments for aging" actually reflects a societal stigma attached to aging and a related lack of social concern for the older population. Further, the presence of specialized environments for aging reduces the moral imperative to expand the application of knowledge from Environmental Gerontology to the broader environment. Policy makers can argue that the needs of older people are addressed by those specialized environments and resist making the general community amenable to healthy aging. I believe that universal design is the key toward achieving an environment that is age friendly everywhere and I wish we had thought about it in 1968. The general community environment (social and physical) in the United States was and still is clearly inhospitable to aging, so it is no wonder that age segregated settings are popular for many older people with the means to live in them. Interestingly, despite the benefits of age segregation, the preference to live in such settings is not shared by the majority of older citizens. When we finally got around to asking them what they would prefer, we found that, for the most part, they want to remain where they are, not move to age segregated settings (e.g., AARP, 2014).

As the concept of universal design has evolved and intersected with other ideas, it is also clear that environmental design is not the sole answer to achieving an age-friendly society or community. We also need to use universal design to reinvent products, policies, programs, and services. In particular, we need to start practicing "service design." As the digital world expanded and permeated all our activities, product designers found an opportunity to design "user interfaces" and become "interaction designers." They quickly learned that design thinking can be applied to more than just objects and places. Service design, which owes its origins to "systems thinking," is an emerging field in which a socio-physical system like public transit is reconceived as a service provided through a combination of policies, practices, software, products, and environments. Environmental gerontology needs to embrace this new paradigm.

Perhaps the most obvious success of service design is Apple Computer. The invention of a new way of buying and playing music, a smartphone operating system that was easy to use with gestures (and, increasingly speech), and a lightweight portable computer that everyone could start using as soon as they opened the box, saved the company from oblivion, and is revolutionizing the way we live. The company was the first to integrate accessibility features into its operating system and, learning from that, introduced many other features that allow customers to customize their products for individual needs and preferences. One of the most interesting examples of service design practiced by Apple is the design of their retail stores, which have revolutionized the concept of "store." The stores include direct access to working products, provide free basic education and assistance in use of the products by knowledgeable staff, offer personalized shopping service for all customers, and eliminate cashiers (and the lines) entirely. They even have chairs! If you visit an Apple Store during work hours you will likely see a lot of retired people. Older people are some of their best customers. In fact, Samsung, their leading competitor, developed an advertising campaign implying that iPhones were for older people not the young and hip (Martellaro, 2012). Imagine if a public transit system did service design like Apple.

The IDeA Center, which I founded in 1984 and still direct, is dedicated to increasing the adoption of universal design. Our main sponsor, NIDILRR, is a major sponsor of rehabilitation technology research. They fund many large center grants in this field, called RERCs, modeled after the National Science Foundation's, Engineering Research Center grants. The RERCs focused originally solely on rehabilitation technology like design of wheelchairs. But, due to their insightful staff and leadership, NIDILRR has also been the major sponsor of U.S. research and development efforts in universal design. Several RERCs have projects focused on universal design as well as rehabilitation technology.

In 1999, I led the team that obtained our first large center grant, the Rehabilitation Engineering Center on Universal Design and the Built Environment, a $5 million, 5-year effort. Since then we have, through competition every 5 years, been refunded four times. Our major partner has been the Intelligent Design for Adaptation, Design and Technology (iDAPT) team at Toronto Rehabilitation Institute (Toronto Rehabilitation Institute, 2016). They have expertise in rehabilitation technology that complements our own expertise in environmental design. Geoff Fernie, the vice president for research at TRI, and creator of the iDAPT team is a human factors engineer with a long history of work in aging. He and his colleagues obtained significant funding from the Canadian government to build a unique research facility, unmatched in the United States. Under the RERC umbrella, they have developed threads of research in stair safety and walking surfaces. They also have other threads of research in health-care products, home aids, and driving.

Since 2009, we have also partnered with CMU's Robotics Institute to win the RERC on Accessible Public Transportation, now in its second cycle. Personally, this second grant has been very rewarding because my son Aaron, an expert in human computer interaction and transportation, is the Principal Investigator and I direct the major subgrant to the IDeA Center. Aaron leads a research team at the Robotics Institute studying intelligent transportation, human interaction with robots, and access to cloud computing. Their work in the RERC focuses on IT applications while ours is focused on the design of transit vehicles. Our large multiyear grants have established the IDeA Center as the premier R&D center on accessibility and universal design in North America.

Major achievements at the IDeA Center include:

- Research on the diffusion of "visitable" housing and development of consensus standards adopted into ICC/ANSI A117.1 (Maisel, 2010; Maisel, Smith, & Steinfeld, 2008; Steinfeld & White, 2010).
- Completion of a 10-year anthropometry study of wheeled mobility users. The findings are now being used to update the accessibility standards we developed in the 1970s to address both demographic changes and technological changes in the industry (Steinfeld, Maisel, Feathers, & D'Souza, 2010).
- Producing tools to help apply the findings of the anthropometry research in design standards development (see Figure 16.5 and D'Souza, Paquet, Steinfeld, & Feathers, 2010).
- Development of a usability testing program, funded by both our grants and manufacturers, for evaluating both existing and prototype products based on universal design characteristics (Lenker, Feathers, Nasarwanji, & Paquet, 2008; Lenker, Narsarwanji, Paquet, & Feathers, 2008, 2011; Paquet, Lenker, Feathers, & Nasarwanji, 2008; Paquet, Nasarwanji, Lenker & Feathers, 2008).
- Development of an updated definition of universal design and *The Goals of Universal Design*, which more clearly articulates the outcomes of universal design and ties design to bodies of scientific knowledge (Steinfeld & Maisel, 2012).
- Establishment of a research program on cold weather streetscape design that is leading to innovation in design and maintenance of outdoor walkways (Hsu et al., 2016; Hsu, Li, Dutta, & Fernie, 2015; Li, Ravindran, Katchky, Dutta, & Fernie, 2015).
- Establishment of a research program on stair safety, including both field and laboratory research (Kim & Steinfeld, 2016; Novak, Komisar, Maki, & Fernie, 2014).
- Development of innovative products with business partners, including home prototypes designed for all ages (Steinfeld & White, 2010) and touch sensitive interactive models (Landau, n.d.).

The IDeA Center has produced three publications that are having an impact in education, research and practice. *Measuring Enabling Environments* (Steinfeld & Danford, 1999) is an edited volume of research focused on measuring the

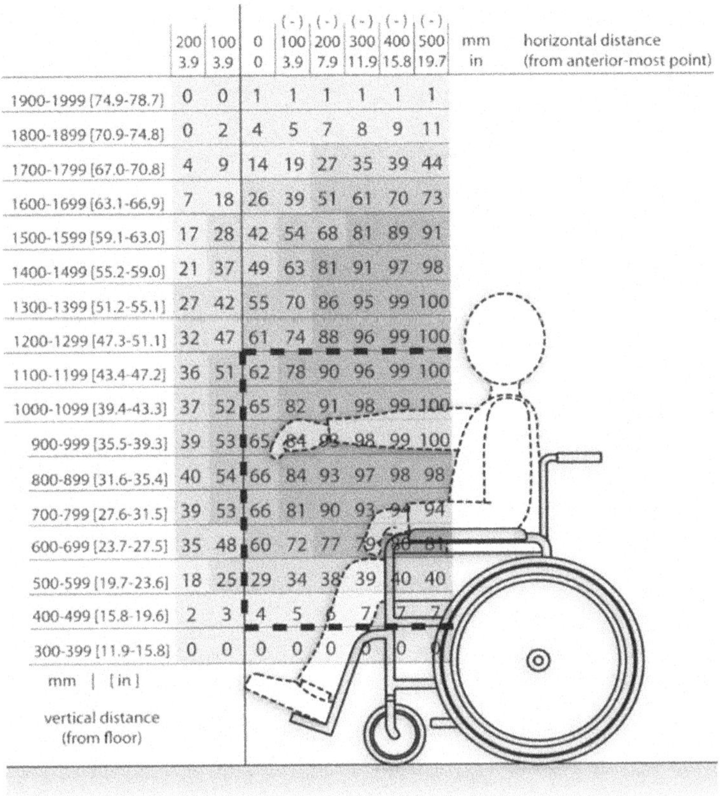

vertical distance (from floor) mm | [in]	200 / 3.9	100 / 3.9	0 / 0	(-) 100 / 3.9	(-) 200 / 7.9	(-) 300 / 11.9	(-) 400 / 15.8	(-) 500 / 19.7
1900-1999 [74.9-78.7]	0	0	1	1	1	1	1	1
1800-1899 [70.9-74.8]	0	2	4	5	7	8	9	11
1700-1799 [67.0-70.8]	4	9	14	19	27	35	39	44
1600-1699 [63.1-66.9]	7	18	26	39	51	61	70	73
1500-1599 [59.1-63.0]	17	28	42	54	68	81	89	91
1400-1499 [55.2-59.0]	21	37	49	63	81	91	97	98
1300-1399 [51.2-55.1]	27	42	55	70	86	95	99	100
1200-1299 [47.3-51.1]	32	47	61	74	88	96	99	100
1100-1199 [43.4-47.2]	36	51	62	78	90	96	99	100
1000-1099 [39.4-43.3]	37	52	65	82	91	98	99	100
900-999 [35.5-39.3]	39	53	65	84	93	98	99	100
800-899 [31.6-35.4]	40	54	66	84	93	97	98	98
700-799 [27.6-31.5]	39	53	66	81	90	93	94	94
600-699 [23.7-27.5]	35	48	60	72	77	79	80	81
500-599 [19.7-23.6]	18	25	29	34	38	39	40	40
400-499 [15.8-19.6]	2	3	4	5	6	7	7	7
300-399 [11.9-15.8]	0	0	0	0	0	0	0	0

FIGURE 16.5 Accommodation model for forward reaching abilities. The illustration plots the abilities of wheeled mobility users on a grid so that designers and standards developers can identify the extent to which a particular dimension, for example, the maximum height and distance of reach targets, accommodates wheelchair users for the task of reaching over the front of a wheelchair. Note that the current standard for forward reach, indicated by the dashed line, only accommodates about 65% of the 500 wheeled mobility users we studied. This model is one of the several ones derived from an anthropometric study of wheeled mobility users.
Source: Steinfeld et al. (2010).

impact of environments on the functional abilities of people with disabilities. *Inclusive Design: A Pattern Book* (Steinfeld & White, 2010) describes the concepts of visitable housing and "life-span housing," which enables people to age in place (see Figure 16.6). It includes the rationale for making one to three family housing accessible, design guidelines, construction details, and examples of how visitability and life-span design can be applied in many different housing styles and types, including high density urban housing. *Universal Design: Creating Inclusive Environments* (Steinfeld & Maisel, 2012), is the first comprehensive textbook on

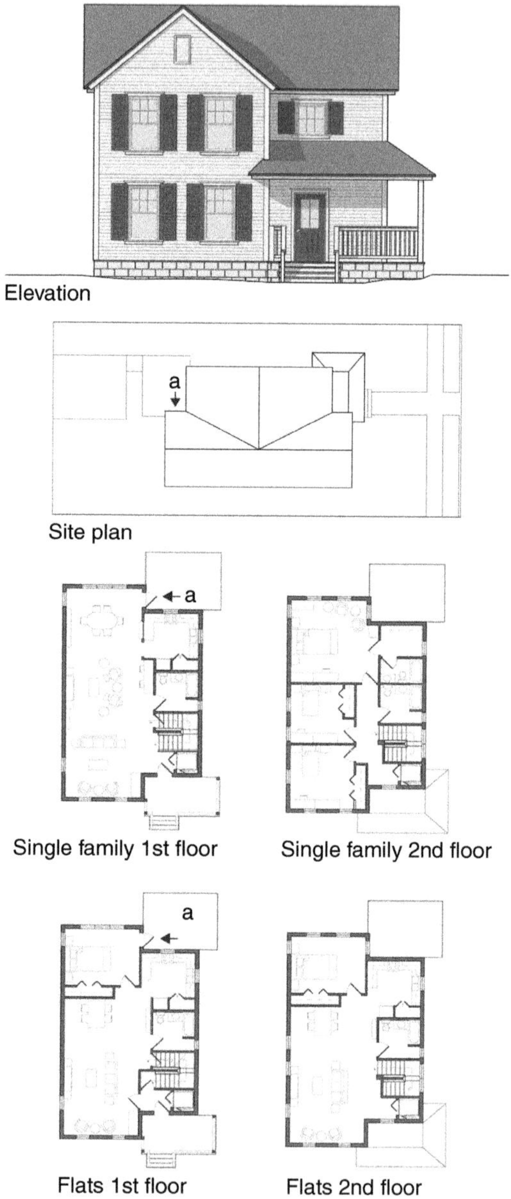

FIGURE 16.6 Life-span house design. This single family house design has an on-grade entry at the rear (a) and basic accessibility (visitability) to the rooms on the first floor from a rear deck or patio. There is a space that can be converted to a bedroom and full bathroom on the first floor, room for installing an elevator and other features for aging in place. The house can easily be converted to two flats when to provide rental income as shown in the second set of floor plans. Steinfeld and White (2010).

universal design with material relevant to many design disciplines. There are two other books in the final stages of completion. One is the first comprehensive texts on accessible public transportation and the other is a concise reference book for architects on universal/inclusive design.

It is important to note that the IDeA Center does more than R&D. We are also engaged in architectural and planning practice and education. As the IDeA Center developed, we were approached to offer design services to local community organizations who could not find the level of expertise we had in accessible design. This fit with my long-standing interest in home renovation or home adaptation as it is referred to in the rehabilitation community. Danise Levine, an architect and graduate of our program is the assistant director of the Center—our second full-time professional staff member. She developed a service program that is an important aspect of our work. We have designed over 700 housing adaptations (see Figure 16.7) in the western New York area and beyond as well as many custom built single family accessible homes in all price ranges. This work has expanded into a thriving consulting practice in accessibility design reviews, field audits, expert witness consulting, and due diligence evaluations. More recently, we led the establishment of the Age Friendly Erie County Initiative in partnership with the County Commission on Aging and the State AARP. We are also working with local advocates of improved streetscapes and bicycling opportunities, affordable housing providers and a children's museum.

It should also be noted that I picked up some important experience in architectural practice along the way. I did become a licensed architect and

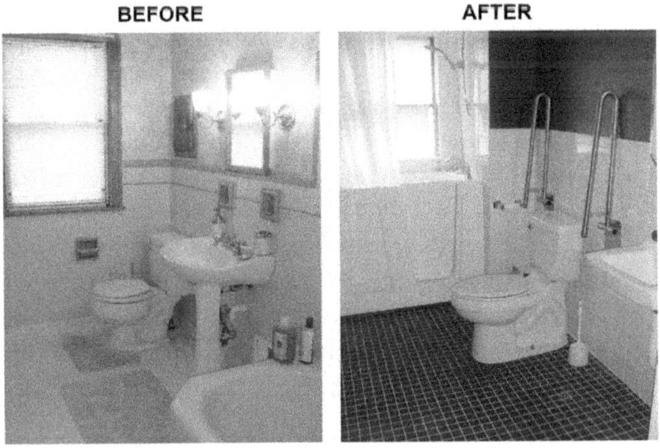

FIGURE 16.7 Housing adaptation. Before and after photographs show a typical example of the home adaptations the IDeA Center designs for families and elders.

fulfilled my boyhood dreams of designing buildings. These included retail stores, a health clinic, three multifamily housing projects, a physical rehabilitation center for older people, a vacation house, a synagogue, and several renovations. This work in practice was secondary to my scholarly activities and its realization depended mostly on working with established firms, but it was important because it informed my teaching, gave me insight into the knowledge needs in practice as well as providing the experience that lends authority to my opinions and recommendations.

TAKING STOCK

From the start of my career, I wanted to influence the shape of the built environment; that is what architects do! Although I started off wanting to enter the traditional career of architecture, my exposure to the social turmoil of the 1960s, combined with my upbringing in a family committed to social progress and respect of elders, made me receptive to the opportunity offered by the gerontology fellowship. Receiving the fellowship in 1963 was empowering because it gave me the feeling that I could make a difference. I think that all of the early gerontology fellows in architecture and planning, like Tom Byerts, Robert Newcomer, Gerald Weisman, Paul Windley, and Uriel Cohen, had this feeling that we were the vanguard of our generation in the field of aging and environment and were preparing ourselves to have an impact on society.

When I left graduate school, I was very motivated to make a difference and sought out opportunities to do so. I did not want any old job in architecture. Working at NBS offered exposure to standards development that prepared me for conceiving the research project on the ANSI Standards. The nurturing environment of the All University Gerontology Center and Walter Beatty's mentorship, prepared me for leading a major research project at an early age. The Gerontology Society's project on Environmental Gerontology gave me the resources to gain a deep knowledge of accessibility and demonstrate the impact that accessible environments could have. In fact, when I hand delivered my proposal in response to HUD's RFP, I arranged appointments at HUD to show their Policy Development and Research staff the self-instructional module. I had no idea that one of the people who I showed it to was in charge of the RFP. So, in that way, the Gerontology Society contributed to the improvements in the accessibility standards, the development of the adaptable housing concept and all the advocacy work that was done to support adoption of the new standards.

The School of Architecture and Planning at the University at Buffalo proved to be fertile ground for expanding my career and developing an extensive sponsored research program. I found many great colleagues and a supportive work environment here. I came to Buffalo because the Dean, Harold Cohen, and the Chair of the Architecture Department, the late George Anselvicius, were both visionaries and understood the importance of developing pedagogy related to design for social issues, or social justice as we would call it today. John Eberhard, the founding Dean, wanted to establish a program that would challenge the traditional practice of architecture and demonstrate the value of research and social action. Cohen and Anselvicius were given the mission of attaining accreditation but they did not abandon those original goals. Although it was a struggle because we did not receive any hard funding from the University or private philanthropists, gradually, my colleagues and I have become the most significant research unit of the School and one of the leading and longest lasting research units in the University. Along the way, HUD, the U.S. Access Board, the National Endowment for the Arts and NIDDILR all have funded our work. NIDDILR, in particular, has championed R&D in universal design.

In the early 2000s, our department decided to establish four concentrations within our graduate programs as "Graduate Research Groups" (GRG). The late Scott Danford, an environmental psychologist, Beth Tauke, a graphic designer, and I were the core faculty of the Inclusive Design GRG.[2] We were later joined by Korydon Smith, an architect and Jordana Maisel, an urban planner and human factors researcher, and Sue Weidemann, an environmental psychologist with extensive experience in housing and workplace research. She was enticed out of retirement to join us part time. Our research group is quite popular with the students and their work is of a high level, so we are attracting more and more good students. We have developed a full curriculum including studios, survey, methods and theory courses. Advanced students now can work with the IDeA Center through three PhD programs in Planning, Rehabilitation Sciences and Industrial Engineering (Human Factors). And, Beth Tauke teaches a very popular large lecture classes open to all undergraduates called Diversity and Design. It has been very satisfying to me to see this all come together. I hope that the move from marginality to mainstream in our department reflects a broader trend in academia and the profession.

One disappointment in my career is that there has never been a critical mass of gerontologists at UB. I would have welcomed more involvement with an active local community of gerontologists who had interests in Environmental

[2]The term inclusive design tends to be viewed as design for social justice with a focus on reducing income inequity and discrimination; universal design tends to be associated with design for usability and social participation. We reconceptualized universal design to encompass all these issues and the closely related goal, design for health promotion.

Gerontology. So, my contribution to the field has been from the "outside." I think it is important that environmental gerontologists reach out to other interest groups and form collaborations, avoiding an insular approach to research and teaching. Universal design is a good conceptual framework for bringing design professionals concerned with human centered design together with academics in other disciplines. I would like to focus more on critical issues of aging because now I can speak with real authority as a "user expert."

LOOKING AHEAD

The near future for me in research and development is pretty well mapped out since we have one major grant with two years left (accessible public transportation) and one with three (universal design and the built environment). Our work in transportation is focused on improving the accessibility of buses and bus service (see Figure 16.8). This is a critical issue for the aging population and the country's public transportation agencies. The rapidly aging population will increase the demand for mandated paratransit service that is 10 times more expensive than fixed route service, but, our political leaders on the whole do not see the value of putting more funding into public transportation. Thus, providers are faced with rising demand for expensive service that cannot be met with the

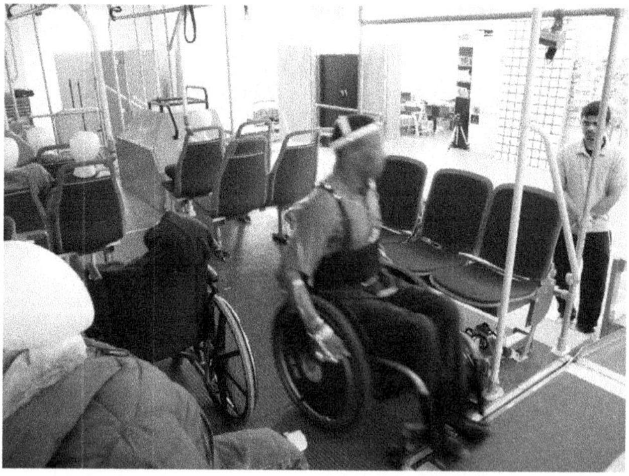

FIGURE 16.8 Full scale simulation of a low-floor transit bus. We built a full-scale simulation of a low-floor bus in our laboratory to study clearances, ramp slope, securement systems, seating layouts, and entry locations. The results are being used in federal rule making on accessible transportation.

resources available and that diverts resources away from general transit service. We are working on several projects to reduce reliance on paratransit. The first is to understand how safety and security of the pedestrian route to and from fixed route service affects dependence on paratransit. The second is to improve the design of small transit vehicles and IT services. On one hand, improving pedestrian access to communities can make fixed route service more accessible and support active living for older people. On the other hand, ride sharing services are enabling new modes of service using smaller vehicles. For older people, this can provide a viable option to driving and paratransit.

In the built environment, our main R&D focus is launching a recognition program. In winter of 2017 we will launch an interactive website to help owners and designers adopt universal design for public buildings, benchmark their work, and document their achievements. Related research activities are geared to improving and expanding the evidence base for universal design. One important aspect of this initiative is translating knowledge about design for disability and aging into design strategies for universal design. Since universal design has a much broader scope than accessible design, it encompasses the knowledge base of Environmental Gerontology. I am leading the team that will expand recognition program into housing. I am also leading our product development activities, including helping to advance our usability testing work. We believe it is critical to test innovative products, ideally at the prototype stage of development, to ensure that people with disabilities and older people will be able to use them effectively. Some companies seem to agree and we hope more will down the road.

I spend a lot of my time managing and expanding our organization and teaching activities. The IDeA Center currently has seven full time staff in a variety of fields and seven faculty who work part time on projects. Key staff at the Center deserve acknowledgment. Danise Levine, an architect, is the assistant director and runs our design and consultation services program. Jordana Maisel, an urban planner with a PhD in industrial engineering—human factors, is director of research. Beth Tauke and Korydon Smith are key faculty colleagues in architecture. There are several other architecture faculty who teach studio and elective courses related to our GRG. Vic Paquet and Jim Lenker, are faculty colleagues in industrial engineering and rehabilitation science. Before I retire, I am working to ensure that the Center can sustain itself for decades into the future by long range planning with school administrators, helping to diversify the sources of sponsored funding, finding philanthropic support and transitioning leadership to my colleagues.

Earlier, I noted that there would not be any need for "environments for aging" if the entire community were designed to be age friendly. It is my personal belief that this observation frames the main challenge for environmental gerontologists over the next 20 years. Even a rich country like the United States does not have the resources to build enough specialized environments to meet the needs of its aging population. The vast majority of our older citizens want to remain living where they are. We need to take a critical look at policy and practices of the past and present. Why did more than 75,000 people move from their communities to live in The Villages, an age restricted community north of Orlando in the middle of nowhere that is only half-heartedly designed for aging in place? What does the new generation of older people who are very clear about their desire to age in place really want? Are their desires realistic? Are there ways to bridge the gap between desire and reality? I think that one way is to make the knowledge from our research mainstream and that the conceptual framework of universal design is the way to accomplish this. I hope that other environmental gerontologists will join us in our efforts to build a community of practice around this idea.

As first world societies become more diverse, we must also pay more attention to differences across the aging population. This includes paying more attention to subcultural groups, for example, the LGBT community, the homeless, minority group elders, and veterans. Aside from disability and aging, increasing social diversity is the other major driver of universal design. A major challenge is addressing disability and aging in the poorer societies of our world. I believe that universal design, practiced in an affordable way, is the means to take on that challenge, because, otherwise, supportive environments for older people will only be available for the wealthy in those countries.

It is critically important that we be strong advocates for evidence-based practice. The design professions are moving so fast that they barely have enough time to think let alone do research. So, we need to find ways to bring knowledge from research to practice quickly. I think more collaboration between the research community and design practices is the only way to reduce the time between discovery and application of knowledge. For academics, bringing research to practice faster may also require changing the modes of publication. In the fast-moving field of computer science, peer reviewed journal articles are not the preferred method of publication because the articles are obsolete before they are published. Peer reviewed conference proceedings are more important for knowledge transfer. In medicine, developing practice guidelines from research evidence using consensus is a method used to bring the complex findings of research to application in clinical practice. Perhaps these are useful models for the Environmental Gerontology community. Finding ways to use information technology to collect data in real time is another. If we could collect data while people use buildings and communities like we do on how they use the Internet, we would have vast amounts of data to mine; it would allow research to be more cost effective. Finally, since anyone can say they are an expert in aging, especially if they have grey hair, developing a credentialing system might be a good idea. We have a plan for that in mind as we move forward with our recognition program.

REFERENCES

AARP. (2014). *Livable communities baby boomer facts and figures*. Retrieved from http://www.aarp.org/livable-communities/info-2014/livable-communities-facts-and-figures.html

Bieri, C., Triolo, R., Danford, G. S., & Steinfeld, E. (2000). A functional performance measure for effort and assistance required for sit-to-stand and standing pivot transfer maneuvers. *Journal of Spinal Cord Medicine, 23*(4), 3.

Carp, F. (1975). Impact of improved housing on morale and life satisfaction. *The Gerontologist, 15*(6), 511–515.

Danford, G. S., & Steinfeld, E. (1999). Measuring the influence of physical environments on the behaviors of people with impairments. In E. Steinfeld & G. S. Danford (Eds.), *Measuring enabling environments* (pp. 111–136). New York, NY: Kluwer Academic – Plenum.

D'Souza, C., Paquet, V., Steinfeld, E., & Feathers, D. (2010). *Anthropometric data visualization tools to improve accessibility of built environments* (pp. 707–716). Proceedings of 3rd International Conference on Applied Human Factors and Ergonomics, AHFE International. Boca Raton, FL: Taylor & Francis, Ltd.

Golant, S. M. (2015). Should older Americans live in places segregated from the young? Retrieved from https://theconversation.com/should-older-americans-live-in-places-segregated-from-the-young-47340

Hardin, M. C., Eribas, R. A., & Poster, C. (2006). *From the studio to the streets: Service-learning in planning and architecture*. Sterling, VA: Stylus Publishing.

Hsu, J., Li, Y., Dutta, T., & Fernie, G. (2015). Assessing the performance of winter footwear using a new maximum achievable incline method. *Applied Ergonomics, 50*, 218–225.

Hsu, J., Shaw, R., Novak, A., Li, Y., Ormerod, M., Newton, R., et al. (2016). Slip resistance of winter footwear on snow and ice measured using maximum achievable incline. *Ergonomics, 59*(5), 717–728.

Kim, K., & Steinfeld, E. (2016). An evaluation of stairway designs featured in architectual record between 2000 and 2012. *International Journal of Architectural Research: ArchNet-IJAR, 10*(1), 96–112.

Landau, S. (n.d.). *Interactive wayfinding for the visually impaired*. Retrieved from https://segd.org/interactive-wayfinding-visually-impaired

Lenker, J. A., Narsarwanji, M., Paquet, V., & Feathers, D., (2008). *Usability of consumer products in the home by adult wheelchair users*. Proceedings of the 2nd International Conference on Applied Human Factors and Ergonomics, Las Vegas, Nevada.

Lenker, J., Feathers, D., Nasarwanji, M., & Paquet, V. (2008). *Perspectives of elders on product usability in the home.* Proceedings of the International Conference on Aging, Disability and Independence, St. Petersburg, Florida.

Lenker, J., Nasarwanji, M., Paquet, V., & Feathers, D. (2011). A tool for rapid assessment of product usability and universal design: Development and preliminary psychometric testing. *WORK: A Journal of Prevention, Assessment, and Rehabilitation, 39*(2), 141–150.

Li, Y., Ravindran, S., Katchky, A., Dutta, T., & Fernie, G. (2015). *Effects of icy surfaces on gait parameters in young and older people.* 37th Annual International Conference of the IEEE Engineering in Medicine and Biology Society (EMBS), Milan, Italy.

Mace, R. (1985). *Universal design: Barrier free environments for everyone.* Los Angeles, CA: Designers West.

Maisel, J. (2010). The evolution of universal design in housing in the United States: Toward visitability and pattern books. In W. Preiser & K. Smith (Eds.), *Universal design handbook* (2nd ed.). New York, NY: McGraw Hill.

Maisel, J., Smith, E., & Steinfeld, E. (2008). *Increasing home access: Designing for visitability*. Washington, DC: AARP Public Policy Institute.

Martellaro, J. (2012). *Samsung says the iPhone is for old folks. Really?* Retrieved from https://www.macobserver.com/tmo/article/samsung-says-the-iphone-is-for-old-folks.-really

Novak, A. C., Komisar, V., Maki, B. E., & Fernie, G. R. (2014). *Age-related differences in dynamic balance control during stair descent and effect of varying step geometry.* National Fall Prevention Conference, Toronto, Canada.

Paquet, V., Lenker, J., Feathers, J., & Nasarwanji, M. (2008). *Incorporating the principles of universal design into assessment of product usability.* Proceedings of the 2nd International Conference on Applied Human Factors and Ergonomics, Las Vegas, Nevada.

Paquet, V., Nasarwanji, M., Lenker, J., & Feathers, D. (2008). *Incorporation of universal design into mainstream consumer product design processes.* International Conference on Aging, Disability and Independence, St. Petersburg, Florida.

Rosow, I. (1967). *The social integration of the aged.* New York, NY: The Free Press.

Steinfeld, E. (1973). Physical planning for increased cross-generation contact. In W. Preiser (Ed.), *Environmental design research* (Vol. 1). Stroudsburg, PA: Hutchinson and Ross.

Steinfeld, E. (1977). Human factors research on building standards for accessibility to disabled people. *The Behavioral Basis of Design Book 1: Selected Papers*. Stroudsburg, PA: Dowden, Hutchinson and Ross.

Steinfeld, E. (1979a). Barrier free design begins to react to legislation, research. *Architectural Record, 165*(3), 69–71.

Steinfeld, E. (1979b). Designing barrier-free toilet rooms within old and new buildings. *Architectural Record, 166*(5), 57–59.

Steinfeld, E. (1979c). Designing entrances and internal circulation to meet barrier-free goals. *Architectural Record, 166*(1), 65–67.

Steinfeld, E. (1979d). Designing the site to meet barrier-free goals. *Architectural Record, 65*(5), 69–71.
Steinfeld, E. (1980a). Designing adaptable housing to meet barrier-free design goals. *Architectural Record, 167*(3), 57–61.
Steinfeld, E. (1980b). Designing barrier-free communications in building. *Architectural Record, 167*(8), 51.
Steinfeld, E. (1981). The scope of residential repair and renovation services and models of service delivery. In M. Powell Lawton & S. L. Hoover (Eds.), *Community housing choices for the older American* (pp. 201–220). New York, NY: Springer Publishing.
Steinfeld, E. (1987). Adaptable housing for older people. In V. Regnier & J. Pynoos (Eds.), *Housing for the aged: Satisfactions and preferences* (pp. 307–340). New York, NY: Elsevier.
Steinfeld, E., & Danford, G. S. (1997). Environment as a mediating factor in functional assessment. In S. Dittmar & G. Gresham (Eds.), *Functional assessment and outcome measures for the rehabilitation health professional* (pp. 37–56). Maryland: Aspen.
Steinfeld, E., & Danford, G. S. (1999). *Measuring enabling environments*. New York, NY: Kluwer Academic/Plenum.
Steinfeld, E., & Maisel, J. (2012). *Universal design: Creating inclusive environments*. Hoboken, NJ: Wiley.
Steinfeld, E., & Schroeder, S. (1976). *Barrier-free design for the elderly and disabled.* New York, NY: All-University Gerontology Center and Center for Instructional Development, Syracuse University.
Steinfeld, E., & White, J. (2010). *Inclusive housing: A pattern book*. New York, NY: W. W. Norton.
Steinfeld, E., Maisel, J., Feathers, D., & D'Souza, C. (2010). Anthropometry and standards for wheeled mobility: An international comparison. *Assistive Technology, 22*(1), 51–67.
Story, M. F. (1998). Maximizing usability: The principles of universal design. *Assistive Technology, 10*(1), 4–12.
Toronto Rehabilitation Institute. (2016). *iDAPT Team*. Retrieved from http://www.idapt.com
Veblen, T. (1912). *The theory of the leisure class*. London, UK: McMillan.

Index

Note: Page references followed by "*f*" and "*t*" denote figures and tables

AARP Public Policy Institute, 52
Academy of Neuroscience for Architecture (ANFA), 264
accommodative adaptive strategy, 66
activities of daily living (IADL), 27
additive home modification, 157
Administration on Aging (AoA) training grant, 243
Adult Lives and Patterns of Aging in an Urban Setting program, 61
Advancing Better Living for Elders (ABLE) clinical trial, 101
Age Friendly Erie County Initiative, 293
age-related vision impairment, 20–21
Age-segregated housing environments, 280–281
American Association of Retired Persons (AARP), 242
American Institute of Architects/American Hospital Association (AIA-AHA) Fellowship in Health Facilities Design, 220
American National Standards Institute (ANSI), 283
American Occupational Therapy Foundation conference, 45
assimilative adaptive strategy, 66
auto-ethnographic methodological approach. *See* Rowles's life course perspective

Barrier Free Design Committee, 282, 283
behavioral home modification, 157
Berlin Aging Study (BASE), 20–21
Bronfenbrenner's bio-ecological model, 31

Calkins, Margaret, 12
  assistive wardrobe design, 230, 231*f*
  building and program, 221
  Centers for Medicare & Medicaid Services, 228
  conducting and dissemination applied research, 225
  construction cost approach, 229–230
  Corinne Dolan Alzheimer Center, 218, 219
  design research, 223
  early educational period
    AIA/AHA fellowship opportunity, 220
    architecture program, 219–220
    design work, 218
    EDRA conference, 221
    environmental psychology, 218–219
    environmental research, 221–222
    environment-behavior program, 220
    Lawton's Competence-Press Model, 220
  enhanced shared room design, 228–229, 229*f*

Calkins, Margaret (*cont.*)
environment design, dementia individuals, 223
evidence-based design practice, 223–224
future research, 234–235
IDEAS, 226–227
life-cycle costing model, 229
Life Safety Code, 227, 228
Management of Aging Services program, 232
Mayer-Rothschild Foundation, 233
Memory Care Assisted Living, 230–231
person-centered care, 226
PhD program, 225
program coordinator, 232
specialized memory care program, 234
Caregiver Appraisal of Function and Upset (CAFU), 104
Center for Innovative Care in Aging, 100
Centre for Environmental and Social Studies in Ageing (CESSA), 136
Community Aging in Place, Advancing Better Living for Elders (CAPABLE) program, 159
community-dwelling elders, 8
Community Ecology and the Adaptation of Older Persons study, 61
Corinne Dolan Alzheimer Center, 221
critical gerontology, 169–170
culturalized press-competence approaches, 83–85

deviation-amplifying approach, 193

ecology theory of aging (ETA), 26
ecopsychosocial (EPS) interventions, 271–272
Elliot Program in Health Care Design, 232
ENABLE-AGE project, 22–23, 116–118
"Enabler" concept, 285
Environmental Design Research Association (EDRA), 221, 260
environmental pro-activity hypothesis, 99
exosystems, 31

Fair Housing Accessibility Guidelines, 285
Fair Housing Amendments Act of 1998, 156
Fall Prevention Center of Excellence (FPCE), 159
Family housing project, 262
Functional Independence Measure, 286
FUTURAGE project, 124–125

gerontological press-competence approach, 78
Gerontological Society-based project, 243
Gerontological Society of America (GSA), 58, 283
Gitlin's reflective essay
action-oriented research, 93, 97
Advancing Better Living for Elders clinical trial, 101–102
anthropology and social psychology, 96–97
bio-psycho-social-environmental paradigm, 93
caregiver interventions, 102–103
Center for Innovative Care in Aging, 100
chronicity and familial adaptation, 96
engagement as pill/prescription, 102
environmental gerontology
competence environmental press model, 92, 98
evidence-based programs, 95
intervention research, 92
multicomponent and multimodal interventions, 92–93
persistent passion, 91
quality of life, 92

environmental pro-activity hypothesis, 99
home environmental modification oriented interventions, 103–105
intellectual development, 95, 98
lack of adequate housing stock, 99
Lawton's good life model, 93–94, 94*f*
occupational therapists, 98–99
personal award and recognition, 103
person-directed/person-centered program, 101
psychological frameworks, 96
reflective research practitioner, 90–91
small behavioral and home environmental adaptations, 101
social-environmental framework, 100–101
socio-historical-political analysis, 97
socio-psychological-environmental approaches, 8–9
Golant's residential normalcy theory, 6, 7
assistant professor position, 60–61
Community Ecology and the Adaptation of Older Persons study, 61
community ecology study, 62
coping/adaptive process
action-oriented adaptive process, 65
age-related declines, 65
cognitive-relational theory, 65
dual process coping framework, 66–67
ecology of aging, 65
individual-environmental congruence, 66
intellectual and emotional stimulation, 65
outcomes, 67–67
incongruent residential environments, 68
individual–environment interactions, 68
Kahana's congruence model, 68
Lawton's environmental docility hypothesis, 68
master's program, 59
PhD program, 59–60
residential satisfaction, 64–65
subjective environments of older people, 62
theoretical model, 63, 63*f*
undergraduate education, 58
UNL's survey research program, 61
validation, 57–58
Growing Older program, 137

Hearthstone Assisted Living Residences, 263
Home Environmental Assessment Protocol (HEAP), 104
Home environmental modification oriented interventions, 103–105
Home modification (HM), 157–159
HOPE model for dementia, 270–271, 271*f*
Housing and Environment for Aging Project, 186
Housing and Urban Development (HUD), 241
Housing Enabler instrument, 115–116, 116*f*

Image-presentation-test (I-P-T) process, 266
Inclusive Design and Environmental Access (IDeA), 286
Inclusive Design: A Pattern Book, 291
Incongruent residential environments, 68
Independent Living Movement, 279
INNOVAGE project, 23
Innovative Designs in Environments for an Aging Society (IDEAS), 226–227
Inquiry by Design, 262

Intelligent Design for Adaptation, Design and Technology (iDAPT) team, 289
International Building Code, 285
International Network on Population Ageing and Urbanisation (INPAU), 176
Introduction to Environmental Design Research, 278
Iwarsson, Susanne
- biography, 110
- environmental gerontology
  - challenges and research tasks, 124–126
  - research contribution, 123–124
- housing accessibility assessments
  - Ecological Theory of Aging, 115
  - Enabler concept, 115–116
  - European ENABLE-AGE project, 116–118
- occupational therapist, 9
  - achievements, 114–115
  - community-based OT, 113
  - early life experiences, 110–111
  - geriatric long-term care, 112
  - higher academic training, 112
  - hospital-based OT, 112
  - interdisciplinary research environment, 112–113
  - PhD graduation, 114
  - primary health care, 112
  - promotions, 114
  - public health, 112
  - theories of aging, 112
- out-of-home environments, 118
- research focus
  - cross-national research, 120–121
  - entrepreneurship and innovation, 122
  - home and health interactions, 119–120
  - individual housing adaptation, 121
  - interdisciplinary approach, 120
  - multifaceted development, 119
  - user participation, 122

Kahana's congruence model, 68

Lawton's Competence-Press Model, 220
Lawton's environmental docility hypothesis, 68
Life Span Developmental Psychology program, 185
life-span house design, 291, 292*f*
life-span theory of control, 27

Macrosystems, 31
Management of Aging Services program, 232
Massachusetts Institute of Technology (MIT) conference, 260
Mayer-Rothschild Foundation, 233
Measuring Enabling Environments, 290
Memory Care Assisted Living, 230–231
Mesosystems, 31
Metropolitan Toronto Area Region Transportation Study, 60
Microsystems, 31

National Association for Mental Health (MIND), 135
National Fire Protection Association's Life Safety Code (LSC), 227
National Institute for Disability, Independent Living and Rehabilitation Research (NIDILRR), 286
National Institute of Mental Health (NIMH)-funded 2-year face-to-face interview study, 187
National Long Term Care Insurance program, 158
Naturally occurring retirement communities (NORCs) research, 154

Netherlands Institute for Advanced Study (NIAS), 262
New ANSI Standard Project, 283

Peace's home thoughts, 9
British Society of Gerontology, 134
care homes, 135–136, 141
CESSA, 136
community development worker, 1411
domestic life and home working, 136–137
environmental experience, 139–140
environmental gerontologist
environmental gerontology, 142–143
facets of life wheel, 138*f*
family background, 132
Graham's in-depth qualitative approach, 134
Growing Older program, 137
housing management, 137
independent care home services, 141
kitchen designer and lighting expert, 140
life-course approach, 137
long-term care, 141
option recognition concept, 143
P-E interaction, 140
PhD program, 133–134
post-doc researcher, 135
research officer, 135
school life, 132
social geographer, 132
TiKL study, 140
undergraduation, 133
Perceived Change for the Better Index (PCI), 104
Person–environment (P-E) assessment approach, 20, 24–25
activities of daily living, 27
agency-belonging approach, 29
behavioral life-span development, 26–27
cohort effect, 31
comprehensive model, 30*f*
ecology theory of aging, 26, 32
ENABLE-AGE project, 30
environmental docility, 27
goal-engagement/disengagement process of aging, 29
life-span theory of control, 27
physical environment, 6, 26
place attachment and identity, 28
residential satisfaction, 28
secondary compensatory control strategies, 27
selective optimization with compensation, 32
Person–environment exchange, 5–6
Philadelphia Geriatric Center (PGC), 73
Phillipson, Chris, 10
age-friendly city development, 176
antipsychiatry movement, 166
biography, 165–166
community and environmental research
economic recession, 170
environment of kin, 171
social change and urban neighborhoods, 171–172
UK ESCR, 170
community service volunteer, 166
critical gerontology, 169–170
family and community life research, 172–173
family background, 166
full-time education, 166
future research agenda, 176–177
globalization and belonging, 175
migration and transnational ties, 173–175
socialization, 166
sociological training
community-related interventions, 168
doctoral research, 168–169
undergraduate degree, 167–168

place therapy, 193
Professional Environmental Assessment Protocol, 225
Program of All-Inclusive Care for the Elderly (PACE), 158
psychological action theory, 19
Pynoos, Jon, 9
  advocacy planning, 149
  assistant director, 149
  background and design interest, 148
  Board Member of Menorah Housing Foundation, 161
  contributions, 161
  Executive Director, 151
  executive director, 151
  federally assisted housing, 150–151
  future research, 161–162
  housing for elderly
    fall prevention, 159–160
    federally funded Section 202 program, 153
    home and community-based services, 156–157
    home modification, 157–159, 158*f*
    housing options, 154
    international perspective, 155–156
  interdisciplinary research, 153
  Minuteman program, 151–152
  PhD dissertation, 150
  social justice and context, 153
  translational research, 152–153

Readiness to Change index, 104
Registered Homes Act 1984, 141
Regnier, Victor, 12
  academic and practice community, 240
  academic exposure, 241
  budding architect, 241
  environmental design, 240
  evidence-based research explorations, 240
  graduate studies, 242
  professional experiences, 240
  school experiences, 241
  tenured position, University of Illinois, 244
  USC Andrus Gerontology Center
    AoA training grant, 243
    architectural programs, 243
    cognitive mapping, 243
    Gerontological Society-based project, 243
    NIMH-funded project, 243
    Powell's national study of public housing, 242–243
    research and practice, 243–246
Rehabilitation Engineering Research Center (RERC), 286
residential comfort zone, 64
residential mastery zones, 64
Residential normalcy theory. *See* Golant's residential normalcy theory
residential satisfaction, 28
Rothschild/Pioneer Network Life Safety Code Task Force, 227
Rowles's life course perspective
  ageing friendly communities movement, 52
  biography, 40
  bodily orientation, 42*f*, 42–43
  doctoral dissertation, 41, 48–49
  emotion and fantasy, 43
  environmental docility hypothesis, 47–48
  ethnographic approach, 50
  hypothesis of changing emphasis, 44
  in-depth interviewing and event analyses, 44–45
  local field director, 41
  making and Theoretical model, 46–47, 47*f*
  nuclear-family-oriented middle-class suburban settings, 50

person-environment relationships, 7, 40–41, 51
physical use of space, 42
systematic listening and relistening, 41
Rubinstein, Robert, 7
biographical approach, 79–80
biography, 73
culture of living alone, 80–81
current day approaches, 85–87
doctoral dissertation work
cultural themes, 75
data gathering, 76
habitus, 77–78
horticulturalists, 75
psychoanalytic types of projections, 77
gerontological press-competence approach, 78
graduate school orientations, 74
miniaturization, 6, 81
older persons and environment, 78–79
personal meaning system
environmentally sensitive design, 82
meaning-referents and contexts, 82
present-day constructed life story, 82
vs. press-competence approaches, 83–85
spiritual/religious beliefs, 82
Philadelphia Geriatric Center, 73, 78, 82

Scheidt, Rick, 10
academic appointment, 184
aging study, Kansas towns
captives of decline, 194
crumbling buildings, 194
"deviation-amplifying" approach, 193
environmental stress, 192–193
ethnographic interviewing, 192
housing-related theory, 192
in-depth collective case study, 192
informed contextual model, 190
Lawton's Philadelphia Geriatric Scale, 187–188
living arrangements, 188
microenvironmental NIMH-funded follow-up, 187
multilayered environmental proposal, 191
NIMH-grant proposal, 191
place therapy, 193
psychological wellbeing, 187, 189
regression models, 189–190
rural economy, 191
self-funded research effort, 194
service utilization and activity profiles, 189
Andrus Gerontology Center, 185–186
Barker's "behavior setting" construct, 183–184
campus-based teaching duties, 184–185
future research, 195
language of stigmatization research, 184
Lewin's theory, 184
life-span developmental psychologist, 186–187
Life Span Developmental Psychology program, 185
social psychology program, 184
Schwarz, Benyamin, 11
basic vs. applied research
architectural background, 208
collaborative research-informed practice, 209–210
design and construction process, 210
journal editor, 210–211
physical environment, 208
research-aware practice, 209
Chesler's School of Sociology, 206
early childhood, 202–203
intellectual growth, 206

Schwarz, Benyamin (*cont.*)
life in kibbutz
communal education system, 204
housing arrangement, 204–205
life-changing hallway conversation, 206
multigenerational community, 203
physical and mental disabilities, 205
regional day-care center for elderly people, 204, 205*f*
supportive old people's home, 205
long-term care settings, 211–212
PhD degree, 207
significance of place, 212–214
secondary compensatory control (SCC) strategies, 27
selective optimization with compensation (SOC), 32
social insideness, 175
social learning theory, 18, 24
social-physical environments over time (SPOT) model, 22
Steinfeld's broader community environment
adaptable housing, 285
age restricted community, 298
age-segregated housing environments, 280–281
architectural practice, 293–294
assistantship, 280
Barrier Free Design Committee, 282, 283
biography, 277–278
building standards, 282–283
day-long "Life Seeing" tour, 280
doctorate program in architecture, 279–280
Eastman's course, 278–279
"Enabler" concept, 285
gerontology fellowship, 279
iDAPT team, 289
IDeA Center, 286, 290
achievements, 290
architectural and planning practice, 293
housing adaptation, 293*f*
organization and teaching activities, 299
PhD programs, 295
publications, 290–293
Introduction to Environmental Design Research, 278
multidisciplinary education, 279
multidisciplinary gerontology center, 283–284
New ANSI Standard Project, 13, 283, 285
NIDILRR center, 286, 289
planning and urbanism, 280
Progressive Architecture Research Award, 285
Rehabilitation Engineering Research Center, 286, 289
research community and design practices, 298
research position, 282
Research Recognition Award, 285
service design practicing, 288
small transit vehicles and IT service design, 297
social action approach, 13, 278
social justice design, 295
transportation work, 296
undergraduate experiences, 278
universal design, 287*f*, 288, 296
work study job, 278
subtractive home modification, 157
symbolic anthropology, 74

Task Management Simplification Index (TMSI), 104
Therapeutic Environments Screen Scale, 225

transformative home modification, 157
Transitions in Kitchen Living (TiKL) study, 140

UK Economic and Social Research Council (ESRC), 170
Universal Design: Creating Inclusive Environment, 291
University of Nebraska-Lincoln (UNL) Gallup Research Center, 61
Urban Field Service (UFS), 149
Usability Rating Scale (URS), 286*f*
U.S. Department of Housing and Urban Development (HUD), 283

Wahl's psychological aging
  academic development, 19
  age-related hearing impairment research, 21
  age-related vision impairment research, 20–21
  ambulatory assessment, 23
  awareness of age-related change, 23
  BASE-related involvement, 20–21
  ENABLE-AGE project, 22–23
  environmental sphere, 25
  environmental thinking, 19
  INNOVAGE project, 23
  issue of ecological validity, 23–24
  and Margret's research
    dependency in old age, 19
    research unit, 18
    social learning theory, 18, 24
  P-E assessment approach (*see* Person-environment assessment approach)
  physical-spatial part, environment, 19
  Powell's influence, 19
  professional life, 18
  psychological action theory, 19
  psychology program, 18
  scientific coordinator, 20
  SPOT model, 22
  transaction and co-construction concepts, 25
  Vern's theory, 19

Zeiral Developmental Spiral, 265–266
Zeisel, John
  assistant professor position, 262
  environmental psychology, 262
  environment–behavior studies, 12
    Alexander's approach, 260
    design for aging, 269
    design for dementia, 269–270, 272–273
    design research and decisions, 267, 272
    ecopsychosocial interventions, 271–272
    evidence-based design, 261
    family housing project, 262
    HOPE model for dementia, 270–271, 271*f*
    iconic pattern language, 260
    Italian working class residents, 259
    neurosciences, 267–268, 268*f*
    PhD thesis, 260
    triangulation of methods, 266–267
    Zeiral Developmental Spiral, 265*f*, 265–266, 272
  graduate degree, 258–259
  Hearthstone Assisted Living Residences, 263
  practical research experience, 259
  professional life, 258

www.ingramcontent.com/pod-product-compliance
Ingram Content Group UK Ltd.
Pitfield, Milton Keynes, MK11 3LW, UK
UKHW021845100926
8556IPUK00019B/1065

9 780826 179869